The Current Status of
Cardiac Surgery

The Current Status of Cardiac Surgery

Edited by
D. B. Longmore, FRCS, LRCP, MB, BS

Consultant Clinical Physiologist
National Heart Hospital, London

MTP
Medical and Technical Publishing Co. Ltd.

Published by
MTP
Medical and Technical Publishing Co. Ltd.,
St. Leonard's House, St. Leonardgate,
Lancaster,
England
Copyright 1975 D. B. Longmore
Softcover reprint of the hardcover 1st edition 1975

ISBN-13:978-94-011-6614-0   e-ISBN-13:978-94-011-6612-6
DOI: 10.1007/978-94-011-6612-6

First published 1975

Contents

Preface *D. B. Longmore*

Part 1   Cardiac Transplantation

1. Introduction *D. B. Longmore*   3
2. Transplantation of other organs *R. Y. Calne*   6
3. Logistics of organ acquisition *J. J. Van Rood*   12
4. The significance of tissue typing and matching in cardiac transplantation *J. R. Batchelor*   17
5. Vascular lesions in experimental transplantation *J. F. Mowbray*   20
6. Cardiac transplantation today *P. K. Caves*   28
7. The place of transplantation *Ch. Dubost*   40

Part 2   Fallot's Tetralogy

8. The surgical anatomy of Fallot's tetralogy *R. H. Anderson and A. E. Becker*   49
9. Angiographic aspects of Fallot's tetralogy in infants *J. F. N. Taylor and G. R. Graham*   62
10. The present indications of palliation in Fallot's tetralogy *D. Waterston*   69
11. Total correction after previous Blalock-Taussig shunt *M. F. Sturridge*   71
12. Total correction after the Brock procedure *S. C. Lennox*   73
13. Radical corrective surgery after Waterston shunts *Jane Somerville and Rosa Barbosa*   78
14. Current concepts in the management of Fallot's tetralogy *A. Starr*   84
15. Primary total correction of Fallot's tetralogy under the age of two years. *M. H. Yacoub*   95
16. Correction of tetralogy of Fallot *W. Klinner*   103
17. Revaluation after total correction of Fallot's tetralogy *F. Fontan and A. Choussat*   104
18. The need for homograft reconstruction of the right ventricular outflow tract in Fallot's tetralogy *D. N. Ross*   117

Part 3 Prosthetic Valves

19. The design characteristics of heart valves *K. Reid* 123
20. Echocardiographic studies following mitral valve replacement *D. G. Gibson* 127
21. Myocardial preservation during aortic valve replacement *R. N. Sapsford* 133
22. The cage ball prosthesis *A. Starr* 144
23. Five years experience with the Björk-Shiley disc valve in aortic, mitral and tricuspid valvular disease *V. Björk* 160
24. The Australian experience with prosthetic valves *H. D. Sutherland* 179
25. The use of Starr-Edwards composite seat valves (models 2320 and 6320) in the aortic and mitral positions *W. P. Cleland* 192
26. Mitral valve replacement *S. C. Lennox* 196
27. The use of Starr-Edwards valves (model 1260) *M. F. Sturridge* 198
28. The use of Braunwald Cutter valves: Part 1 *J. E. C. Wright* 200
29. Experience with the Björk-Shiley prosthesis: Part I *J. G. Bennett* 202
30. Experience with the Björk-Shiley prosthesis: Part II *G. H. Smith* 204
31. The use of the Braunwald Cutter valve: Part II *J. K. Ross* 206

Part 4 Tissue Valve Replacement and Repair

32. Viability of homografts and problems of long-term storage *N. Al-Janabi* 209
33. Problems of sterilisation in homograft preparation *Eunice Lockey* 215
34 Tissue valve preparation. *A. Carpentier, J. Relland and Ch. Dubost* 219
35. Mechanical characteristics of vena cava and a technique for its use, unsupported, for mitral valve replacement *B. T. Williams* 226
36. Homograft and autograft replacement of the aortic valve *D. N. Ross* 234
37. Experience with heterografts *C. G. Duran* 246
38. Homograft replacement of the mitral valve *M. H. Yacoub* 253
39. Experience with tissue heart valves *Marian I. Ionescu* 260
40. Late results of cardiac valve replacement with autologous fascia lata *D. J. Parker* 272
41. Reconstructive valve surgery *A. Carpentier, J. Relland and Ch. Dubost* 279

Part 5 Open-Heart Surgery under One Year of Age

42. Open-heart surgery in the first year of life *J. Stark* 293
43. Experience with infant perfusions *A. Starr* 298
44. Management of ventricular septal defects in infants *A. J. Furst* 302
45. Total surgical correction of total anomalous pulmonary venous drainage in infancy *F. Midgley* 307

46. Operative treatment of patients with transposition of the great arteries in infancy *J. Stark*   312

47. Treatment of valvar stenosis *A. Rees*   319

Part 6 Post-Operative Care following Cardio-thoracic Surgery

48. Osmolar balance after open-intracardiac operations in children *P. B. Deverall*   325

49. Peripheral temperature measurement as an aid to postoperative care *H. R. Matthews*   330

50. Atrial pressure measurement after open-heart surgery *R. D. Bradley* 337

51. Assessment of left ventricular function and simultaneous measurements of pressure and dimension *D. G. Gibson*   339

52. Measurement of cardiac output in infants and young children using thermodilution *A. Rees*   344

53. Cardiac output and its derivatives using an implantable electro-magnetic flow probe and intra-cardiac manometers *B. T. Williams, A. F. Rickards and J. H. Chamberlain*   347

54. The place of the computer and automation in postoperative care *T. D. Preston*   357

Part 7 Ischaemic Heart Disease

55. Selection of patients for coronary artery surgery *J. L. Waddy*   367

56. Pre and postoperative investigation *R. Balcon*   372

57. Problems of technique in aorto-coronary bypass operations *J. E. C. Wright*   374

58. The coronary bypass operation *A. Starr*   381

59. Coronary endarterectomy *C. Hahn, N. Radovanovic and B. Faidutti* 386

60. Postoperative blood flow in auto-coronary saphenous vein bypass grafts *B. T. Williams, A. F. Rickards, J. F. C. Wright and C. A. Barefoot*   396

61. Pathological aspects of ischaemic heart disease *E. G. J. Olsen*   401

62. The intra-aortic balloon pump *R. J. Donnelly*   406

63. Infarctectomy *C. Hahn, E. Hauf and B. Faidutti*   413

64. Surgical treatment of left ventricular aneurysm *H. H. Bentall*   415

65. Management of postinfarction mitral regurgitation *M. H. Yacoub*   420

66. The treatment of postinfarction VSD *B. N. Pickering*   426

Part 8 Results of Surgery in Rare Congenital Heart Disease

67. Results of surgery in rare congenital heart disease *Ch. Dubost*   435

Part 9 Discussion

   Index   489

List of Contributors

N. Al-Janabi, PhD
Senior Biologist, Surgical Department, National Heart Hospital; Honorary Lecturer, Cardio-Thoracic Institute, London

R. H. Anderson, FRCS, MD
Department of Paediatrics, Cardio-thoracic Institute, Brompton Hospital, London

R. Balcon, MRCS, LRCP, MB, BS
Consultant Cardiologist, London Chest Hospital; Consultant Cardiologist, Southend General Hospital, England

Rosa Barbosa, MD
181, Voluntaris Da, Patria Apto 201, Rio de Janeoro, Brazil

C. A. Barefoot, MD
Carolina Electronics, King, North Carolina 27021, USA

J. R. Batchelor, MRCS, LRCP, BChir, MB, MD
Professor, McIndoe Research Unit, Queen Victoria Hospital, East Grinstead, Sussex, England

A. E. Becker, FRCS, MD
Department of Cardiology and Experimental Physiology, Amsterdam

J. G. Bennett, FRCS
Senior Registrar, Brompton Hospital, London

H. H. Bentall, FRCS, LRCP, MB, BS
Professor of Cardiac Surgery, Royal Postgraduate Medical School; Consultant Thoracic Surgeon, Hammersmith Hospital, London

V. O. Björk, MD
Professor of Cardiac Surgery, Royal Postgraduate Medical School, Consultant Thoracic Surgeon, Hammersmith Hospital, London

R. D. Bradley, MB, BS
Consultant Physiologist, St Thomas's Hospital, London

R. Y. Calne, FRCS, LRCP, MD, BS, MS
Professor of Surgery, University of Cambridge, England

A. Carpentier, MD
Professor of Cardiac Surgery, Hôpital Broussais, Paris, France

P. K. Caves, FRCS, MD
Senior Lecturer in Cardiac Surgery, Royal Infirmary, Edinburgh, Scotland

J. H. Chamberlain, MB, BS, MRCP
Consultant Clinical Physiologist, Guy's Hospital, London

A. Chousset
Hopital Du Tondu, Bordeaux, France

W. P. Cleland, FRCP, FRCS
Director of Department of Surgery, Institute of Diseases of the Chest, London; Consultant Surgeon, Brompton Hospital, London; Senior Lecturer in Thoracic Surgery, Royal Postgraduate Medical School, London

P. B. Deverall, FRCS, LRCP, MB, BS
Consultant Cardio-Thoracic Surgeon, Leeds General Hospital; Lecturer in Thoracic Surgery, University of Leeds, England

R. J. Donnelly, FRCS, MB, BS
Consultant Cardio-thoracic Surgeon, Broadgreen Hospital, Liverpool

Ch. Dubost, MD
Professor de Clinique Chirurgicale Cardio-Vasculaire, Chirurgien de L'Hôpital Broussais, Paris, France

C. M. G. Durran, MD
Jefe Servicio Cardiovascular Centro Médico Nacional "Marques de Valdecilla", Universidad de Santander, Spain.

B. Faidutti, MD
Clinique Universitaire de Chirurgie Cardio-Vasculaire, 1121 Geneva 4, Switzerland

A. F. Fontan, MD
Professor of Cardiac Surgery, Hopital du Tondu, Bordeaux, France

A. J. Furst, MD
Senior Surgical Registrar, The Hospital for Sick Children, London

D. G. Gibson, BChir, MB
Consultant Cardiologist, Brompton Hospital, London

G. R. Graham, MD
Consultant in Clinical Physiology, The Hospital for Sick Children, London

C. Hahn, MD
Professor, Surgical Department, Hopital Cantonal, Clinique Universitaire de Chirurgie Cardio-Vasculaire, 1121 Geneva 4, Switzerland

E. Hauf, MD
Clinique Universitaire de Chirurgie Cardio-Vasculaire, 1121 Geneva 4, Switzerland

Marian I. Ionescu, FRCS
Consultant Thoracic Surgeon, Leeds General Infirmary, England

W. Klinner, MD
Professor of Surgery, Herzchirugische Klinik der University München

S. C. Lennox, FRCS, LRCP, MB, MS
Consultant Surgeon, The Brompton Hospital, London

Eunice Lockey, Bsc, MD, FRCPath
Consultant Pathologist, The National Heart Hospital, London

B. Longmore, FRCS, LRCP, MB, MS
Consultant Physiologist, The National Heart Hospital, London

H. R. Matthews, FRCS, LRCP, MB, BS
Senior Surgical Registrar, Broadgreen Hospital, Liverpool, England

F. Midgley, FRCS
Senior Surgical Registrar, The Hospital for Sick Children, London

J. F. Mowbray, BChir, MB
Reader in Immunopathy, St. Mary's Hospital, London

E. G. J. Olsen, MRCS, LRCP, MB, BS, MD
Consultant Pathologist, The National Heart Hospital, London

D. J. Parker, FRCS, MRCP, MB, CHB
Senior Lecturer, Honorary Consultant Surgeon, Cardio-Thoracic Institute; Consultant Thoracic Surgeon, The National Heart Hospital, London

B. N. Pickering, FRCS, LRCP, MB, BS
ConsultantCardio-thoracic Surgeon, Colindale Hospital, London

T. D. Preston, FRCS, BChir, MB
Computer Director, Westminster Hospital, London

N. Radovanovic, MD
Clinique Universitaire de Chirurgie Cardio-Vasculaire, 1121 Geneva 4, Switzerland

A. Rees, FRCS
Senior Surgical Registrar, The Brompton Hospital, London

K. Reid, FRCS
Senior Surgical Registrar, National Heart Hospital, London

A. F. Rickards, MD, MRCP
Consultant Cardiologist, National Heart Hospital, London

D. N. Ross, FRCS, MB, CHB
Director, Department of Surgery, Institute of Cardiology; Consultant Surgeon, The National Heart Hospital & Guy's Hospital, London

J. K. Ross MS, FRCS
Thoracic Surgeon, Southampton Chest Hospital R. N. Sapsford, FRCS, MB, CHB Senior Surgical Registrar, The Hospital for Sick Children, London

Current Status of Cardiac Surgery

G. H. Smith, FRCS, LRCP, MB, BS
Consultant Cardio-vascular Surgeon, Northern General & United Sheffield Hospitals, Sheffield,, England

J. Somerville, MB, MRCP
Consultant Cardiologist, The National Heart Hospital, London

J. Stark, FRCS
Consultant Thoracic Surgeon, The Hospital for Sick Children, London

A. Starr, MD
Professor of Surgery, Chief of Cardio-Pulmonary Surgery, University of Oregon Medical School, USA

M. F. Sturridge, FRCS, MB, BS, MS
Consultant Thoracic Surgeon, London Chest Hospital and Middlesex Hospital, London

H. D. Sutherland, MS̄, FRCS, FRĀCS
Consultant Surgeon, Royal Adelaide Hospital, South Australia

J. F. N. Taylor, MRCS, MRCP, MB
Senior Research Fellow, Paediatric Cardiology, The Hospital for Sick Children, London

J. J. Van Rood, MD
Professor, Surgical Department, Oegtgeest, Nr Leiden, The Netherlands

J. L. Waddy, FARCS
Cardiologist, Royal Adelaide Hospital, South Australia

D. J. Waterston, FRCS, MB, BCH
Consultant Surgeon, The Hospital for Sick Children, London

B. T. Williams, FRCS
Consultant Cardio-thoracic Surgeon, St Thomas's Hospital, London

J. E. C. Wright, MRCS, LRCP, MB, BS
Consultant Cardio-Thoracic Surgeon, London Chest Hospital and Southend General Hospital; Honorary Consultant, The Italian Hospital, London

M. H. Yacoub, FRCS, LRCP
Consultant Thoracic Surgeon, Harefield Hospital and The National Heart Hospital, London

Acknowledgements

The tremendous success of the 1974 cardiac surgical course was due to two main factors. Firstly, Dr Albert Starr who was Moderator and whose attendance at every session was of immeasurable value. He was able to make these great contributions because the organisers and the secretariat had produced an impeccable and well-planned course.

Many of the contributors were extremely helpful and co-operated on the production of the edited version of the course and I wish to thank those who helped with the editorial work and who gave so much time and effort.

This book could not have been produced without generous help from ICI and encouragement from Mr. Beale of ICI. It would also have been impossible to produce in its present form without the generosity of MTP. An enormous amount of hard work has been undertaken by Miss M. Smith at the National Heart Hospital and the editorial staff of Medical and Technical Publishing Company. Finally, I would like to take the opportunity to thank all those who have helped during the transcription and preparation and who have overcome problems due to postal strikes throughout Europe.

Preface

This book consists of an edited report of the proceedings of the Fifth Cardiac Surgical Course run by the Royal Post-Graduate Medical School, The Institute of Cardiology. The Institute of Diseases of the Chest, The Institute of Child Health, The National Heart Hospital, The Brompton Hospital, The Hammersmith Hospital and Great Ormond Street Children's Hospital. These organisations encompass most of the major London hospitals associated with cardiac surgery.

The course has been run annually, its aim being to help young men and women who are training in the specialised field of cardiac surgery. Thus this book consists of the proceedings of a teaching course rather than of a symposium, the 60 authors having been charged with the task of teaching rather than displaying their results or discussing their latest ideas and the proceedings reflect an interesting appraisal of the current status of cardiac surgery. The speakers were chosen from all over the world, because they were leaders in their field or because they have access to up to date and reliable information, and I am grateful to all the lecturers for their cooperation in the production of this volume.

Ten thousand surgical cases are reported. These figures are drawn from experience in the United Kingdom, France, Germany, Switzerland, the United States of America, Australia and New Zealand. The reader may be surprised to find that only a handful of experiments are described. This does not necessarily mean that cardiac surgery has passed the stage when its exponents spend a proportion of their time in the experimental laboratory, but regrettably, it does mean that a lot of the experimentation has now to be done in the operating theatre, using the human subject as the final arbiter for the safety and efficiency of any procedure. This is the current situation with regard to the ideal method of replacing the aortic valve.

Although routine major cardiac surgery is only just over a decade old the exponential growth of the discipline has now ceased, the principles are established and the era of extravagant claims for its advances and results has passed. It was the fact that cardiac surgery has now attained this stable state that led to the decision that this particular year of the

Cardiac Surgical course should be published. The book is not intended to be comprehensive and there are areas in which it is impossible to use it as a reference work, but where subjects are dealt with they are comprehensively covered and up to date.

Part 1

Cardiac Transplantation

1
Introduction

D. B. Longmore

It is important to remember before discussing in depth this particular aspect of heart disease that we are still faced with many major deficiencies in the surgical treatment of cardiac disease. Approximately half of the deaths in the United Kingdom and the United States of America were cardiovascular and of these approximately 17 % were under the age of sixty-five (Figure 1.1). Many of these people could have been treated by surgical means and yet examination of the number of operations done in that year shows that only approximately 1% of these people received surgical care. The figures for heart replacement are even more unsatisfactory; in the whole world only a handful of patients had their hearts replaced. Many young people who were otherwise fit have died simply because they did not have enough myocardium to support their circulation. What is perhaps worse than this failure to apply heart transplantation has been its unfavourable reception. It is a reasonable and satisfactory procedure with good results for this early stage in its development, despite the horrendous mortality rate which daunted the first replacements of the aortic valve and the early disastrous attempts to repair complex congenital difficulties of tetralogy of Fallot. It would be better if the new was compared with the established and not with the theoretical, and if more consideration was given to the fate of the patient with terminal heart failure.

Homotransplantation is only one of the possible methods of replacing the heart, as the heart can also be replaced by mechanical or biological methods. However, very little of the past expenditure on the mechanical heart has been of value as it is difficult to insert, is mechanically unreliable, will not incorporate with the living tissue, is difficult to design in such a manner that it will not damage blood, is not easy to control by linking it to physiological mechanisms and furthermore it is not possible to power it satisfactorily with a clean implanted power source. Of the three biological alternatives there are:

1. Man to man transplantation with its major ethical and immunological problems.
2. Animal to man transplantation with greater immunological differ-

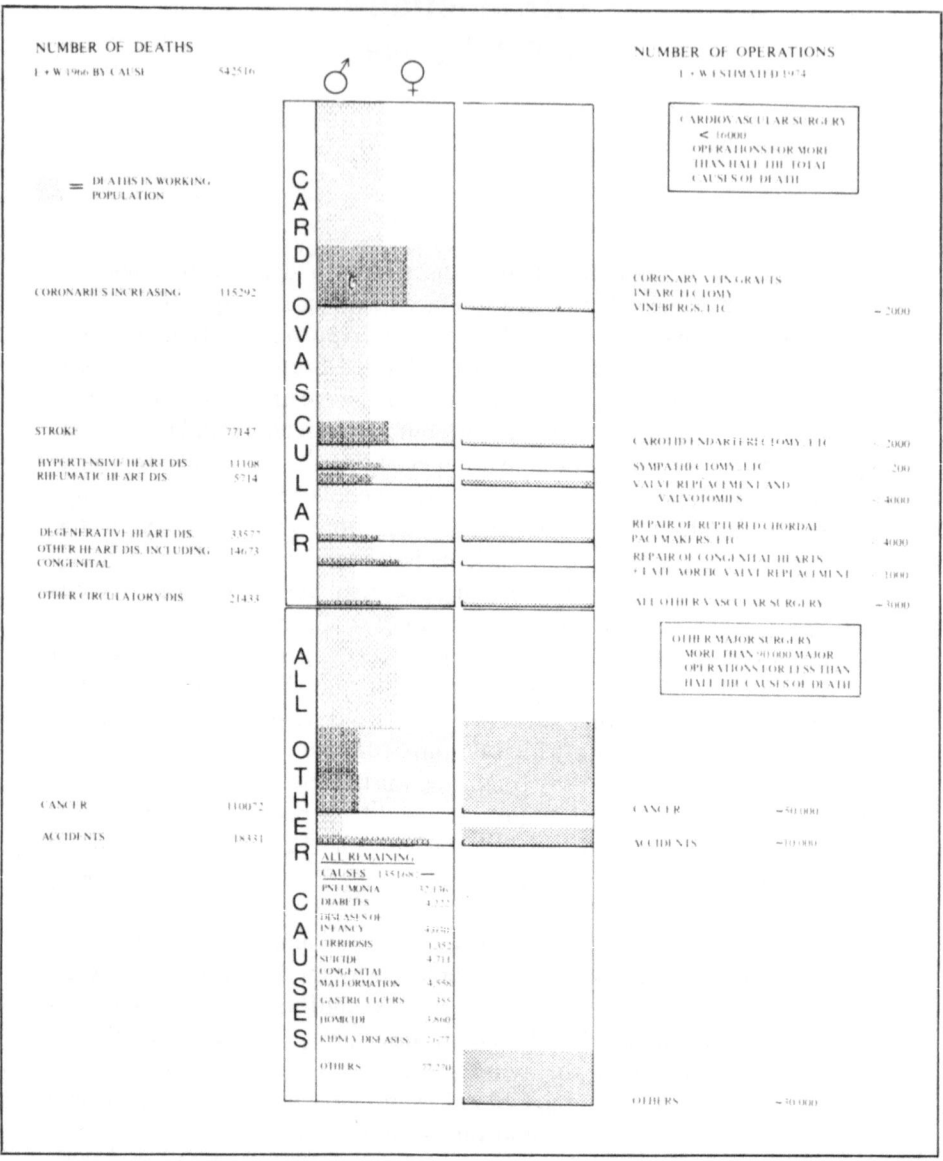

Figure 1.1 To show the currently small contribution of cardiac and vascular surgery to cardiovascular disease even when compared to deaths under the age of 65

ences and the added problem of biochemical differences.

3. The use of foetal tissues to cause the adult cells in the myocardium to revert to a stage at which cell differentation and repair can occur.

It is well known that some human organs such as the liver have enormous powers of regeneration and yet a myocardial infarction is surrounded by only a few mitotic figures and these abortive attempts at repair soon give way to the formation of a scar. However, recent experimental work suggests that there is sufficient information encoded in the nucleus to reform any cell and it is known that foetal cells have the ability to influence the tissues around them. It has already been demonstrated that a foetal heart can be banked for up to forty days in organ culture and will remain beating in this period. This means that the already weakly antigenic foetal tissues can be tissue typed. All species studied so far behave in a similar manner and it has been possible to assemble composite foetal hearts from pieces of animal hearts, thus crossing the species barrier. The performance of these foetal hearts is so predictable that they can be used for testing effects of drugs, anaesthetic gases and other environmental factors at various stages of development. Furthermore experiments on infarcts in dogs indicate that it may be possible to repair the infarcted adult heart.

The foetal tissues available from the very large number of abortions which are done might have certain advantages. It is human material which can resist anoxia well, which can be stored and is readily available. Because of the wide availability it can be tissue typed and matched without the pressure of time, whereas the selection of human heart donors does not allow the luxury of good tissue matching. Foetal tissues have certain other biological advantages. They are less antigenic and they have the ability to modify the response of tissue around them. All this means that if adult cells still contain the information required to replicate and repair themselves it might be found possible to use foetal implants to cause the adult cells around the infarct to continue their attempts at cell division and to form new vascular beds and new heart muscle instead of scar tissue.

I hope that all readers will bear in mind two main facts.

1. That contemporary cardiac surgery by no means encompasses all the potential surgically treatable cases.
2. Within the field of heart replacement we have only scratched the surface of one of four possible alternative methods; at least another two show sufficient promise to warrant some further research efforts.

2
Transplantation of other organs
R. Y. Calne

CLINICAL KIDNEY GRAFTING

Transplantation of the kidney is the major field of clinical transplantation, more than 20 000 cases having been reported to the Transplant Registry. The kidney has a tremendous advantage in the field of transplantation because the organ function can be replaced by regular dialysis. A patient who is moribund can be restored to reasonable health and then treated with a transplant and if the graft does not function immediately, the patient can be tided over until the kidney takes over. If the kidney never functions, then the transplant can be removed and the patient goes back to dialysis and can receive another transplant. In our own experience we have transplanted some 300 kidneys and 30 of these have been second or even third transplants.

The results of kidney transplantation are quite encouraging, despite the fact that the percentage of survivals has not improved in the past five years. With identical twins the results are excellent since there can be no rejection. The figure for one year survival of transplants is 90%, for two years is 86% and the figure for the longest survival is now 18 years. Grafts between close blood-relatives give good results; 75% functioning at one year and 70% at two years. The figure for the longest survival in these cases is nearly 15 years. With grafts between HLA-typed identical sibling donors, the results are even better. With cadaver donors, the results overall are much worse, graft survival being 55% at one year, 48% at two years and the figure for the longest survival is now eleven years. With cadaver transplants, added to the greater incompatibility, there is also the likelihood that the kidneys have been damaged severely by ischaemia.

We have recently analysed the degree of rehabilitation of patients with satisfactory functioning transplants in our unit. We were gratified to find that the overall degree of full rehabilitation is 90%. So 90% of patients who have had a functionary transplant are restored back to full work, often heavy work in the case of men, to housework in the case of women, or to school in the case of children. The patients themselves feel that this new lease of life that they get must be used to its full. If one speaks to patients with good kidney transplants many will point out that this extra time was a bonus due to transplantation and therefore life is more enjoyable. Of course kidney transplant patients have the advantage of some security since if the kidney goes wrong they can get another kidney or go back onto dialysis.

There is one 'spin off' in the transplantation of a kidney which may have application to other organs, even the heart, and that is so-called 'workbench surgery'. There have been a number of reports by different authors on using this technique. I have been rather fortunate in now having five patients with hypernephroma of a single kidney or hypernephroma of both kidneys occurring at the same time. In one of them, an old man with a small tumour, I was able to remove the tumour without removing the kidney, so it was an *in situ* partial nephrectomy. In the other cases, the tumours were so large that they involved the main vessels and were close to the renal pelvis. Satisfactory dissection would have been very difficult due to poor access and the danger of producing traumatic and ischaemic damage. The kidneys were therefore removed and cooled by a standard method in a dish with cold saline and then at relative leisure the tumours were removed and the kidneys were retransplanted in the iliac fossae. With these grafts of course there is no rejection and so far all four patients have done well.

CLINICAL LIVER GRAFTING

Two types of conditions are suitable for liver grafting; benign parenchymatous diseases and primary malignancy of the liver, but the results here are worse than for heart grafting. Two hundred grafts have been performed and at the end of last year there were only 15 patients living, the figure for the longest survival being five years. Dr Starzel has the largest series of more than 60 cases. Of the 16 patients he followed-up for a year, six were alive, giving a 38% one year survival. This of course is very much better than the overall results. In the Cambridge-Kings' series, 35 orthotopic allografts have been performed. Twenty-six patients have survived the early postoperative period and 12 have left hospital. Four patients are now alive at five years, one year, three months and one month.

There are certain difficulties in liver grafting. The patient may be very ill, as physicians tend to refer patients for this kind of surgery when they are taking their 'last breath'. Furthermore, there is a serious shortage of donor livers but the situation is not quite as bad as for heart grafting because one can wait until the circulation in the donor has ceased. In America, most donors used are the so-called 'heart-beating cadavers', with established brain death. In the United Kingdom, organs are not removed until the circulation has stopped, but the availability of donors is very poor. The liver is more difficult to preserve than the kidney and can only be kept satisfactorily for a few hours. The last two livers that we transplanted were removed from a hospital sixty miles from Cambridge and then kept in cold ice and brought to Cambridge where they were transplanted after more than five hours of ischaemia. However, they both functioned well and continue to function.

In addition, the operation can be difficult. The liver produces most coagulating factors and there may be serious defects of coagulation. The

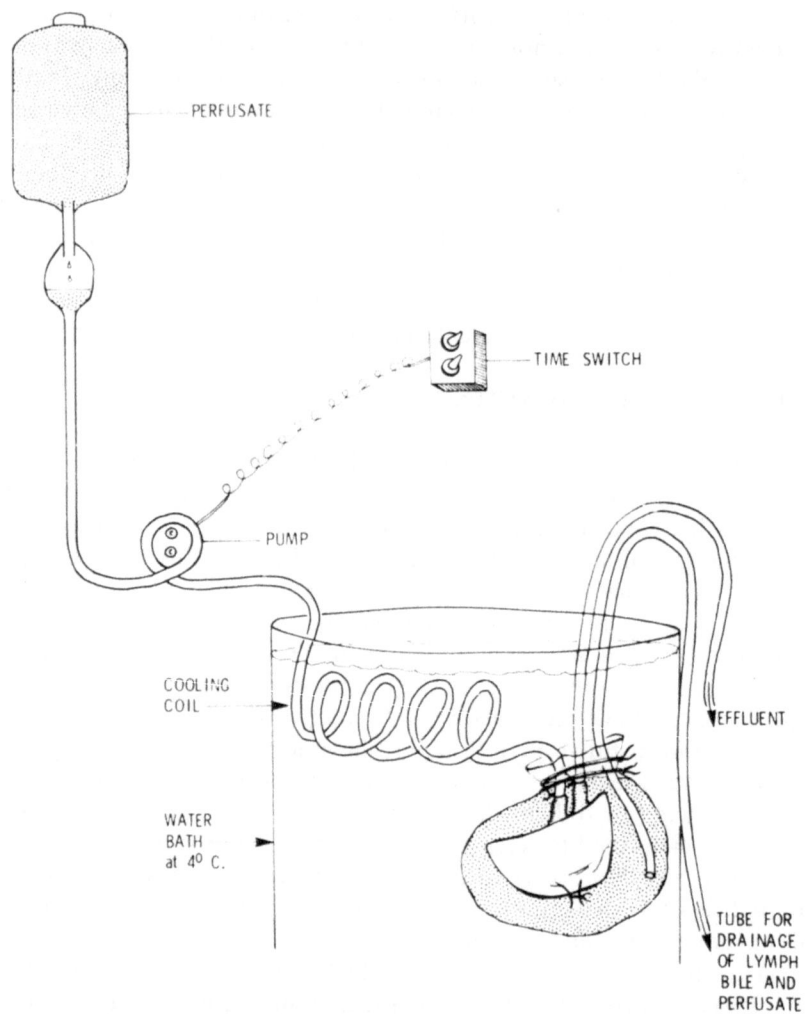

Figure 2.1 Diagram of single passage 'squirt' hypothermic perfusion of the liver. Every 5 min, a bolus of 20 ml is pumped through the portal vein at a pressure of 30–40 mm Hg

only way in which they can be countered is to give the patient a new liver which will synthesise new coagulating factors. The liver when it is ischaemic loses potassium and when it recovers it needs potassium, so the potassium in the vascular spaces when the liver is transplanted may flood into the circulation and cause cardiac arrest. If this is avoided by discarding the initial effluent, then the liver, deficient in potassium, may draw potassium out of the blood and cause dangerous hypokalaemia in the postoperative period. Potassium supplements must therefore be given. Thus, acidosis and hypoglycaemia may be a consequence of the ischaemically-damaged liver and there may also be hypothermia due to the large cold organ that is grafted. Added to these matters are infection, rejection and drug toxicity, common to all kinds of grafting.

SURGERY

In both the donor and the recipient, the operation is performed through the abdomen, through a bilateral subcostal incision. The donor liver is cooled *in situ* by perfusion through the portal vein, with drainage via the

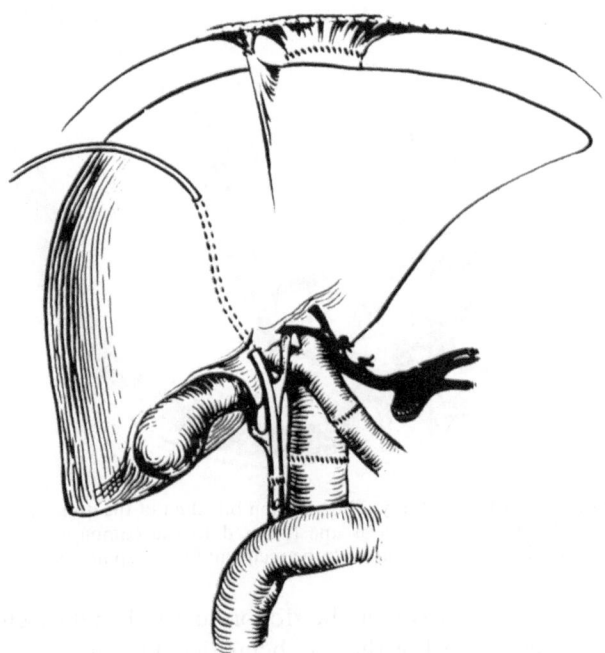

Figure 2.2 Biliary drainage using end to end common bile duct to common bile duct anastomosis over transhepatic shunt brought out through the right lobe of the liver

vena cava (it can be cooled using an extracorporeal circuit, Figure 2.1). The recipient's liver is removed and the inferior vena cava clamped above and below the liver. The new liver is inserted orthotopically, anastomosing the inferior vena cava above the liver and the portal vein, the hepatic artery and inferior vena cava below the liver.

Most technical complications have been with biliary drainage (Figure 2.2). It is of interest that with kidney grafts most troubles occur with the ureteric drainage, with the pancreas the drainage of pancreatic juice and with the lung, drainage of the bronchus. Vascular anastomoses seldom give trouble. End to end bile duct anastomosis over a T tube is a technique that Starzel originally described, and is probably the best one to use. Another technique used, when transplanting a child's liver into an adult, is to fillet the liver off the vena cava, clamping the hepatic veins and leaving the vena cava intact, then inserting the new liver orthotopically,

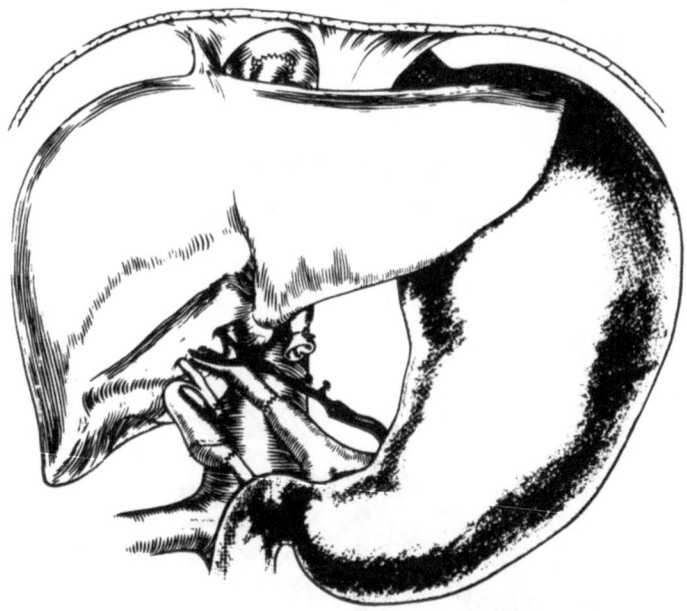

Figure 2.3 Cholecystocholedocostomy. The common bile duct of the donor is ligated below the cystic duct and the gall bladder is anastomosed to the common bile duct of the recipient, allowing biliary drainage through the recipient Oddi's sphincter

anastomosing the vena cava of the donor to the hepatic veins of the recipient, the vena cava below the liver being tied. On three occasions bile has been drained by anastomosing the donor's gall bladder to the recipient's common bile duct, preserving the sphincter of Oddi (Figure 2.3).

The fact that it is possible to live for more than five years with normal function in an orthotopically transplanted liver means that this procedure must eventually flourish. Kidney grafting is now established treatment, and liver and heart are likely to be the next two organs to be grafted as routine practice. However, the results of grafting other organs have been disappointing, e.g. the figure for the longest survival of a functioning pancreatic transplant is two years. In this case, the pancreatic juice was drained by joining the pancreatic duct to the recipient's ureter. The figure for the longest survival of a lung transplant is only 9 months. The lung appears to be highly susceptible to rejection. The intestine is also aggressively rejected, the figure for the longest survival being 76 days.

EXPERIMENTAL STUDIES

There is a spectrum of susceptibility to rejection which has not received a great deal of attention until recently. Skin is more likely to be rejected early than the heart and kidney, whilst the liver suffers least. These differences can be shown in the pig. Skin grafts between tissue typed identical sibling donor pigs last 10 days, whilst from mismatched pigs the grafts live five to six days. The benefit that accrues from tissue typing is a mere four or five days extra life of the graft. Kidney grafting however between similarly selected litter-mate pigs behave quite differently. 60% of the animals survive for a very long period of time—weeks or months instead of days, and some animals are alive beyond two years without any immunosuppression, whereas most of the mismatched sibling litter-mates reject kidney grafts in two weeks.

In a small series of orthotopic heart grafting in the pig, two animals lived nearly five months and two animals are currently alive at two months. The remaining ten animals rejected their grafts between five days and two weeks. Since the donors were litter-mates it would appear that in the pig the heart and kidney have similar immunogenecity.

Liver grafts in the pig can survive for several years without immuno-suppression. Pigs grafted at three months grow and the livers grow, and sows can be fully fertile after orthotopic liver grafting. These phenomena are not fully understood but may eventually have relevance to clinical transplantation.

3
Logistics of organ acquisition
J. J. Van Rood

This chapter presents a combination of the extrapolation of experience in Eurotransplant with kidney transplantation and an exercise in theory. Three areas will be considered.

1. The discrepancy between the number of patients in need of a heart transplant and the number of donors available.
2. The possibilities of heart–organ exchange between heart transplant centres and possibilities of heart preservation.
3. The evidence of the Dutch transplant group relating to the importance of tissue typing in experimental heart grafting.

THE NUMBER OF PATIENTS IN NEED OF AN ORGAN TRANSPLANT AND THE NUMBER OF POTENTIAL DONORS AVAILABLE

The situation in Holland has been taken as a point of reference. Here there are 13 million inhabitants and 3000 deaths/annum are caused by car accidents. There are also several hundreds of deaths due to brain tumour and subarachnoid bleeding etc. In all, the number of donors available—that is the theoretical maximum number of donors which could possibly be used—is 1000, or 80 donors/million inhabitants/year. This figure is the theoretical maximum possible attainable and is by no means the actual number which have been obtained (Figure 3.1).

Lately, many people in Holland under the direction of Schippers of Eurotransplant, and Terpstra, the transplantation surgeon, have made a systematic attempt to make the public and the medical profession more transplantation minded. An analysis of the situation in Holland, Germany and to a lesser extent in Belgium, confirmed what others have said before and that is that there is still a very strong reluctance, especially in the medical profession, to follow-up potential donors.

Reasons for reluctance
1. It is contrary to our philosophy.
2. There is no financial reward. (Until recently this was so in Holland

but it has now been changed and there is work going on in other countries to rectify the situation.)
3. There is no scientific reward.
4. It is extremely time consuming.
5. There is an understandable reluctance to talk to the family.
6. There are worries about the legal aspects.
7. Quite a few people have had an unpleasant experience with previous donations.

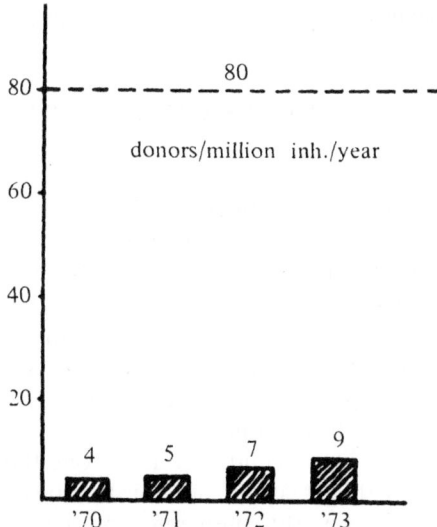

Figure 3.1 The differences between the theoretical maximum number of donors attainable in Holland and the actual numbers obtained between 1970 and 1973

However, there is now a much better understanding of the facts. The newspapers in Holland have helped with £100 000 of free advertising to educate the lay public. One of the advertisements shows the entrance to a cemetery and the caption reads. Sometimes there is new life after death: for 700 Dutchmen to be precise . The next one shows you another pamphlet, 'The second life of your kidneys'. which implores you to write a codicil and carry a card with you giving permission to use the organs after death. Through these efforts during the last six months the number of donors has increased by about 50"₀. Nevertheless, even if these numbers continue to increase there will never be enough donors for the potential number of heart transplant patients, although there might be enough for kidney patients. The reason for the shortage of donors for heart transplants is as follows – the number of patients dying from ischaemic heart disease in Holland is 24 000 annually – about 2000/million inhabitants/year.

Even when considering only the patients who die under 50 years of age, this is still 1000 patients/year/million inhabitants. This means that it would be impossible to even start to help all the patients who would be potential benefactors from such treatment.

This discrepancy between available material and potential donors is an important point which should be stressed. When heart transplantation is reintroduced in Holland this undeniable fact must be taken into account before raising hopes in patients which cannot be fulfilled. The conclusion is that there will never be enough donors to help all the patients in need of a heart transplant.

ORGANS EXCHANGE BETWEEN HEART TRANSPLANT CENTRES

In the United States a donor is sometimes flown *in toto* to the recipient. This procedure has been discussed in the Netherlands by several government committees and by the committee of the Netherlands Red Cross, but the general concensus of opinion was that this was a rather undesirable procedure and would not be acceptable in the Netherlands. However, it would not be the first time that the experts were pessimistic about what the public would accept, only to be proved wrong. Time will show what is the case with regard to heart donors.

In Eurotransplant we have found that about one-third of the kidneys are transplanted at the donor centre, one-third in the donor country and one-third abroad. However, this data refers to a paired organ and of course is not necessarily valid for the heart, but it does indicate that there is a willingness to share organs.

HEART PRESERVATION

A machine in which the heart could be preserved would be something of great potential. Work in this field has been carried out in Amsterdam by the Cardiologist, Durrer, who has now perfected a perfusion system in which the heart can maintain normal contraction and ECG waves *in vitro* for periods of up to 12 hours (Figure 3.2). However, retransplantations have not been done. Therefore, it appears that organ exchange seems rather a doubtful possibility in Europe but the prospects for preservation might be hopeful as a means of expediting organ exchange.

IS HLA MATCHING NECESSARY?

This topic will be dealt with in depth by Professor Batchelor (Chapter 4).

but as an introduction, certain experiments performed by the Rotterdam-Leiden Experimental Surgery Group can be discussed. This group has

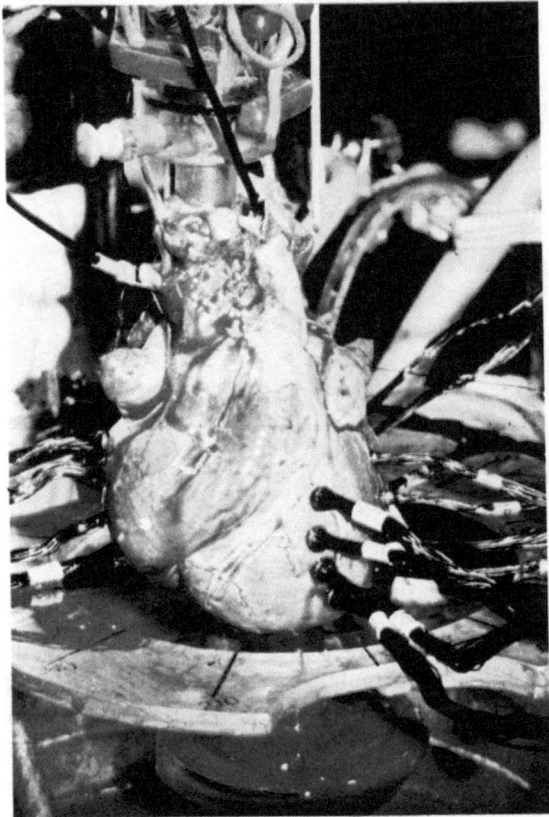

Figure 3.2 The heart in an experimental perfusion apparatus. The perfusion fluid is red blood cells and dextran

shown that if heart transplants are exchanged between mismatched beagles all are rejected between 8 and 12 days (Figure 3.3). However, similar to the rejection of skin, kidney and small bowel the matched DLA identical sibling shows that in each case survival is much more prolonged. In the heart, the DLA identical siblings have, without any immunosuppression, by far the longest survival time, but this is the type of experiment that would not be performed in humans.

In heart transplantation, if we can manage to match for HLA the benefits might be expected to be very good and better, for instance, than kidney grafting. In some transplant centres the unconvincing results of

HLA matching of kidney graft survival have led to the conclusion that HLA matching is only of minor importance for kidney graft prognosis. However, the vastly superior prognosis of HLA identical siblings kidney grafts unequivocally proves that HLA is of major importance. If such

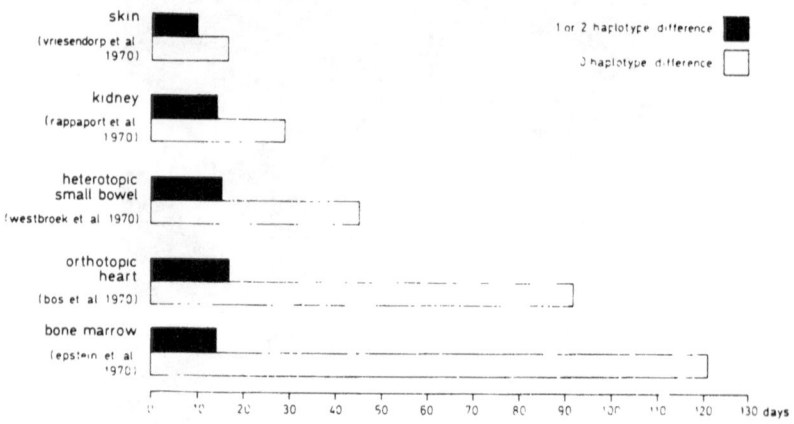

Figure 3.3 Mean graft survival times in identical and non-identical littermates (without immunosuppressive therapy)

good results can not be attained in unrelated donor–recipient combinations then HLA can not be of minor importance. It should be realised that it is quite difficult to match for this complicated system and that matching for the serological recognisable antigens as has been done so far is not the whole answer and that it might be necessary to match for other structures, perhaps those coded for by the MLC locus. If it is possible to do this then it can be expected that the results on heart transplantation can be significantly improved by matching for HLA and the benefit might be even greater than for kidney transplantation.

4

The significance of tissue typing and matching in cardiac transplantation

J. R. Batchelor

When considering the possible importance of matching donors and recipients for antigens of the HLA system in cardiac transplantation, the clinician may wish to look at the experience accumulated by kidney transplant units. There has been considerable study of the significance of HLA matching in kidney transplantation and although some issues are still argued there are also considerable areas of agreement. One of the areas of agreement is in the significance of HLA matching when donor and recipient are related. Statistically significant correlations have been observed between graft survival and the degrees of donor–recipient matching; for example in a recent study[1] soon to be published 90% of grafts from HLA identical siblings were functioning at one year, only 67% were functioning at this time in cases where the donor differed by one HLA haplotype and where the donor differed by two haplotypes, graft survival at one year was 59%. Whether these results are due directly to the effect of HLA antigens, or to the products of a closely linked locus or loci is still not certain.

One major reason for raising this doubt is that in cadaveric kidney transplant, where donor and recipient are unrelated, general agreement on the significance of HLA matching has not been reached. Early studies indicated a direct correlation between matching and graft survival[2-4] or matching and histological evidence of rejection.[5] But later, Terasaki and his colleagues analysing the pooled results of many American centres concluded that HLA matching did not influence the clinical results of cadaver kidney transplantation. It is beyond dispute and within every transplantation unit's experience that there are many instances of good clinical results being obtained in the face of a three or four HLA antigen mismatches. More recently an extensive study by the London Hospital Group and Dausset and his colleagues has provided compelling evidence in favour of a correlation between matching and graft survival.[6] This study on 918 patients showed a clear match-related rank order of the cadaver kidney grafts surviving. At two years 70% of those receiving four antigen-matched grafts had functioning kindeys whereas graft survival was 34% in those which were transplanted with kidneys showing only one or no antigens compatible. It was also observed that the effect of the second series antigens was stronger, but not significantly so, than that caused by the first series antigens. Similar studies by other European centres have usually shown some correlation between HLA matching and graft survival, but often the effect was confined to a particular subgroup of patients such as patients who were not Group O[7] or patients known to have been previously sensitised against HLA antigens.[8] The results on approximately 150 cadaver grafts performed by the kidney transplant unit for Guy's and King's College Hospitals also show a direct correlation between matching and graft survival.

Why then has there been varied experience in the results of matching? One possibility briefly mentioned earlier is that another locus or loci closely linked to HLA has an important influence on compatibility. At present, the evidence on this possibility is inconclusive. The author's own view is that the evidence indicating that HLA antigens in general influence graft survival is strong. However, in kidney transplantation there are many other factors of equal and sometimes greater importance which help to determine whether a graft survives or not. It is therefore hardly surprising that the degree of HLA compatibility does not always produce an observable effect.

Some of the other known factors are listed below:

1. General condition of patient, e.g. well dialysed or not, presence of severe complications, etc.
2. Variable therapeutic index of currently used immunosuppressive drugs in different patients.
3. Strength and type of immunological reactivity shown by different individual recipients.
4. Previous immunisation against HLA antigens.
5. Quality of donor organ.
6. Quality of patient care.

In the case of cardiac allotransplantation, both the experience of Shumway's group and common sense would suggest that there are factors other than HLA compatibility which determine or at least greatly influence the clinical outcome. Griepp et al.[9] reported that HLA compatibility did not influence survival rates but that it did have a significant effect upon the combined frequency and severity of rejection episodes. Obviously, if the opportunity of transplanting a well-matched heart graft arises it should not be ignored, but in most clinical circumstances choice of donor material is so restricted that the opportunity will rarely arise.

A final comment is due on the question of previous immunisation. In experimental systems, depending upon the exact circumstances, previous immunisation may have no apparent effect, cause hyperacute or accelerated rejection, or prolong graft survival (enhancement). At present in kidney transplantation, a graft is not transplanted into a recipient known to have circulating HLA antibodies against that graft. A similar policy is prudent in cardiac transplantation. However experimental examples of enhancement of heart allografts are well-documented, and if a clinically safe protocol can be devised it may be necessary to know the HLA antigens of donor and recipient in order to put the protocol into practice.

References

1. Opelz, G., Mickey, M. R. and Terasaki, P. I. (1974). *Transplantation*, (in press)
2. Patel, R., Mickey, M. R. and Terasaki, P. I. (1968). *New Engl. J. Med.*, **279**, 501
3. Batchelor, J. R. and Joysey, V. C. (1969). *Lancet*, **i**, 790
4. Batchelor, J. R., Joysey, V. C. and Crome, P. E. (1971). *Transplant. Proc.*, **3**, 133
5. Morris, P. J., Kincaid-Smith, P., Ting, A., Stocker, J. W. and Marshall, V. C. (1968). *Lancet*, **ii**, 803
6. Dausset, J., Festenstein, H., Hors, J., Oliver, R. T. D., Paris, A. M. I. and Sachs, J. A. (1973). *Data presented at meeting of British Transplantation Society*
7. Joysey, V. C., Roger, J. H., Evans, D. B. and Herbertson, B. M. (1973). *Nature (London)*, **246**, 163
8. van Hooff, J. P., Schippers, H. M. A., van der Steen, G. J. and van Rood, J. J. (1972). *Lancet*, **ii**, 1385
9. Griepp, R. B., Dong, E., Stinson, E. B. and Shumway, N. E. (1973). *Transplant. Proc.*, **5**, 835
10. Jenkins, A. McL. and Woodruff, M. F. A. (1971). *Transplantation*, **12**, 57

5
Vascular lesions in experimental transplantation
J. F. Mowbray

The rejection in cardiac transplants is, as it is in kidneys, very largely a vascular event. Thus the major reason for the pause for thought after the initial flood of enthusiasm for cardiac transplantation was because of the loss of hearts within the period of 9 to 15 months after transplantation by the development of severe immunologically-mediated vessel damage in the transplants. In an attempt to prevent this Dr Shumway has pushed the immunosuppression to the point where vascular lesions are not desperately important in his series compared with losses of

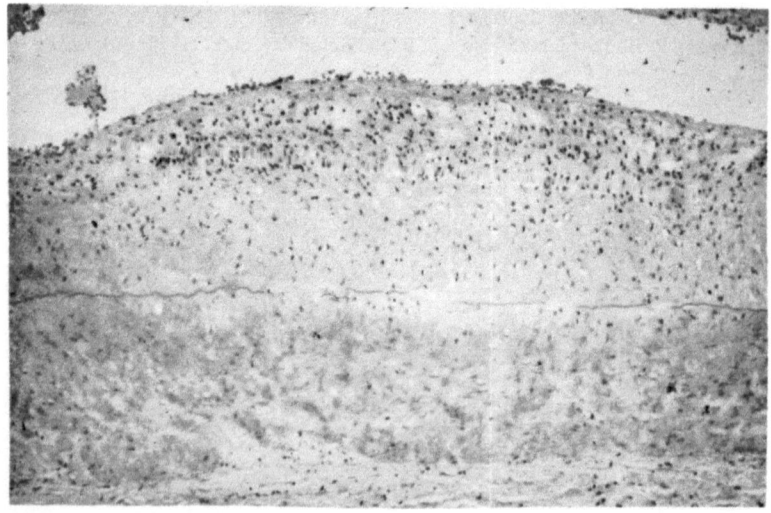

Figure 5.1 The left coronary artery of a human cardiac transplant 16 days after transplantation

patients from the consequences of heavy immunosuppression. These vascular lesions can be produced very readily in normal vessels by exposure to transplantation antibody. The immunosuppressive agents that are used may ameliorate very considerably the natural history of the vascular damage produced by antibody; in a similar way the same drugs

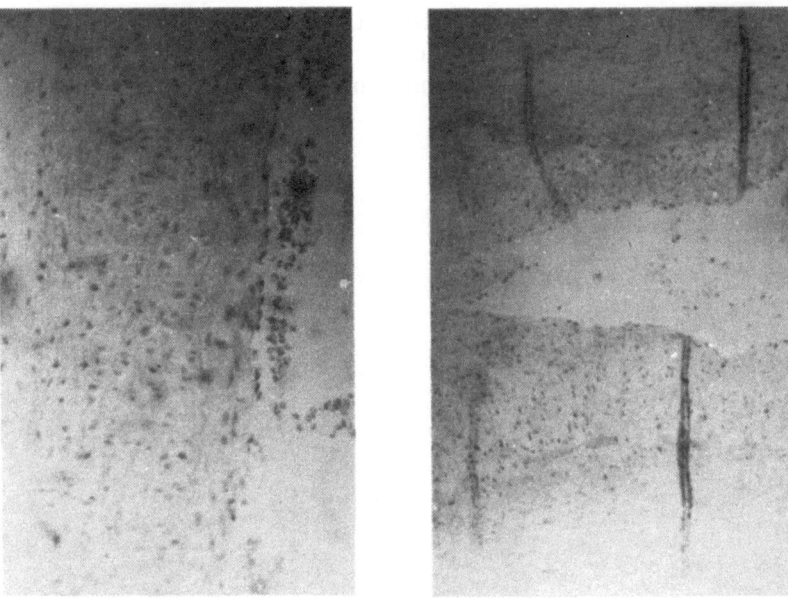

Figure 5.2(a) A normal rabbit carotid artery (b) A rabbit carotid artery injected with antibody four weeks after injury

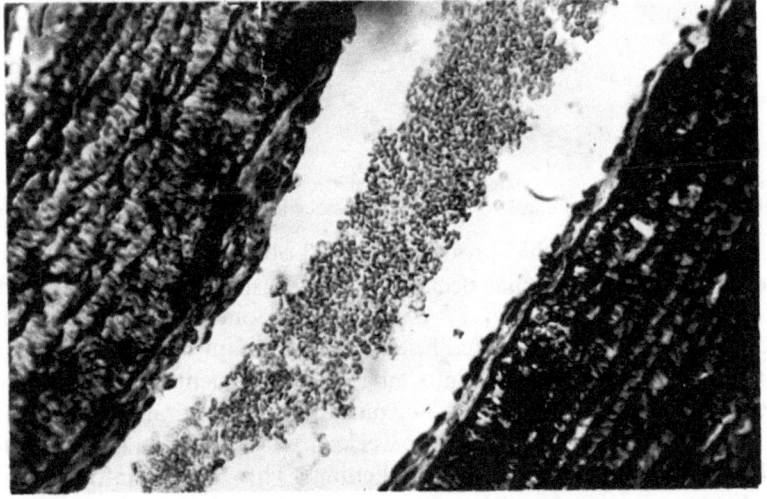

Figure 5.3 A rabbit carotid artery after injection of the animal's own serum

can influence the development of atheroma in vessels that are injured by other means.

Figure 5.1 demonstrates the lesion that can occur in the vessels of a cardiac transplant. It shows the left coronary artery of a human cardiac transplant 16 days after transplantation. Intimal thickening has occurred

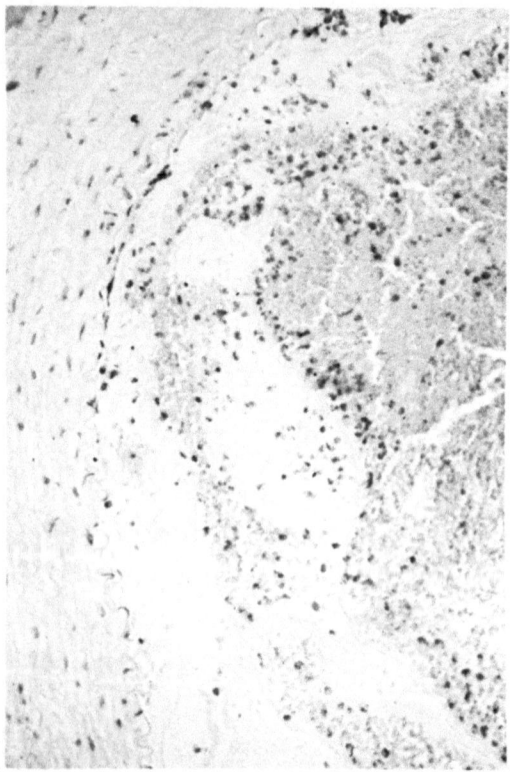

Figure 5.4 A rabbit carotid artery with ragged irregular platelet thrombi lying on the walls of the vessel and a number of polymorphs associated with the outside of the lesion

to a degree which would produce material obstruction to blood flow in the artery. This process has occurred after transplantation of the heart of a 19-year-old and is a very common phenomenon in transplanted kidneys as well as transplanted hearts. In an attempt to mimic this lesion, antibody has been injected into an isolated segment of rabbit carotid artery. Figure 5.2a shows a normal rabbit artery and Figure 5.2b shows one which was injected four weeks after injury. The injected artery exhibits considerable intimal thickening. This atheromatous intimal thickening was produced by putting transplantation antibody between two bulldog clamps, allowing three minutes for it to fix to the vessel wall and then removing the clamps and leaving it for a month.

If antibody is injected into a vessel in this way, left for three minutes to fix and then left for a further two to four weeks until the mature lesions are present, the animal's own serum can then be injected and will not lead to intimal thickening apart from the trauma which

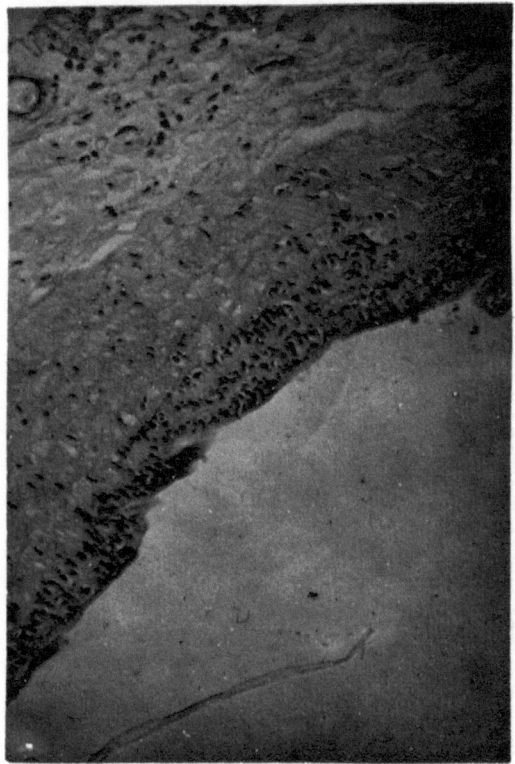

Figure 5.5 Denuded wall of rabbit carotid artery

occasionally produces minor damage (Figure 5.3). If however immune rabbit serum is injected, severe lesions are produced; if rabbit serum which is immune is injected, intimal thickening does not occur. This is a phenomenon related to the ability of transplantation antibody to bind to the transplantation antigens on the endothelium.

When antibody is injected and the vessels are examined five minutes after re-establishing the circulation, ragged irregular platelet thrombii can be seen lying on the walls of the vessels and a number of polymorphs have become associated with the outside of the lesion (Figure 5.4). Within 30 min, an MSB stain shows the wall of the vessel with a platelet thrombus adherent to the endothelium, and many polymorphs which are now starting to migrate through the thrombus to the wall of the vessel can be seen. Within two to four hours they have migrated right into the wall of the vessel, as shown in Figure 5.5, and the thrombus which was on the wall has been stripped off and presumably has passed down the

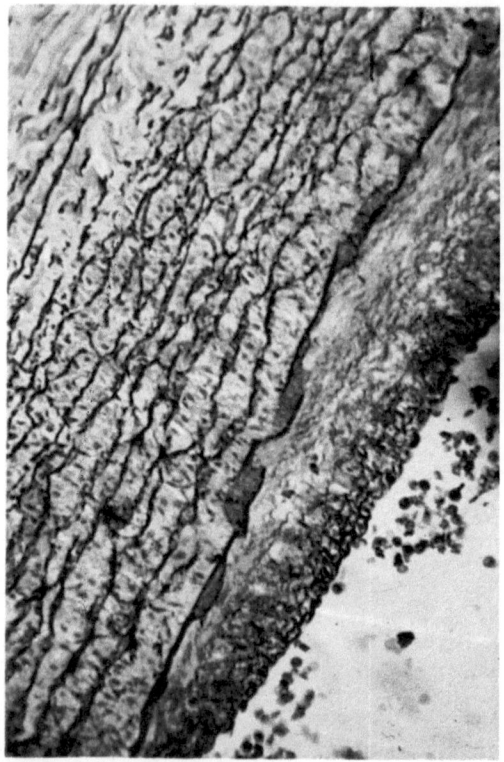

Figure 5.6 The region of the clamp in a rabbit carotid artery

lumen, leaving a few polymorphs in the wall. There is no endothelium on the vessel wall at this time, the thrombus and the endothelium have been stripped, denuding the vessel as a result of binding antibody to the endothelium.

After two to three weeks, the lesions of the kind shown at the start develop. Figure 5.6 shows the region of the clamp, the normal vessel being at the bottom, the injected segment being at the top; the intimal thickening appears in the middle of the injected segment and thins out at the region of the clamp.

These lesions can be mimicked quite easily in peripheral vessels. Hence it is possible to see how effective immunosuppression is in preventing these lesions, and not only immunosuppression, but also certain drugs used to treat the patients. Since the patients are on azathioprine, would azathioprine or steroids interfere with this lesion? In rabbits azathioprine can not be used because rabbits lack the enzyme required to convert

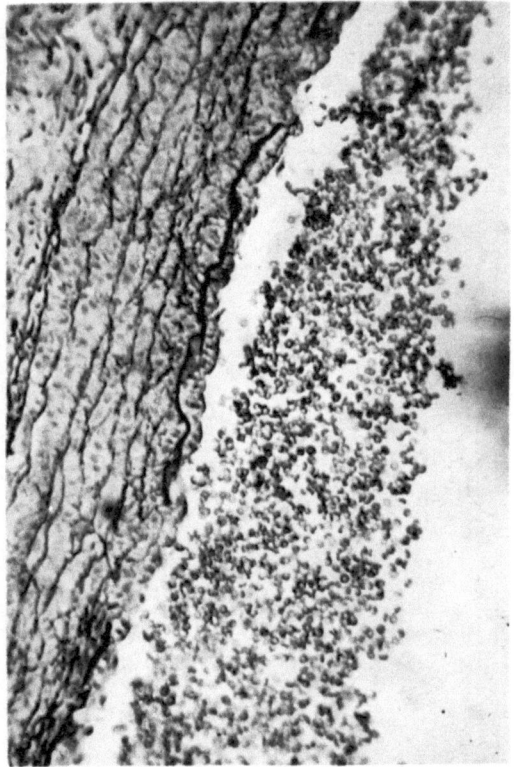

Figure 5.7 A rabbit carotid artery after three weeks of treatment with 6-mercaptopurine

azathioprine into the active 6-mercaptopurine. Therefore, azathioprine's active metabolite is used instead. In rabbits treated with 6-mercaptopurine for three weeks, intimal thickening can be greatly reduced, but not completely abolished (Figure 5.7). This is because the internal elastic lamina is covered with two or three layers of cells thickening the intima. This would presumably also occur in a human patient if treated with a sufficient degree of immunosuppression, i.e. the changes which occur as a result of the antibody being formed could be largely abolished, but not as effectively as using some of the antiplatelet, anti-inflammatory drugs. In particular, sulphinpyrazone or Anturan, which is a very potent agent, completely abolishes any damage to the vessel wall so that there is a layer of endothelium sitting on the internal elastic lamina and no thickening of the intima (Figure 5.8). Thus, one must remember that if treating a cardiac transplant, not only is the strength of the immune response important (that is the strength of response of which the patient is capable and the strength of the antigens in immunising the patient) but in addition,

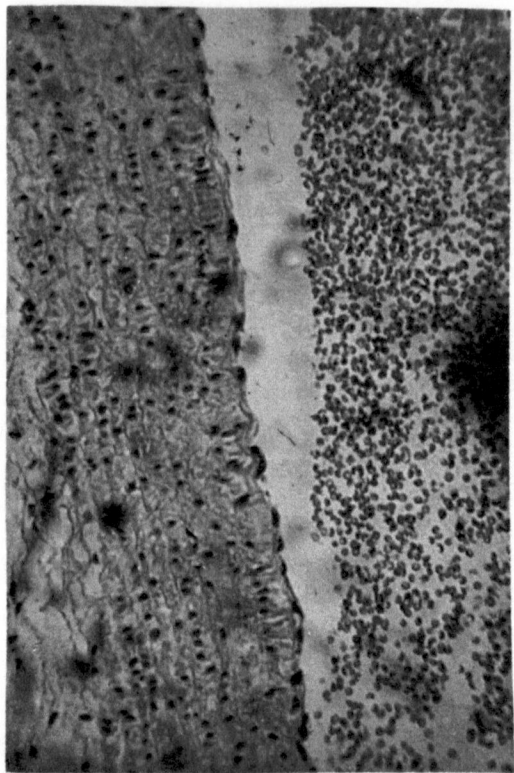

Figure 5.8 A human carotid artery after treatment with sulphinpyrazone (Anturan)

the drugs used are very important. This is a very complex and extremely variable regime – it varies from centre to centre – and a number of agents such as Persantin, cyproheptadine, and other antiplatelet agents have been used in cardiac transplantation to try to prevent the development of severe intimal thickening. By using an experimental technique of this kind, not only can the fact that the antibody causes the damage be demonstrated, but also the efficacy (at least in the test species) of a variety of these drugs can be studied. The use of such specific agents is required to make life for the doctor tolerable in cardiac transplantation as well for the patient. At the moment, using the present regimes, it is extremely difficult to effectively immunosuppress the recipients of cardiac transplantation, since in effective doses, the agents used verge too often on killing the patient. In renal transplantation, where lighter immunosuppression is possible, the patient is rarely killed but even so quite a number of kidneys are lost by this same process.

6
Cardiac transplantation today
P. K. Caves

It is important that we should not dwell on the mistakes and tragedies of the past, or be overawed by some of the problems that remain to be solved in the future. Instead we should appreciate that cardiac transplantation today is a realistic therapeutic modality available for the management of people with end-stage cardiac disease who are in imminent danger of dying and for whom there is no other form of treatment currently available.

After the first heart transplant at the end of 1967 there was an amazing world-wide enthusiasm which very quickly over the next two years changed to generalised disillusionment because of the very poor results which were achieved. Statistics from the World Transplantation Registry show that at Stanford University in Palo Alto, California a steady rate of about 10 – 15 transplants/year has been maintained up to the present time. In the last three years these transplants have represented considerably more than 50% of the total number of transplants done throughout the world. Therefore, all further statistics presented in this chapter will be entirely confined to this group of patients transplanted at Stanford University.

Cardiac transplantation at Stanford University began in 1958, when Dr R. Lower and Dr Shumway successfully transplanted the heart in the orthotopic position in the dog. They decided to continue an experimental study in the laboratory on the subject of heart transplantation and identified the following four problems:

1. Satisfactory surgical technique.
2. Would the heart perform after it was denervated and reimplanted?
3. How could the heart be preserved during the anoxic period of transit from donor to recipient?
4. The problem of homograft rejection.

After the first successful transplantation of the heart in the dog, they very quickly developed a technique which enabled cardiac transplantation in the dog to be performed subsequently on many hundreds of occasions with a very low operative mortality rate. This experimental model was then used over the next few years by Dr E. Dong and others working with Dr Shumway, who found that the physiological changes after transplantation of the denervated heart were perfectly acceptable and that, although the transplanted donor heart responsed in a physiologically abnormal way, it responded in a physiologically appropriate fashion to the demands of exercise. These animals were able to live in an almost normal fashion and at least one had a litter of normal puppies! The problem of the extracorporeal transfer of the graft was solved by cooling the heart in ice-cold saline, a technique which is used by Dr Shumway for the protection of the heart in routine cardiac surgical procedures. However, it was very quickly discovered that the heart, like the kidney and other solid organs, is subject to acute rejection. Could this problem be solved? Before rejection can be treated it has to be diagnosed and by 1965 it was appreciated that, during rejection, a reduction in the QRS complexes of the electrocardiogram occurred and that, if immunosuppression was then given, these changes could be reversed. It was also recognised that rejection is usually episodic in nature and it was these two facts which basically made clinical cardiac transplantation possible. Once these findings were recognised in the dog, it was soon possible with suitable immunosuppression to extend the survival of dogs to more than one year. Thus, by 1967, it was considered that it was justifiable to commence cautiously a clinical heart transplantation programme.

Patients were selected on three criteria: (1) total incapacity with prospect of imminent death (2) full evaluation of incapacity and (3) no possible help from further medication or lesser surgery. Unlike kidney transplantation there is no support device for the heart and therefore the heart can only be transplanted when there is nothing else available which offers any hope. Up to June 1973 61 transplants had been performed in 59 patients, two patients having been transplanted twice. Patients who have had a cardiac transplant since then have not been included in this figure. Table 6.1 shows that the majority of these patients had coronary artery disease and no other surgical procedures were

Table 6.1 The recipient disease

Preoperative diagnosis	
Coronary artery disease	39
Idiopathic cardiomyopathy	17
Post traumatic aneurysm	1
Rheumatic heart disease	2
Total	59

considered of any value. There were two patients with rheumatic heart disease and the others were patients with a cardiomyopathy. Throughout this period, 91 patients were accepted for transplantation, 59 of whom were transplanted after an average waiting time of 30 days. 32 were not

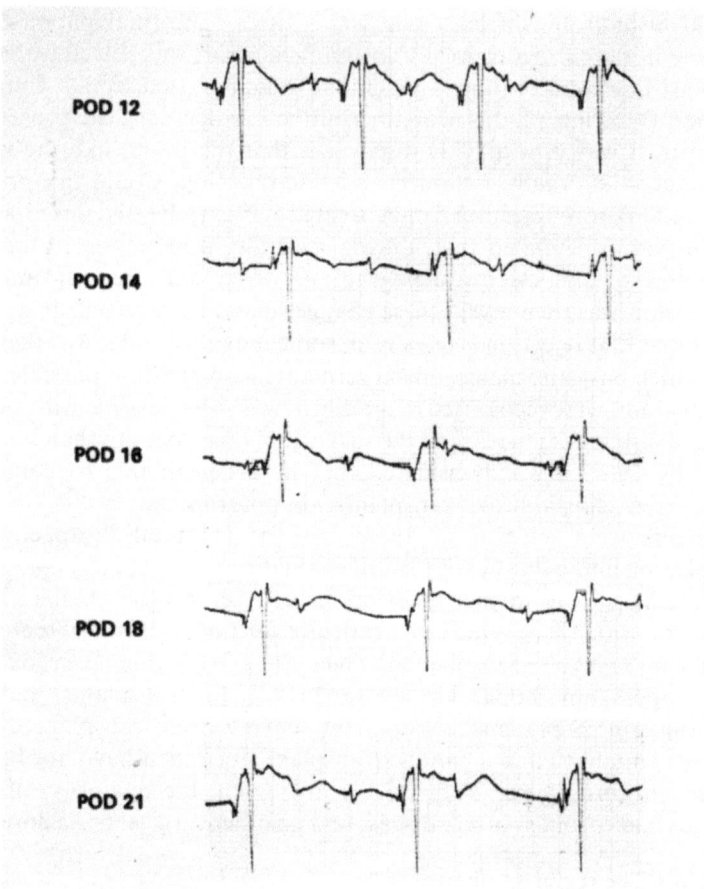

Figure 6.1 Stanford cardiac transplantation atrial electromyogram during acute rejection episode

transplanted and the average survival period of these patients was 39 days which indicates the severity of the pre-existing disease in all prospective recipients.

At operation, the heart is removed leaving the empty pericardial cavity and leaving the posterior walls of the right and left atria and the main pulmonary artery and ascending aorta; it is now considered important to use central cannulation of the venae cavae and of the aorta rather than peripheral cannulation because of the problems of infection which may arise in the groin and neck wounds. It is quite possible to cannulate the inferior and superior venae cavae at the junction of the SVC and the right atrium. The donor heart is preserved during transit in cold saline. In the experimental laboratory it has been possible to keep a heart in cold saline for seven hours and then transplant it into a dog with long-term survival. In the human situation, it is considered essential to give the recipient the best possible chance by taking the heart out of the donor while beating and by keeping the ischaemic time of the donor heart as short as possible – between 45 and 60 min. When the heart is inserted into the pericardial cavity two wires are attached to the right atrium of the donor heart. These are used both for atrial pacing in the postoperative period and also for the recording of surface electromyograms from the heart.

Tissue typing to date has had no influence at all upon the long-term survival of the patients who have been transplanted. It was soon apparent in clinical heart transplantation that the principal determinant of long-term survival would be the ability to accurately diagnose and successfully treat the acute rejection episodes which almost inevitably occurred in the first two to three postoperative months. In the first three years of clinical transplantation, the diagnostic criteria used were: changes in the electrocardiogram; clinical changes – development of a gallop rhythm or impaired cardiac movement and, at one stage, echocardiography, measuring the increased thickness of the ventricular walls which occurred during the rejection process. It is quite obvious that these parameters are functional changes which only occur in the heart after rejection has already started. The search continued, therefore, for a parameter which would enable rejection to be diagnosed before it had done any damage to the graft at all, so that rejection episodes might be more easily reversed and the donor organ left unimpaired. In the last 18 months at Stanford two further indices of rejection have been used. One is the recording of an electrocardiogram from the wires which are attached to the donor atrium. This gives approximately the same kind of changes as are obtained from the standard electrocardiogram leads but is subject to less variation from extraneous factors because it is recorded directly from the surface of the heart. Figure 6.1 shows a rejection episode with a 25% fall in the QRS complexes over the four day period from day 12 to day 16. Immunosuppression was augmented and there was an increase in the QRS complexes over the next five day period of the increased immunosuppression. These records also show the P wave of the recipient atria which have been left behind as well as the ECG of the donor heart.

The other index of rejection that has been used in the last 18 months has been serial biopsy of the transplanted heart itself. This was first tried in the dog laboratory because it seemed that the histological changes of rejection might permit earlier recognition of a rejection episode and enable treatment to be more accurately monitored. One of the greatest

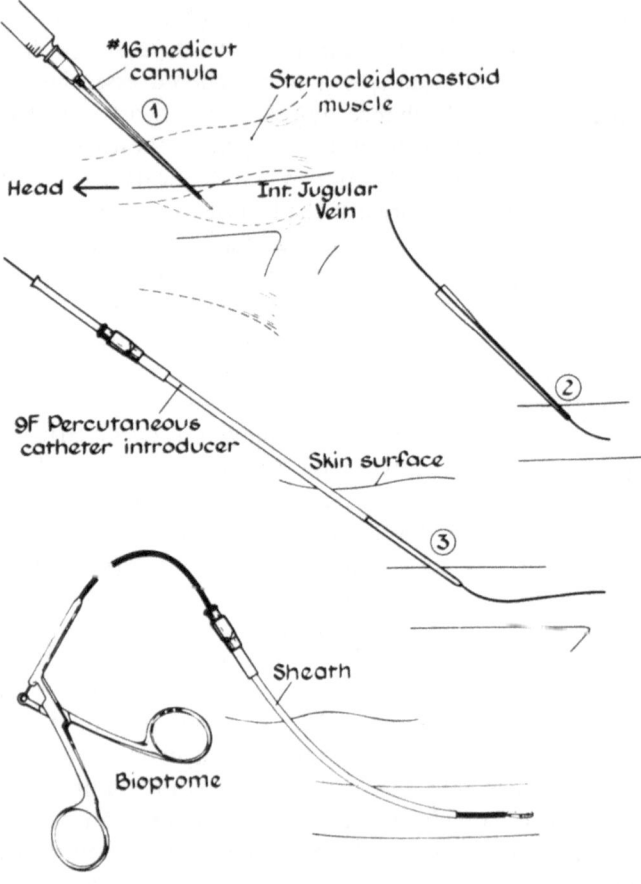

Figure 6.2 Serial biopsy of the heart in man. The insertion of a sheath into the internal jugular vein with a percutaneous technique

problems in human cardiac transplantation is knowing when to reduce immunosuppression after a rejection episode. Although the electrocardiogram may change with the onset of rejection, it does not always return to its pre-rejection characteristics after reversal of the rejection episode. It is therefore obvious when to give the treatment but difficult to know when to stop treatment, and it was thought that biopsies might indicate when the rejection episode had been reversed and therefore when to stop the potentially dangerous treatment.

The use of serial biopsies in dogs after transplantation suggested that very valuable information was obtainable from the biopsies – the problem was to develop a simple, safe technique which would permit serial biopsy of the heart in man. The technique developed was the insertion of a sheath into the internal jugular vein with a percutaneous technique, through which a Konno–Sakakibari bioptome was introduced initially (Figure 6.2). More recently an instrument which essentially consists of movable jaws at one end, like miniature bronchoscopy forceps and a flexible catheter and a handle to open and close the jaws at the other end has been used (Figure 6.3a and b). This is inserted through the internal jugular vein very easily and advanced across the tricuspid valve into the apex of the right ventricle where usually two small bites are taken for histological examination (Figure 6.3c).

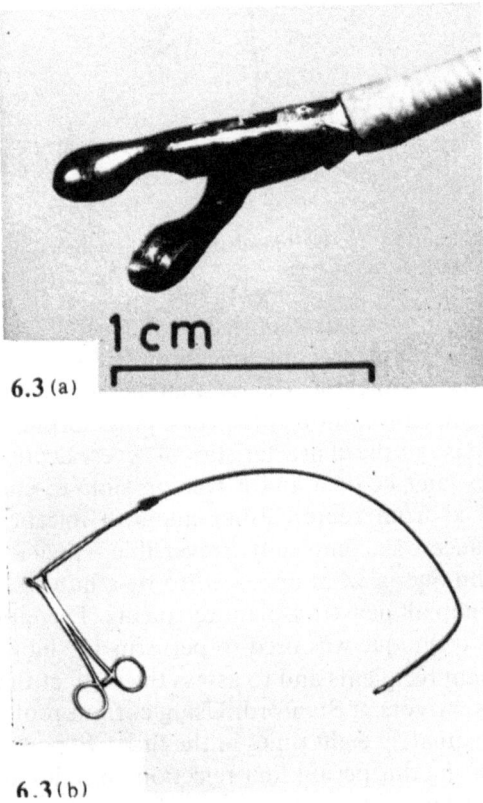

6.3 (a)

6.3 (b)

Figure 6.3 An instrument used in serial biopsy of the heart in man. (a) Movable jaws at one end of the instrument. (b) A flexible catheter and a handle to open and close the jaws at the other end.

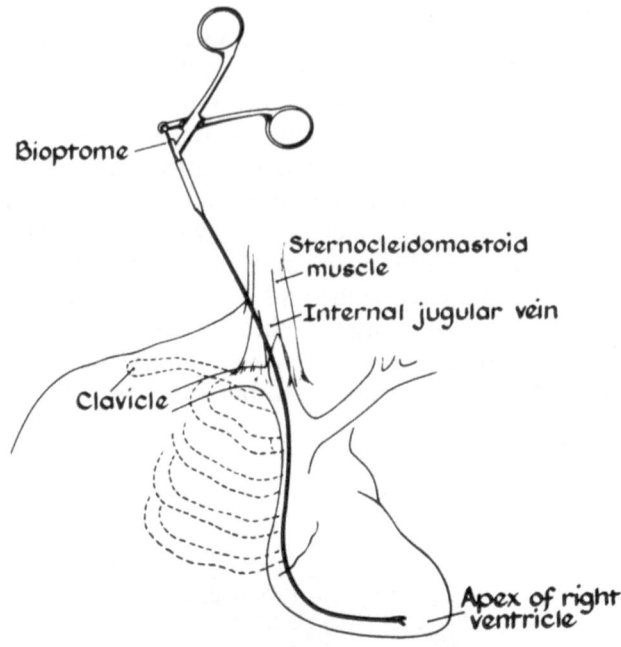

Figure 6.3(c) Insertion of the instrument through the internal jugular vein into the apex of the right ventricle

The first patient who was biopsied in August 1972 underwent what appeared to be totally irreversible rejection 21 days posttransplantation. His biopsy showed only too clearly that he had acute rejection with interstitial oedema, infiltration of red cells, polymorphs and lymphocytes, and myocytolysis; all the characteristics of severe acute rejection (Figure 6.4). Four days later he died and it was possible to confirm at autopsy that he had died from acute cardiac allograft rejection, which in this particular instance was completely irreversible. Having first justified the use of this technique in what appeared to be a hopeless situation it was decided to use it in all new transplant recipients. Therefore, over the next 10 months this technique was used to perform 119 biopsy procedures in 16 new transplant recipients and to assess the state of the myocardium in the long-term survivors at Stanford. Using current protocol, patients are biopsied approximately eight times in the first two postoperative months because it is during this period that rejection episodes are most frequent and serious, and if patients can be successfully kept in good health through the first two postoperative months, then they have an excellent chance of long-term survival. Thus biopsies are performed at regular intervals, first on the 6th postoperative day and then, using the electrocardiogram or the atrial electromyogram, whenever a rejection episode appears imminent. Even if the patient appears to be doing well, a biopsy is performed every seven to 10 days, because the histological changes of rejection sometimes occur three or four days before there are any changes on the electro-

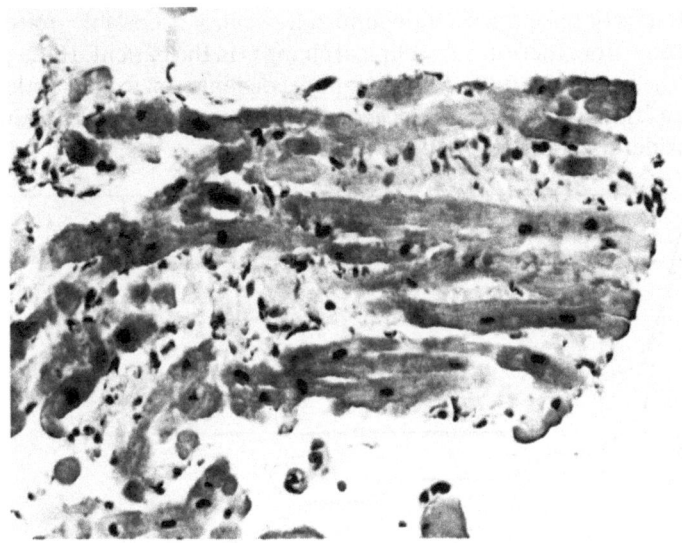

Figure 6.4 The results of a biopsy showing all the characteristics of severe acute rejection

cardiogram. If these early changes can be detected, it might be possible to be more successful in the management of these patients and use smaller amounts of immunosuppression. Figure 6.5 shows the current protocol for the diagnosis of acute rejection. The principal determinant of long-term survival following clinical heart transplantation today is the ability to recognise early acute rejection episodes and to reverse them successfully. Nowadays only three main parameters are used: the electrocardiogram

1. Diagnosis of acute rejection:
    (a) Serial transvenous endomyocardial biopsy
    (b) Electrocardiogram and atrial electromyogram
    (c) Clinical examination
2. Indications for treatment:
    (a) ΣQRS voltage (leads I, II, III, V_1, V_6) decreased > 20%
    (b) Atrial electromyogram QRS voltage decreased > 20%
    (c) Atrial arrhythmias
    (d) Diastolic gallop sound (S_3 or S_4)
    (e) Histological evidence of rejection

Figure 6.5 The current protocol for the diagnosis of acute rejection

and the atrial electromyogram which are recorded twice daily in the first two postoperative months; clinical examination twice daily, and the biopsies as on the previously outlined protocol. The indications for treatment of an acute rejection episode are: histological evidence of rejection, with or without a drop in the QRS voltages or the development of atrial arrhythmias, and clinical signs such as a third heart sound. Note that clinical signs of rejection are now unusual because if possible, rejection is diagnosed before there are any clinical changes in the patient. If the patient gets to the stage of having cardiac failure, oedema, or feeling listless and tired, rejection has probably proceeded too far and his chances of survival are considerably decreased.

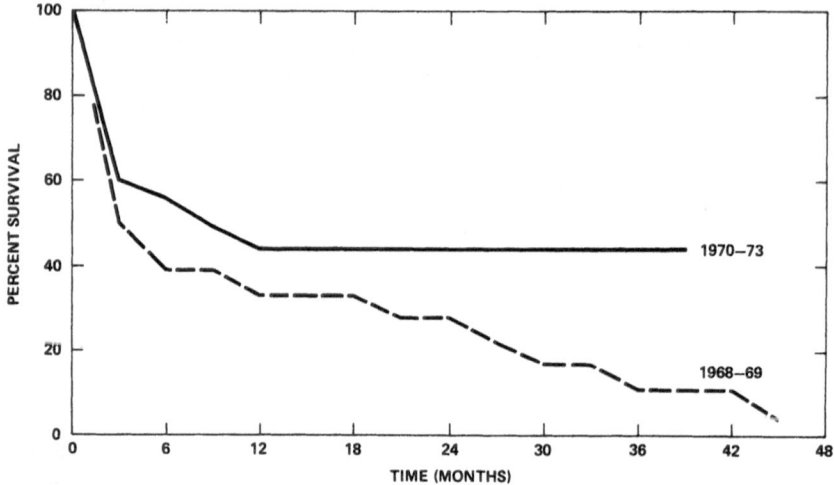

Figure 6.6 Heart transplant survival results at Stanford University, for 1968–1969 and 1970–1973

The basic immunosuppressive regimes were largely as in renal transplantation and consisted of triple therapy with azathioprine, prednisone and antilymphocyte globulin. In the last year and one-half cyclophosphamide has been used in preference to azathioprine and may have given slightly better results. The treatment of an acute rejection episode consists of giving large doses of methylprednisolone for a few days, increasing the basic prednisone while leaving the cyclophosphamide or azathioprine unchanged and sometimes using Actinomycin D. The patient is also heparinised for seven days. In addition the patients are all on long-term anticoagulation with Warfarin and also receive Diparydimol to try to prevent vascular lesions (see Chapter 5).

Figure 6.6 compares the results for the first two years of the programme and the next three and one-half years and shows that there has been an improvement over the years of up to around 50% one-year survival. This 50% mark is approximately the same figure as the survival of cadaveric renal transplants taking the world-wide figures. In the last year the Stanford one-year heart transplant survival has been 57% but these are not really very large changes. However, if the patient survives the first three months, in good health, then the chance of long-term survival is really very good indeed. It is the first two to three post-operative months which are crucial as far as the heart transplant recipient is concerned (Table 6.2).

Table 6.2 Heart transplant survival statistics

Overall

43% – 1 year survival
40% – 2 year survival
28% – 3 year survival

1st programme year	22% 1 year survival
2nd programme year	44% 1 year survival
3rd programme year	50% 1 year survival
4th programme year	42% 1 year survival
5th programme year	53% 1 year survival
6th programme year	57% 1 year survival

3 Month Survivors

76% 1 year survival
71% 2 year survival
50% 3 year survival

The main causes of death in heart transplant recipients are rejection and infection. Since there is no means of mechanical support for the transplanted heart, the heart must function adequately from the moment of transplantation and it is necessary to immunosuppress the patients heavily in the face of repeated rejection episodes. Inevitably, in these patients, deaths occur from the complications of immunosuppressive therapy. Deaths from infection are often really deaths from repeated rejection episodes which had to be treated in order to keep the patient alive. When the infections appear, they have a quite different pattern from hospital infections in non-immunosuppressed patients – the main problems are pulmonary infections with a high incidence of fungal, viral, parasitic and nocardial infections. This high incidence includes rare infections such as aspergillosis, nocardiosis and pneumocystis, as

well as infections with the gram negative bacteria *E. coli* and Klebsielli.
E. coli and Klebsielli.

In order to attempt prevention of these particular pulmonary infections, it is very important to monitor the lungs almost as closely as the
heart. The patients have daily chest X-rays, daily sputum culture and
if there is any suspicion at all of the development of a pulmonary
infection, they are put through a very intensive diagnostic regime in
order to begin the treatment for infection at the earliest possible moment
(Figure 6.7). In the face of an intrapulmonary infection a delay of a matter
of hours may make the difference between the patient's survival or death.

Screening
 1.   Daily PA and lateral chest X-ray films
 2.   Daily sputum culture – routine and fungal
 3.   Twice-daily physical examination

When pulmonary infection suspected
 1.   Immediate transtracheal aspiration of secretions for gram stain, fungal stains and
      cultures
 2.   Whole lung tomograms
 3.   Percutaneous needle biopsy of opacities

Figure 6.7 Diagnosis of pulmonary infections

In the early days, three of the long-term transplant survivors died
between 18 to 36 months and, on examination of the donor hearts, they
had severe coronary artery disease. This coronary artery disease occurred
even in those recipients who had been transplanted initially for idiopathic
cardiomyopathy and was obviously some form of chronic rejection
process resulting in intimal proliferation. It was concluded that this intimal
proliferation was related to acute rejection damage with intimal repair and
regeneration and then deposition of lipid. This finally resulted in coronary
occlusive disease. Since the patients did not get angina in their denervated hearts, the first evidence of chronic rejection was often
arrhythmias, myocardial infarction or sudden death. However, in the
last three and one-half years heparin has been given to patients during
acute rejection episodes and long-term treatment with anticoagulation and
Diparydimol has been instituted. Since this therapy has been introduced
the problem of chronic graft rejection seems to have almost disappeared.

As a result of the Stanford series it has been observed that those
patients who have had previous cardiac bypass surgery have had remarkably better results than the group of patients who have not. Figure
6.8 shows that in a group of 11 patients only one died in the first year.
The number of rejection episodes and amount of immunosuppression
etc. all seemed to be less and it appears that a previous cardiopulmonary bypass operation in some way enhances the possibility of
putting in a donor heart and getting a good result. These figures are not

yet statistically significant but there is certainly a remarkable difference. Furthermore patients over the age of 50 do considerably less well. The recent one-year survival rate for patients under the age of 50 is about 70%. This is because the older patients do not tolerate the immuno-suppression and the serious infections which often ocur in the first three postoperative months.

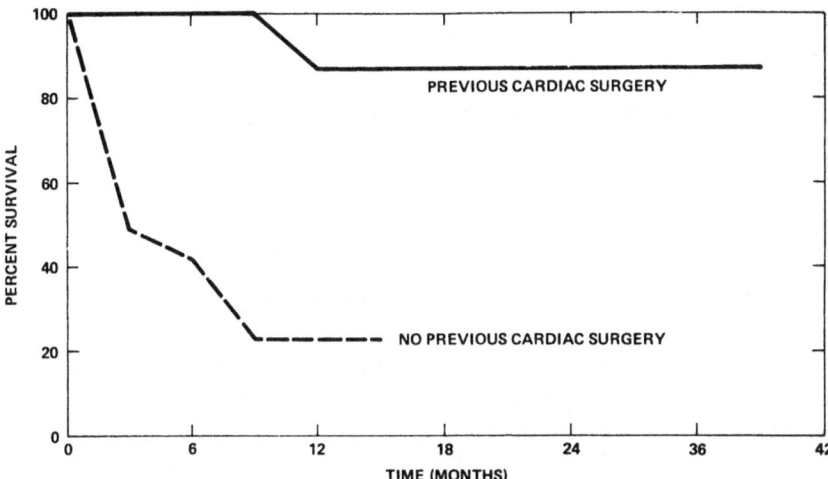

Figure 6.8 The percent survival figures for transplant patients who have had previous cardiac bypass surgery as compared with those who have not

In the first year at Stanford, three patients were transplanted with high pulmonary vascular resistance and all three died from right heart failure within the first three days. Since high pulmonary vascular resistance (> 6 units) was recognised as an absolute contraindication there have been no operative deaths at all in the rest of the series. The absence of infection is very important for long-term survival. Similarly there must be no serious primary or secondary impairment of renal or hepatic function.

In conclusion, it can now be said that following heart transplantation, patients currently have a 55% one-year survival, that survival for several years is possible – the figure for the longest survivor is now over five years – and that excellent functional rehabilitation is possible – many of the Stanford long-term survivors are back at work, full time. How-ever there are remaining problems. These are related to the supply of donor organs, the complications of the immunosuppressivé agents which have to be used at the present time and to chronic graft atherosclerosis, but these remaining problems should not obscure the fact that cardiac transplantation offers, today, the possibility of new life to some patients terminally ill with cardiac disease for whom, otherwise, there is no hope.

7
The place of transplantation
Ch. Dubost

In 1968 in Paris, three attempts at heart transplantation in human patients were made by my team. Several factors arising from these attempts led to the decision that no further attempts would be made.

THE RECIPIENT

Cardiac human transplantation is suitable for treatment of all types of heart diseases but contraindicated in patients with profound extra-cardiac disorders. The ideal patient is the patient without any disease in lungs, kidney, liver or brain, i.e. an ideal recipient would be one with isolated cardiac disease. Coronary heart disease is the most common disease to be dealt with in a programme of heart transplantation. Patients may also present with intractable heart failure after several myocardial infarctions or failure of saphenous vein bypass grafts. The cardiomyopathies and idiopathic cardiomyopathies seem to give less good results in the cardiac transplantations. The average survival figure in 20 patients put forward for transplantation but not operated on is 30 days. This means that all these patients selected for transplantation have a life expectancy of only 30 days, although sometimes a patient can survive for a year of more. Similarly in the group of patients waiting for cardiac transplantation in 1968 in Paris, the majority died soon after they had been selected for transplantation. However, one of them is still alive today – five years later. The selection of the recipient is therefore no easy matter.

THE DONOR

The selection of a donor is a very difficult problem to solve. In France a law was established in April 1968, just before the first cardiac trans-plantation, which includes a definition of cerebral death, i.e. the absence of a spontaneous respiration, the absence of reflexes, the absence of a reading on the electroencephalograph in a normothermic patient receiving no depressive drugs and confirmation of this by cerebral arteriogram. The diagnosis of cerebral death, according to French law, should be documented by a neurosurgical team independent of the team involved in the transplantation operation. This law assumes that cerebral damage is irreversible, but if in the future it is found that brain damage can be successfully treated, then the present definition of cerebral death will be inadequate for the purposes of cardiac transplantation.

HISTOCOMPATIBILITY

Two years ago Dr Shumway abandoned tissue typing and now selects donor hearts on the basis of ABO group compatibility and suitability of size. However, the author believes that tissue typing and matching is very important and would lead to better results.

The procurement of cardiac grafts sets moral and ethical problems. There is an enormous number of potential recipients and a very small number of donors. How are patients selected for transplantation? This is a very important ethical problem and it is very difficult to face. Obviously the surgeon would select the best possible recipient i.e. one without lung, kidney, or liver diseases. Further difficulties lie in the fact that organ banks are still non-existent and this raises the question as to whether the donor or recipient should be sent to the place where there is a heart available for transplantation. Obviously it would be preferable if the heart could be preserved for days or weeks and then used in the place where the recipient is waiting.

REJECTION

Dr Shumway has shown that after heart transplantation several patients have developed a coronary atherosclerosis. However in chronic rejection the involvement of coronary artery branches by intimal proliferation is not similar to the atherosclerotic process. For this reason the efficiency of long-term anticoagulant therapy could be questionable. The anti-rejection drugs are azathioprine, prednisone and antilymphocyte globulins. In cases of rejection the doses are increased with the addition of anticoagulants. This is exactly the programme used in 1968 in Paris in the three cases of human cardiac transplantation, i.e. antilymphocyte globulin, azathioprine and prednisone, and platelets, lymphocytes and leukocytes were counted. The level of prednisone had to be increased in the first patient after seven days because of a pleural effusion but after that the level was decreased and 50 mg prednisone was administered daily.

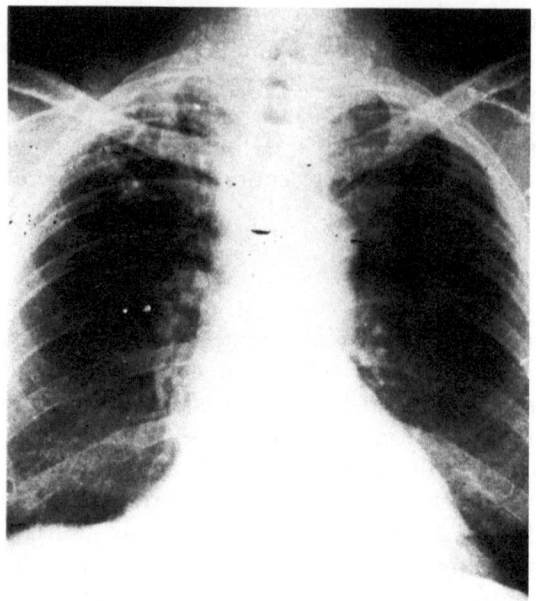

Figure 7.1 Heart and lungs 14 months after operation

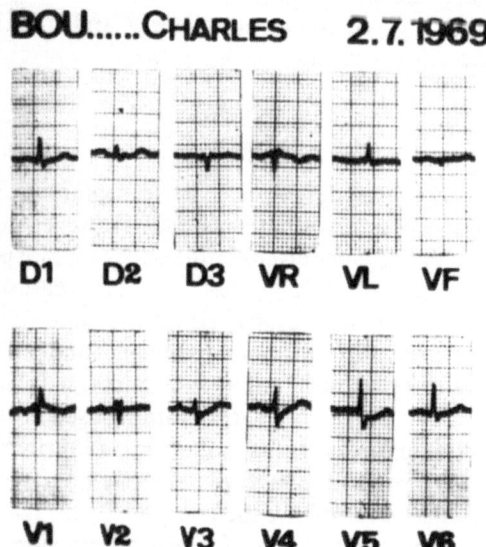

Figure 7.2 Decrease in the voltage at the same time

Figure 7.1 shows an X-ray taken 14 months after the operation of the heart. After 14 months evidence of chronic rejection appeared (Figure 7.2). Despite all efforts this patient died suddenly 18 months after operation. The postmortem angiogram (Figure 7.3) showed that the main coronary branches were not involved in any atherosclerotic process.

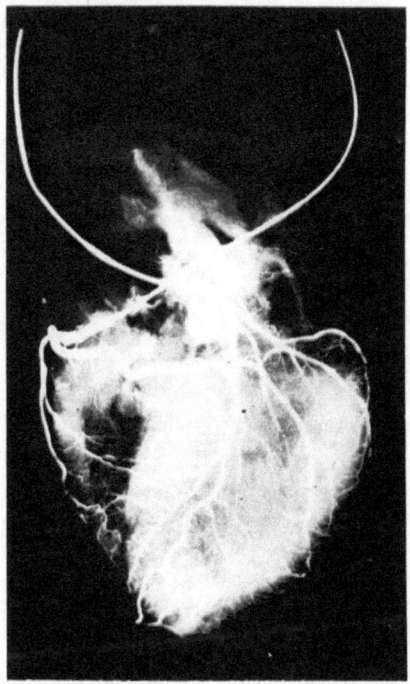

Figure 7.3 Postmortem coronary angiography

However, microscopic examination revealed that there were alterations of the coronary vessels by intimal thickening (Figure 7.4). The postoperative course of the second patient was exactly the same. He was given imuran, antilymphocyte globulin and prednisone and died after 13 months with evidence of chronic rejection. The angiogram (Figure 7.6) showed that he had developed very profound disorders at the level of both coronary arteries. Figure 7.5 shows evidence of very profound rejection in the heart muscle. The third patient died two hours after transplantation of an unknown cause.

At present, world figures for heart transplantation are 227 in 223 recipients. Only 35 are alive with functioning grafts and the figure for the longest survival is 5.2 years. In France, one patient who was operated on in November 1968 is still alive five years and four months after the operation. He is doing well though it is not known why. He has a little decalcification of the spine due to cortisone therapy but he leads quite an acceptable life. Since tissue matching in this patient was poor his success

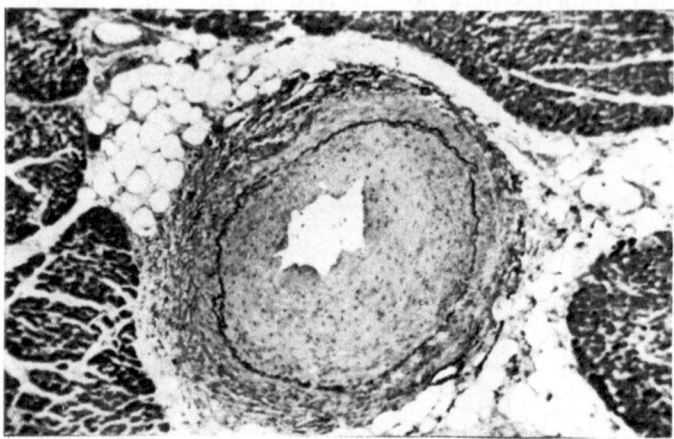

Figure 7.4 Almost complete obstruction of a small coronary branch

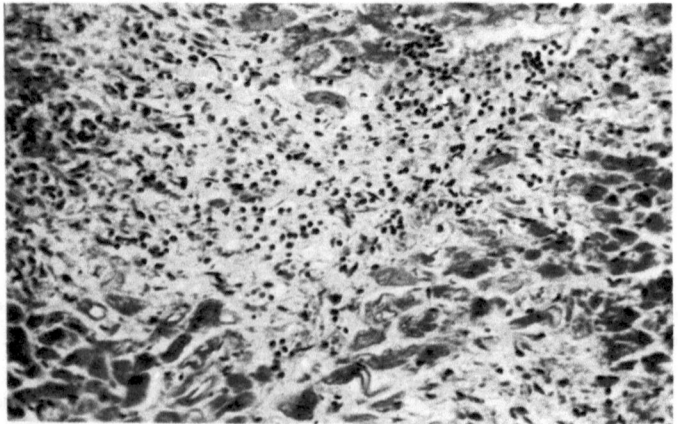

Figure 7.5 Photomicrograph showing massive rejection

lends support to Dr Shumway's theories. In 1973 in France, nine human cardiac transplantations were performed in eight recipients. Only one is alive at the moment 12 months after operation. The technique of human cardiac transplantation is still an experimental one particularly with respect to the problem of taking care of the patient after transplantation. In fact, human cardiac transplantation is no longer a surgical problem and the majority of cardiac surgeons are able to perform it. However, in the author's opinion, a surgeon should not be permitted to perform a

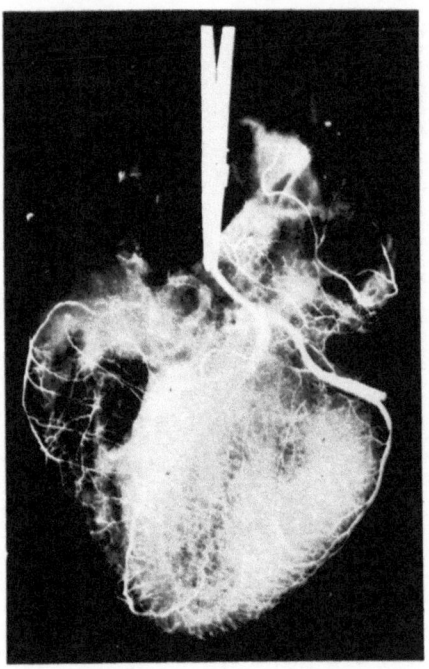

Figure 7.6 Postmortem coronary angiography

transplantation simply because he can and wants to do it. Heart transplantation must be the business of a small number of groups with a profound commitment and with financial backing. The conclusions of Fadali and Soloff appear very sound, i.e. that in every country there should be only one group of physicians, scientists, surgeons. This group should be profoundly devoted to the business of heart transplantation, and should have the facilities for experimentation in order to improve not only the surgical results of heart transplantation but also to simplify post-operative care. To take care of these patients and carry out and interpret biopsies every week inflicts a heavy responsibility on the surgical and medical team. Patients become very hospital-dependent and need intensive daily care. At the present time in France, it would be very hard for any of the cardiac surgery services available to take on this responsibility.

Part 2

Fallot's Tetralogy

8
The surgical anatomy of Fallot's tetralogy
R. H. Anderson and A. E. Becker

Knowledge of cardiac embryogenesis enables the morphology of many anomalous hearts to be interpreted in the light of normal cardiac architecture. This is the case with Fallot's tetralogy and it is therefore pertinent to commence this chapter with a brief review of its development, or rather its maldevelopment.

It has recently been demonstrated by Goor and his associates[1] and confirmed by the authors' own investigations[2] that normal development can be summed up as conal inversion followed by absorption of the posterior conoventricular junction (or bulboventricular ledge) (Figure 8.1a and b). The conal inversion is such that the conotruncal ridges which ultimately septate the conus are laid down in sinistro-anterior and dextro-posterior positions, but following inversion the presumptive aorta is still above the bulbar cavity. It is conal absorption (Figure 8.1b) which is responsible for transferring the aorta to the left ventricle. At the same time this process reorientates the primary interventricular foramen so that it becomes the aortic outflow tract and produces mitral-aortic fibrous continuity. Posterior excursion of the conus septum simultaneously blocks the anterosinistral portion of the newly-formed secondary interventricular foramen. The aorta is then closed from the right ventricle by growth of the endocardial cushions which form the membranous septum. The parietal portion of the conus septum together with the overlying conoventricular flange separate the tricuspid and pulmonary valves in the roof of the right ventricle, forming the crista supraventricularis.

In Fallot's tetralogy it can be postulated that there is lack of normal conal inversion. This is indicated by a counter-clockwise rotation of the conotruncal ridges so that they occupy sinistral and dextral positions (Figure 8.1c). Conal absorption then occurs, but since the presumptive aorta is more right-sided, full reorientation of the primary foramen cannot occur, consequently although there is mitral-aortic fibrous continuity the aorta overrides the septum. Since the aorta is right-sided, conal absorption can also produce aortic-tricuspid fibrous continuity (Figure 8.1d). The single process of 'lack of conal inversion' explains the

49

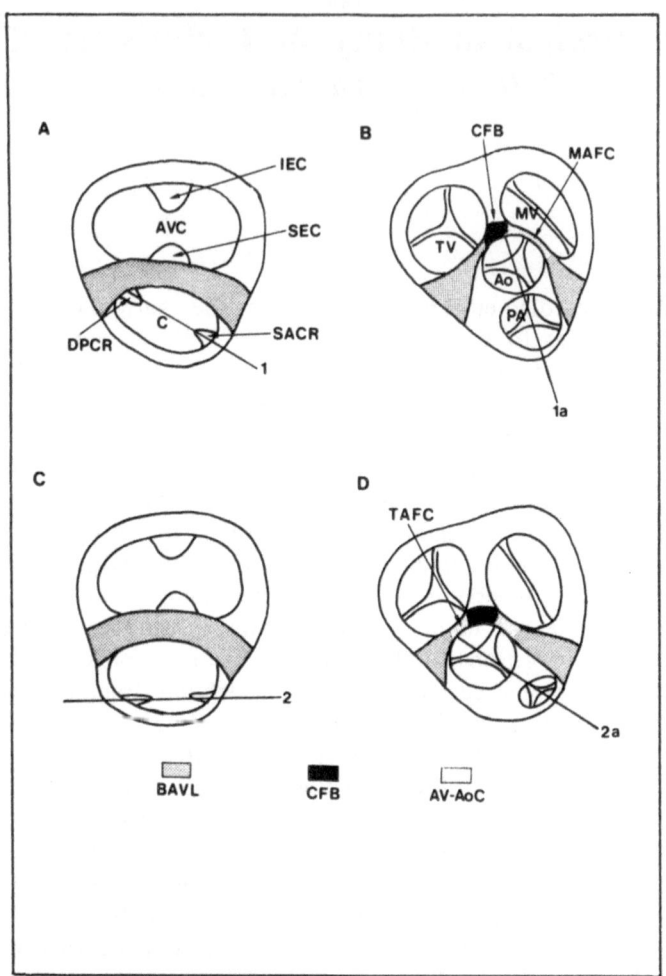

Figure 8.1 The embryogenesis of Fallot's tetralogy. (a) The bulboventricular loop after normal conal inversion. The conal ridges (DPCR, SACR) are in dextro-posterior and sinistro-anterior positions and their orientation is indicated by line 1. The atrioventricular canal (AVC) is being septated by the endocardial cushions (IEC, SEC). (b) The transference of the aorta following absorption of the midportion of the bulboatrioventricular ledge (BAVL). (The bulboatrioventricular ledge is the embryonic structure that is termed the conoventricular flange (CVF) in adult specimens.) This produces aortic-mitral continuity (MAFC) and establishes the central fibrous body (CFB). (c) in Fallot's tetralogy, lack of normal conal inversion results in counter-clockwise rotation of the conal ridges and they are additionally deviated in an anterior deviation. (d) Conal absorption then results in an overriding, dextroposed aorta and produces both aortic-mitral continuity and aortic-tricuspid continuity (TAFC). From Becker *et al.*, by courtesy of *Amer. J. Cardiol.*)

septal defect and aortic dextroposition. However, in order to explain the pulmonary stenosis it is necessary also to postulate anterior deviation of the conus septum, thus producing malseptation of the conus at the expense of the pulmonary artery (Figure 8.1c and d). The right ventricular hypertrophy which completes the classical tetrad is an haemodynamic consequence of these embryonic maldevelopments. Thus the embryogenesis of Fallot's tetralogy can be summed up in terms of conal rotation and anterior deviation of the conus septum.

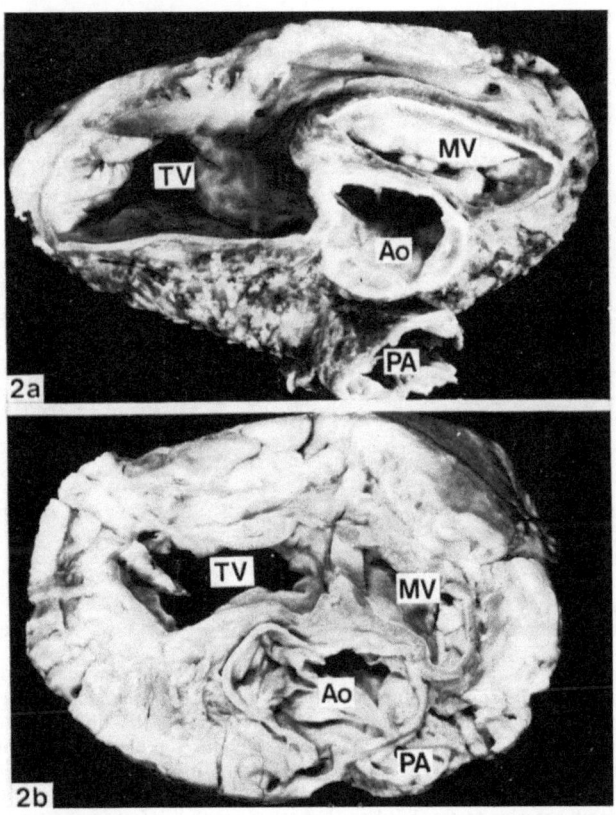

Figure 8.2 (a) The superior aspect of a normal heart. (b) A specimen of Fallot's tetralogy. In the normal heart the aortic valve (Ao) is wedged between tricuspid and mitral valves (TV, MV). In the Fallot specimen the aortic valve is dextroposed and anteriorly deviated. Note also the change in orientation of the aorta relative to the pulmonary artery (PA).

Examination of specimens of Fallot's tetralogy enables us to test the validity of these hypotheses, again comparing them with normal hearts. A superior view of the normal heart dissected to demonstrate the interrelationships of the valve rings illustrates that the aortic valve is deeply wedged between the tricuspid and mitral orifices (Figure 8.2a). This position is a consequence of normal conal absorption following normal conal inversion. It should also be noted that the pulmonary artery is anterior and to the left. In Fallot's tetralogy the aortic valve is deviated anteriorly and to the right, and is no longer in its wedge position (Figure 8.2b). Instead it is related to the front of the tricuspid valve and is also in a more side-by-side relationship with the pulmonary artery.

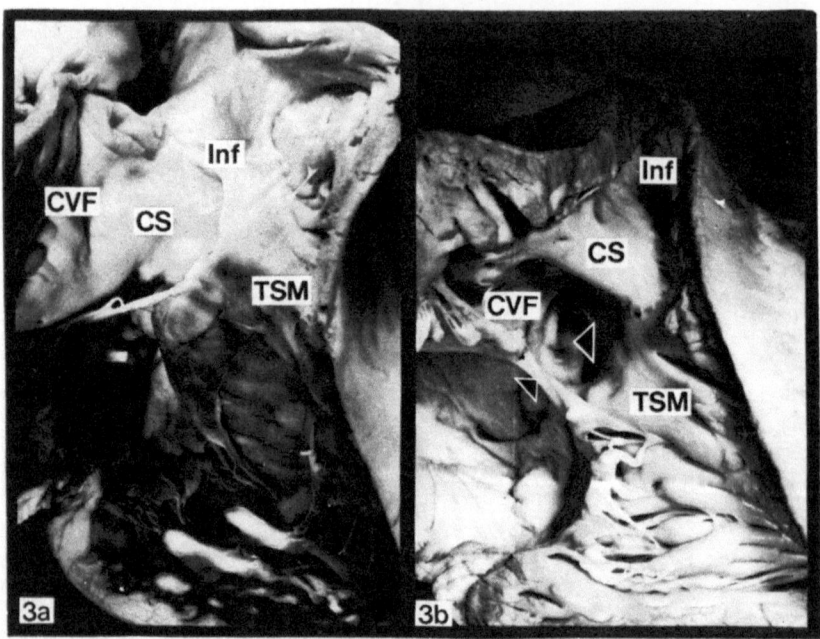

Figure 8.3 (a) The right ventricles of a normal heart. (b) The right ventricle of a Fallot heart. In the normal heart the conus septum (CS) blocks the anterior part of the interventricular foramen and is inserted in the muscular septum between the limbs of the trabecula septo-marginalis (TSM). The parietal part of the conus septum together with the right margin of the CVF form the crista supraventricularis. In the Fallot specimen the conus septum is anteriorly deviated and rotated so that it spans the ventricular cavity. Its septal insertion is now anterior to the TSM so that a wide septal defect is present (arrowed). It is also separated from the CVF which intervenes partially between the tricuspid and aortic valves. However, note the area of aortic-tricuspid continuity (open arrow). Inf-infundibulum

This relationship has been confirmed by two recent geometric studies of hearts exhibiting Fallot's tetralogy[3,4] and is an expression of 'lack of normal conal inversion'.

Examination of the septal aspect of the normal right ventricle shows that inflow and outflow portions of the ventricle are separated by an extensive trabeculation, termed by Tandler the trabecula septomarginalis, but also referred to as the septal band. This structure, which shall be referred to as the TSM, is not part of the conus septum. Superiorly in the normal heart it splits into two limbs and the septal insertion of the conus septum fuses with the muscular septum between them (Figure 8.3a). The conus septum arches from this position to the parietal wall of the ventricle, lying beneath and fused with the right extremity of the conoventricular flange and together with it forming the crista supraventricularis.

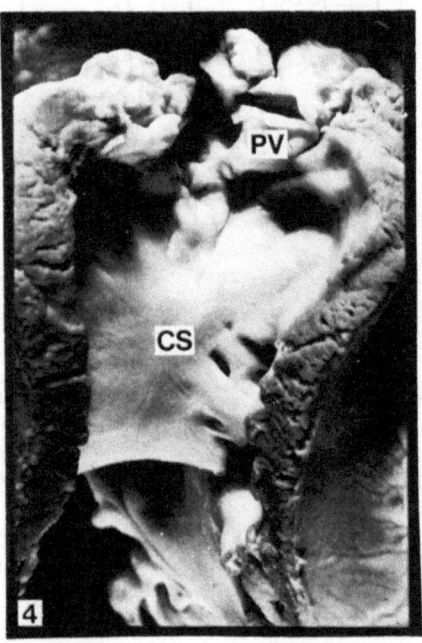

Figure 8.4 Anterior view of the pulmonary infundibulum. It is of normal length, but is constructed due to the anterior deviation of the conus septum (CS). PV – pulmonary valve

In Fallot's tetralogy, owing to the conal rotation, the parietal portion of the conus septum is divorced from the CV flange. In addition the septal insertion is deviated anteriorly (Figure 8.3b). This is indicated by the fact that the septal insertion is anterior to the anterior limb of the TSM, rather than being between the limbs of the structure as in the normal heart. As a consequence of both rotation and anterior deviation the conus septum straddles the right ventricular cavity as a thick muscular bar. The anterior edge of the septum encroaches upon the pulmonary infundibulum, but nonetheless the infundibulum is well-formed and is of normal length (Figure. 8.4). Indeed, the morphometric studies referred to[3,4] demonstrate that infundibular length may even be increased compared with the normal (Figure 8.5), and do not support a recent claim that the infundibulum of Fallot's tetralogy is 'too short, too narrow and too shallow'[5].

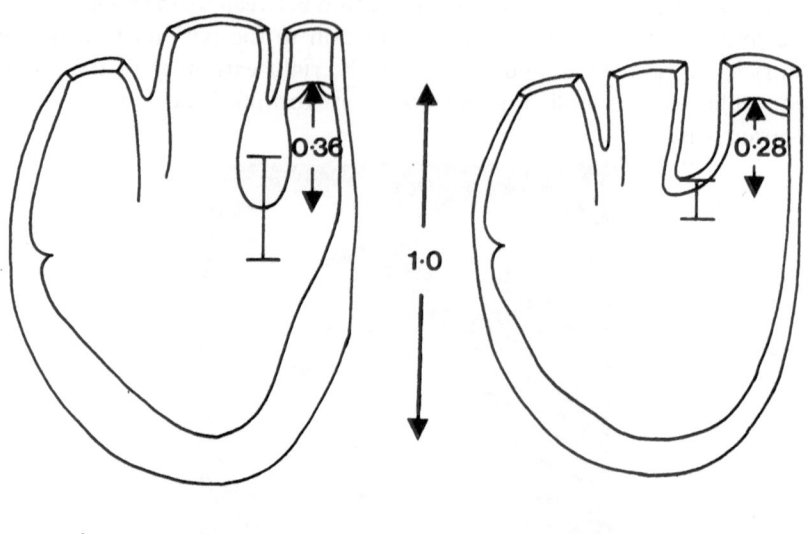

Fallot's Tetralogy   **Normal Hearts**

Figure 8.5 Diagram illustrating the average length of the pulmonary infundibulum as a ratio of right ventricular length in 14 Fallot specimens compared with 10 normal hearts. From Becker *et al.*,[4] by courtesy of *Amer. J. Cardiol.*)

Having established that pathologic observations endorse the embryogenetic hypothesis, the authors are now in a position to give an exact account of the arterial outflow tracts and the associated septal defect in Fallot's tetralogy. The anterior margin of the aortic outflow tract is the deviated conus septum, which fuses with the muscular septum medially, being reinforced by the TSM. Superiorly the aortic valve rises from the conus septum and from the left extremity of the CVF, and then takes origin from the region of mitral-aortic continuity. Owing to the conal absorption this part of the outflow tract is part of the left ventricle. Posteriorly the aortic valve arises from the central fibrous body and in this situation the muscular septum sweeps up to become the posterior interventricular septum. To the right in most specimens there is then a small area where the aortic valve is in continuity with the tricuspid valve and then the aortic valve arises from the right margin of the CVF. This part of the outflow tract is above the right ventricle and the CVF forms the remaining circumference of the aortic valve, fusing anteriorly with the conus septum (Figure 8.6). From a surgical viewpoint, the aortic outflow tract can therefore be considered to represent an additional segment of the right ventricle, intervening between its inflow portions and the infundibulum. In total corrections it is necessary to close the right border

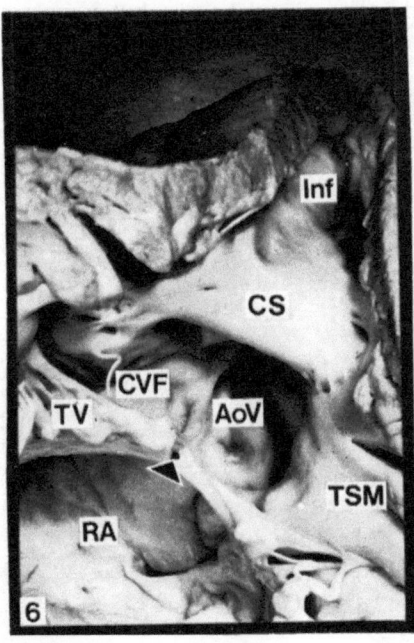

Figure 8.6 Photograph illustrating the aortic segment of the right ventricle in a specimen of Fallot's tetralogy (high power of Figure 8.3b). RA – Right atrium; TV – Tricuspid valve; CVF – Conoventricular flange; AOV – Aortic valve; CS – Conus septum; TSM – Trabecule septomarginalis; Inf – Infundibulum; Arrow – Aortic tricuspid continuity

of the aortic outflow tract, thus restoring its continuity with the left ventricle. The boundaries of this border are mostly muscular, being the CVF superiorly, the conus septum anteriorly and the muscular septum reinforced by the TSM inferiorly. Posteriorly the area of aortic-tricuspid continuity and the central fibrous body complete the margin.

In some specimens, however, this latter area is also muscular, and the origin of this muscle is a source of some controversy. In the authors' opinion (Figure 8.7a and b) the muscle is unabsorbed CVF, as is demonstrated by dissection and sectioning of the muscular ridge. It follows from this that in these specimens both components of the crista supra-ventricularis of the 'normal' right ventricle present above the ventricular cavity as muscular crests. For this reason the authors consider it inappropriate to use the term crista when describing specimens of Fallot's tetralogy.

This term could equally well be applied to either muscle bundle. Instead they recommend the use of 'conus septum' to describe the anterior ridge and 'conoventricular flange' to describe the posterior ridge.

The pulmonary outflow tract or infundibulum, as stated, is of usual length compared with normal hearts, but is narrowed by the anterior deviation of the conus septum. Its posterior boundary is the conus septum,

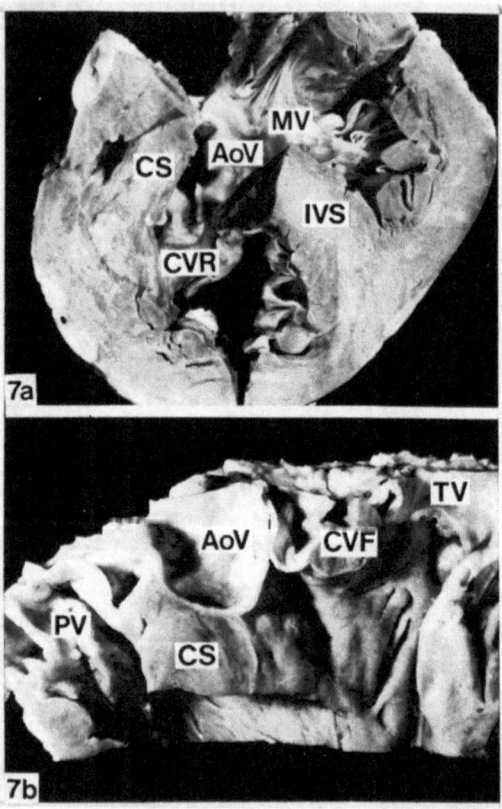

Figure 8.7 Specimen of Fallot's tetralogy with aortic-tricuspid discontinuity. (a) Inferior view exhibiting the muscle bar separating the valves. (b) Section of the right ventricle demonstrating that the bar is an infolding of the heart wall and represents that conoventricular flange (CVF). Abbreviations as for Figure 8.6

and the parietal extension of this structure descends the lateral wall of the ventricle as a well-formed trabecula. In most specimens there are additional trabecula within the infundibulum which further encroach upon its lumen. From examination of pathological specimens it does not appear that the TSM (or septal band) produces much infundibular stenosis and if it

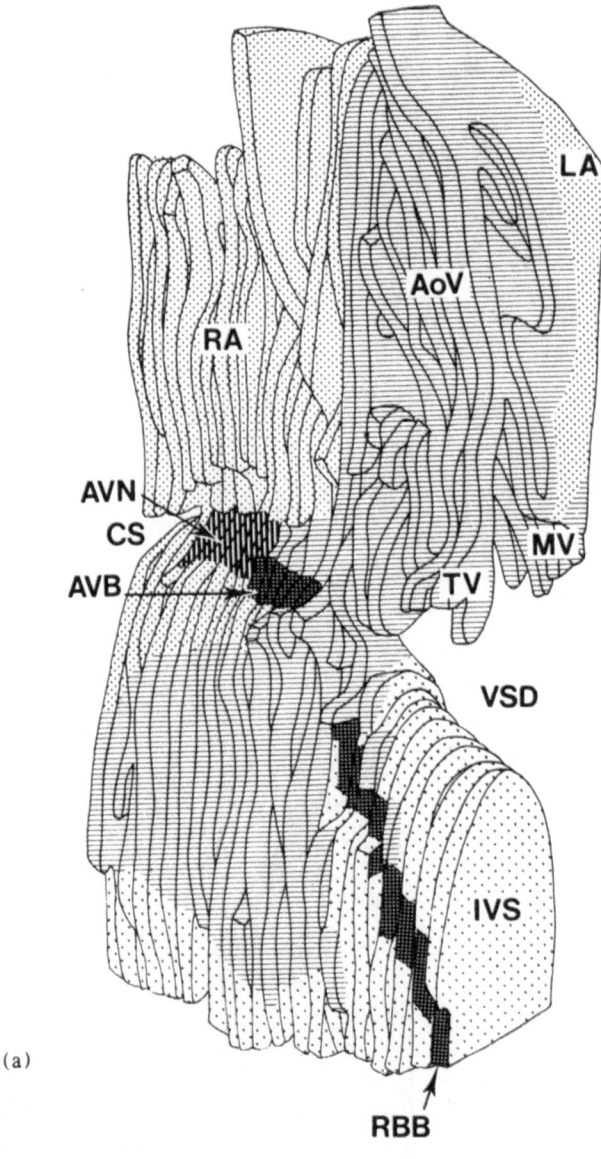

(a)

Figure 8.8 Artist's impression of a reconstruction of the conducting tissue in a specimen of Fallot's tetralogy. The block taken consisted of the posterior margins of the septal defect. (a) A view from the right side. (b) A left-sided view. Although the right bundle is shown subendocardially, it was in an intramyocardial position. AVN – atrioventricular node; AVB – perforating bundle; LBB – left bundle branch; RBB – right bundle branch; IVS – Interventricular septum; TV – tricuspid valve; MV – mitral valve; AoV – Aortic valve; RA – Right atrium; LA – Left atrium

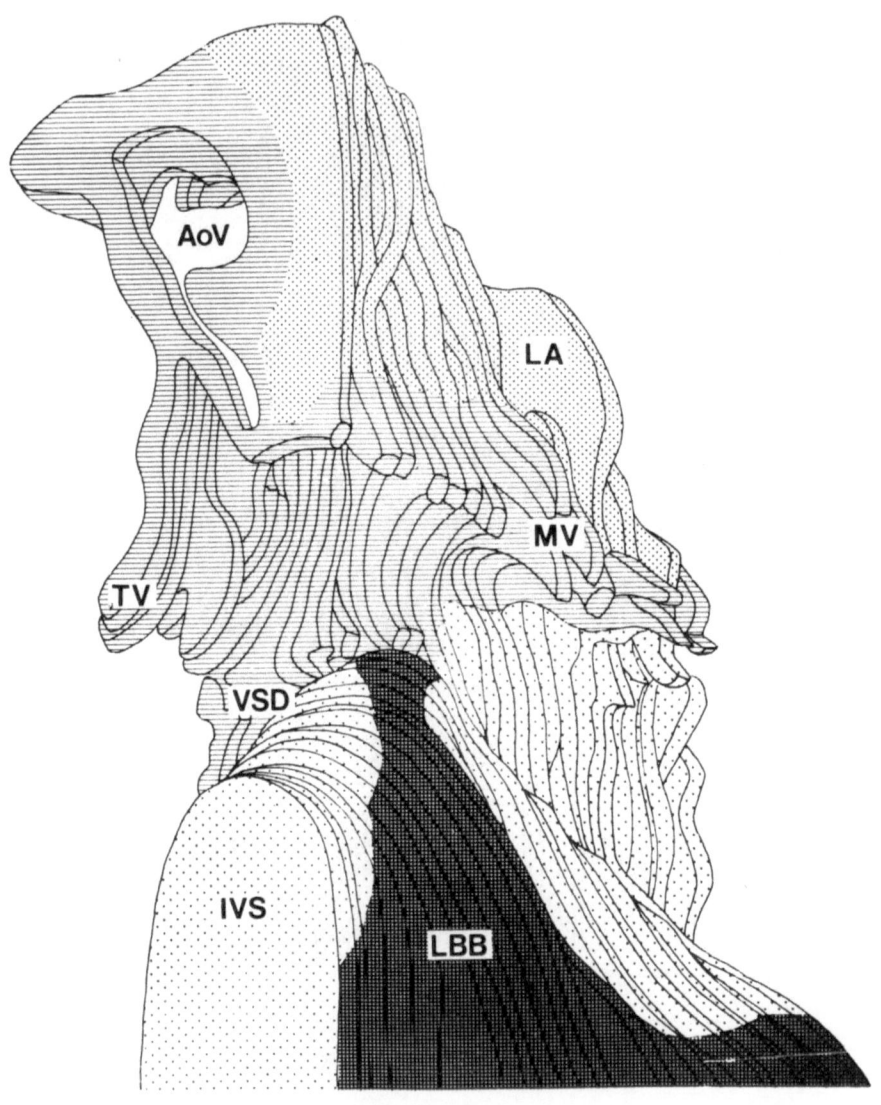

Figure 8.8 (b)   A left-sided view

produced an angiographic feature, it would be a septal feature, not parietal or anterior.

No description of surgical anatomy is complete without an account of the disposition of the atrioventricular conduction tissues. The authors' own observations in this respect represent an endorsement of the excellent and detailed description by Lev.[5] The atrioventricular node is normally formed to the right of the central fibrous body. The penetrating bundle then perforates the fibrous ring in the posterior margin of the defect (Figure 8.8) and descends down the left side of the septum, lying some distance from the surface of the defect. The right bundle branch is given off well beneath the defect margin and penetrates intramyocardially beneath the TSM to the right side of the septum. It then descends as a thin strand between the TSM and the septum, passing directly beneath the conal papillary muscle when present. The posterior radiation of the left

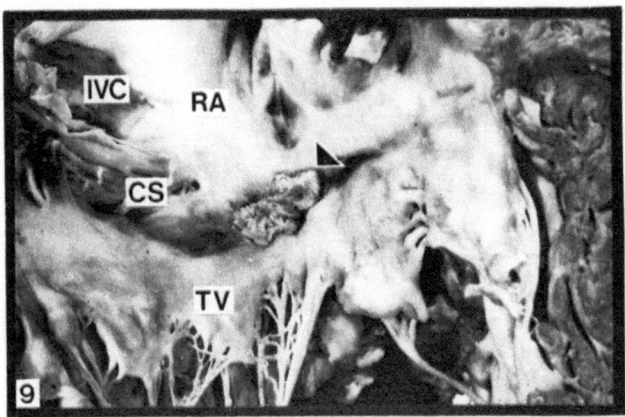

Figure 8.9 Photograph of a specimen of Fallot's Tetralogy in which operative repair produced traumatic heart block. The arrowed Teflon 'pearl' had been sutured into the area of tricuspid – aortic fibrous continuity and the penetrating bundle had been extensively traumatised. RA – Right atrium; IVC – Inferior vena cava; CS – Coronary sinus; TV – Tricuspid valve

bundle is unrelated to the defect, whilst the anterior radiation streams forward a good distance beneath the crest of the septum. The reconstruction (Figure 8.8a and b) demonstrates that the conducting tissues are relatively safe during suturing round the defect. The 'danger area' must be considered as the point where the tricuspid valve joins the central fibrous body, since this marks the point of passage of the penetrating bundle from right to left sides. In one case in the authors' collection a suture inserted at this point produced complete heart block (Figure 8.9).

In conclusion the authors would emphasise that they have described the anatomy of a typical Fallot specimen. However, examination of their specimens indicates that Fallot's tetralogy does not constitute a well-defined entity. It is rather part of a spectrum of bulboventricular malformations and many specimens exhibit features of pseudotruncus, double outlet right ventricle septal defect with overriding aorta. It is the embryogenetic concept outlined at the beginning of the chapter which is the unifying feature of this spectrum (Figure 8.10). It is also significant that a recent investigation has established a spectrum of progression of Fallot's

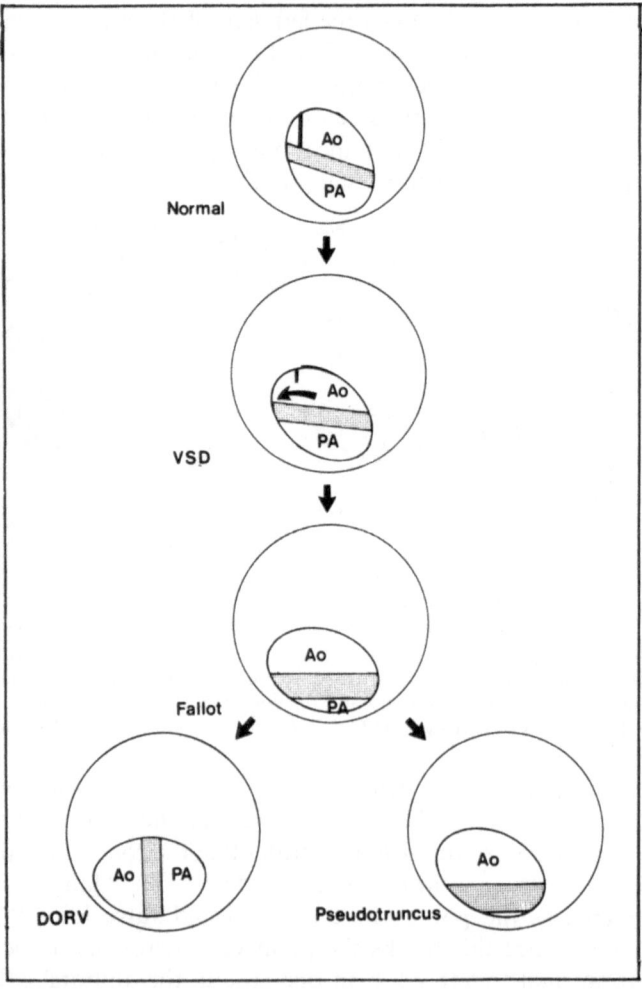

Figure 8.10 Diagram of the spectrum of anomalies to which Fallot's tetralogy belongs. The spectrum is based on 'lack of normal conal inversion' together with anterior deviation of the conus septum. Examination of pathological specimens reveals that intermediate specimens exist between the illustrated forms. (From Becker *et al.*,[4] by courtesy of *Amer. J. Cardiol.*)

tetralogy during life, from acyanotic to cyanotic forms.[6] It may well be that this spectrum is related to increasing pulmonary infundibular stenosis occurring in the presence of a dextroposed aorta (conal rotation). Further studies are necessary to evaluate this possibility.

Acknowledgments

The reconstruction of the conducting tissue was prepared by Mrs Audrey Smith, Institute of Child Health, University of Liverpool. The drawing was by Miss S. Teengs and photographs were produced by Mr R. Verhoeven, both of the University of Amsterdam. R. H. Anderson is in receipt of a grant from the British Heart Foundation.

References

1. Goor, D. A., Dische, R. and Lillehei, C. W. (1972). The conotruncus. I. Its normal inversion and conus absorption. *Circulation*, **46**, 375
2. Anderson, R. H., Wilkinson, J. L., Arnold, R. and Lubkiewicz, K. (1974). The morphogenesis of bulboventricular anomalies. I. Embryogenesis in the normal heart. *Brit. Heart J.*, **36**, 242
3. Goor, D. A., Lillehei, C. W. and Edwards, J. E. (1971). Ventricular septal defects and pulmonic stenosis with and without dextroposition. Anatomic features and embryologic implications. *Chest*, **60**, 117
4. Becker, A. E., Connor, M. and Anderson, R. H. (1974). Tetralogy of Fallot – a morphometric and geometric study. *Amer. J. Cardiol.* **35**, 402
5. Lev, M. (1959). The architecture of the condition system in congenital heart disease. II. Tetralogy of Fallot. *Arch. Pathol.*, **67**, 572
6. Bonchek, L. I., Starr, A., Sunderland, C. O. and Menarke, V. D. (1973). Natural history of tetralogy of Fallot in infancy. *Circulation*, **48**, 392

9
Angiographic aspects of Fallot's tetralogy in infants

J. F. N. Taylor and G. R. Graham

Most infants, i.e. children under the age of one year, investigated at the Hospital for Sick Children over a five year period between 1968 and 1972, presented within the neonatal period with cyanosis (Table 9.1). In the majority the cyanosis or the symptoms of those having 'spells' were

Table 9.1 Clinical features of Fallot's tetralogy in 40 infants

	< 28 days	1–3 months	4–6 months	> 6 months
Cyanosis	24	6	1	
'Spells'		1 (5)	(6)	(1)
Murmur	7			1

Figures in parentheses indicate development of 'spells' in infants who had presented with cyanosis in the first 28 days.

severe enough to warrant cardiac catheterisation and angiography under three months of age (Table 9.2). It is to be noted that 40 of the 1078 infants who were investigated in the five year period indicated, were found to have Fallot's tetralogy. Thus, the incidence amongst infants with congenital heart disease is only 4%. Therefore this is a particularly severe end of a clinical spectrum of disease. With regard to angiocardiography, the right ventricular angiocardiogram of all 40 infants was studied. Figure 9.1a is representative, showing the features that are essentially those of Fallot's tetralogy in any age group. The figures in this chapter are all right ventricular angiograms performed from the saphenous vein with the catheter coming up from below in all. The hypertrophy of the right ventricle is obvious. The very narrow outflow between the body of the right ventricle and pulmonary artery is indicated and the narrow channel or egress is bordered medially by the conus septum and laterally by hypertrophy of the free wall of the top part of the right ventricle or infundibulum. There is also a disorganised and stenotic pulmonary valve, more obvious in the lateral projection (Figure 9.1b). In all the infants studied the aorta was very heavily opacified from the right ventricle. The conclusion was that the degree of obstruction to the normal egress from the right ventricle was fairly severe.

Table 9.2 Cardiac catheterisation in infants with Fallot's tetralogy. (1968–1972)

Age at catheterisation		No.	Percentage
0–28 days		14	35
1–3 months		10	25
4–6 months		11	27
Over 6 months		5	12
	Total	40	

(Total infant catheterisations 1968–1972 = 1078)

The conus septum may be more clearly delineated in some specimens than others. This probably does not represent any major difference in the anatomy; it merely reflects the way the heart is rotated within the chest as a whole and therefore the projection to the X-ray beam differs. The conus septum is a very obvious structure in most of the angiocardiograms from infants with Fallot's tetralogy and it contributes in part to the narrowness of the infundibular region.

The hypertrophy of the anterior part of the free wall part of the right ventricle also contributes to the narrowing of the outflow and is very obvious in some specimens. In a great many cases there is virtually a ring-like constriction at one point within the infundibulum. Figure 9.2a is the lateral angiocardiogram showing a very narrow outflow tract in systole. To evaluate a narrow outflow tract it is probably better to study cineangiocardiograms rather than Elema-angiograms firstly because with the former there are 10 or more times as many frames to examine per second and secondly because with an infant heart rate of 150 or 180 at the time of angiocardiography, there is a much better chance of actually achieving full systole or full diastole. However this study was undertaken from Elema-angiocardiograms. Figure 9.2b shows a full diastole and that the infundibulum is not a static structure, but is very mobile and within the cardiac cycle will exhibit a great variation in size.

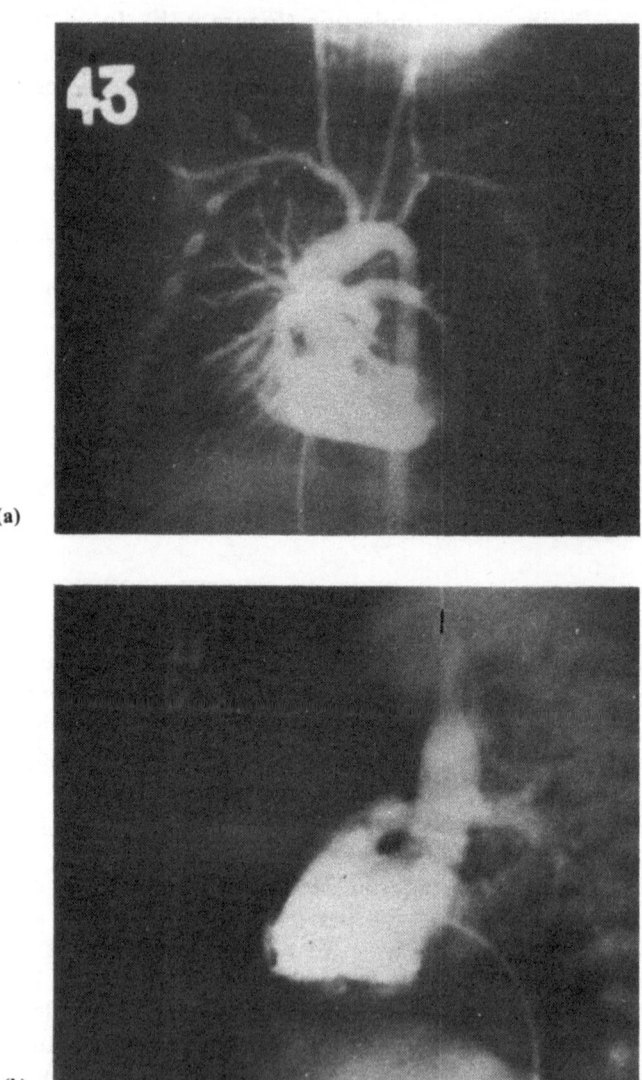

(a)

(b)

Figure 9. 1a Angiogram of a typical Fallot's tetralogy in infancy.
Figure 9. 1b Lateral projection showing the disorganised stenotic pulmonary valve which is less well seen in the anterior projection.

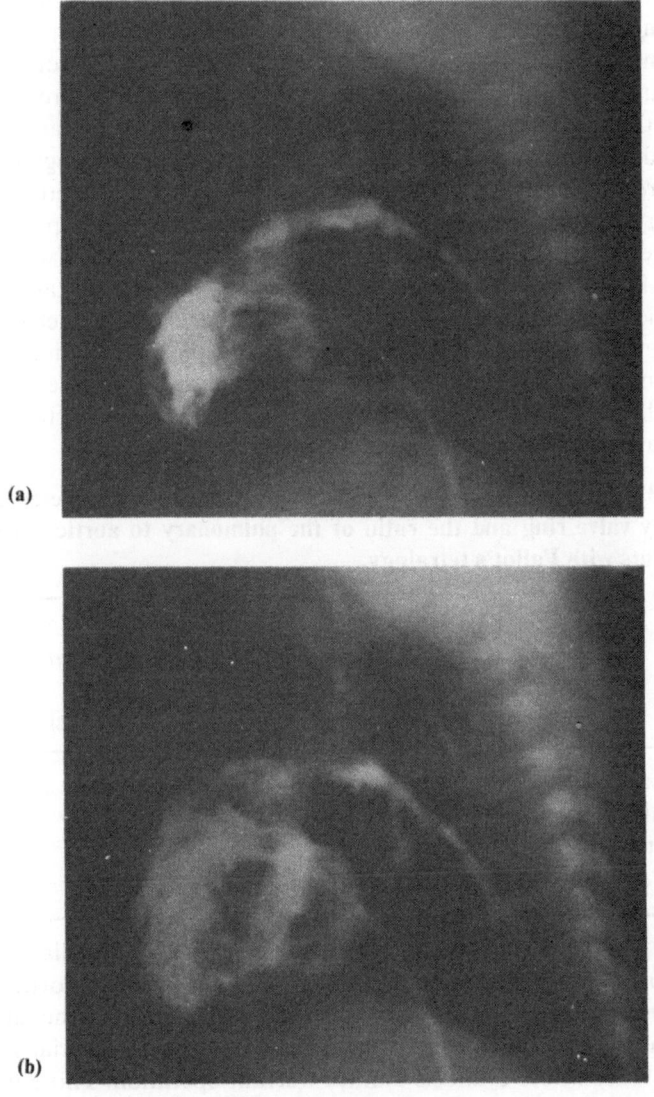

(a)

(b)

Figure 9.2a and **b** The same heart taken during systole and diasystole showing the dynamic changes and the almost complete obstruction during systole

All 40 infants had virtually normal distribution of the pulmonary arteries. There were none in which the upper lobes or any other part of the pulmonary arterial tree was deficient but there were two where the main pulmonary artery was of a very different calibre to the infundibulum. Measurements were taken from the angiocardiograms of the aortic valve ring size and the pulmonary valve ring size and the results expressed as a ratio. As these measurements were taken from angiocardiograms which were not done with a fixed tube-to-film distance and as the angiocardiograms were performed on a series of infants whose age and therefore size varied very considerably, the actual measurements were expressed as percentages of the interpediculate distances. The distances were thus corrected for the magnification and possibly for the different age of the infant. The sclerotic or more dense medial border of the pedicles of the lower thoracic vertebrae can easily be seen on the preinjection angiocardiogram film. Simril and Thurston[1] have shown that the distance between the pedicles and between the 3rd and 9th thoracic vertebrae are constant and are related to age.

Table 9.3 The diameter of the aortic valve ring, the diameter of the pulmonary valve ring and the ratio of the pulmonary to aortic valve ring in 40 infants with Fallot's tetralogy.

	Unoperated group		Operated group (a) cyanosis	(b) spells
Arterial saturation (%)	71	($p=<0.001$)	54	78
Aortic valve ring diameter	101		93	90
Pulmonary valve ring diameter	44		36	42
Ratio P: Ao valve ring diameter	0·42		0·38	0·47

Table 9.3 shows the diameter of the aortic valve ring, the diameter of the pulmonary valve ring and the ratio of the pulmonary to aortic valve ring in the group of 40 infants. The top line indicates the arterial saturation; the cyanosed group obviously had a different arterial saturation from those whose cyanosis did not warrant operation. Those infants who present predominantly with 'spells' had an arterial saturation which was not dissimilar from those who seemed to be managing tolerably well. There is no significant difference in the aortic valve ring diameters of any of the infants, neither is there any significant difference in the pulmonary valve ring diameters of any of the infants. Therefore there is no significant

difference in the pulmonary valve ring size between those infants who run into trouble from cyanosis or from 'spells' and those infants who do not. In other words, figures for the pulmonary valve ring size itself do not enable differentiation of those infants who are going to run into trouble during infancy from those who do not develop symptoms of cyanosis or 'spells' of such severity that one is forced to attempt some operation.

Table 9.4 A comparison between infant valve ring sizes and those of a series of children aged between four and seven years operated on for Fallot's tetralogy in 1972

	No.	PV diameter Mean	PV diameter SD	AoV diameter Mean	AoV diameter SD	PV/AoV diameter Mean	PV/AoV diameter SD
Infants	23	36	9·79	93	14·78	0·38	0·41
Children	11	88	18·83	113	9·90	0·77	0·17
		$p=<0·001$		$p=<0·001$		$p=<0·001$	

A comparison was made between these infant valve ring sizes and those from a series of children aged between four years and seven years of age, who were operated on in the year 1972 for Fallot's tetralogy, but who had not had any previous operations and who had not developed symptoms until childhood (Table 9.4). The pulmonary valve ring is obviously a great deal larger in these children with Fallot's tetralogy than in the infants, but the aortic valve ring is also larger. The possible reasons are not considered here. However the significant fact is that the ratios of the pulmonary valve ring to aortic valve ring diameter of the infants were all under half, and of the children they were all over half. This indicated that all the infants had relatively small pulmonary valve rings compared to a series of children who developed the symptoms later in life. However, within the infant group, although the pulmonary valve ring and aortic valve ring ratio is the same irrespective of when or whether they developed serious symptoms that warrant surgery, it is not possible to pick the difference on these sizes. A major contribution to the obstruction in infants must therefore lie in muscular hypertrophy in the infundibulum. An attempt was made to measure the infundibulum to assess this factor but because it is not a structure which lies at right angles constantly to either the AP or lateral frames and because Elema and not cineangio-cardiograms were being studied, no worthwhile measurements were produced.

CONCLUSIONS

Infants with tetralogy of Fallot who have severe symptoms have more severe obstruction to the outflow from the right ventricle angiographically than those who develop symptoms after infancy. Part of this obstruction would appear to be related to the absolute size of the pulmonary valve mechanism. This study suggests that it is relatively larger in those who develop symptoms later in life. However, within the infancy period (under one year of age) it is not not possible to distinguish those who develop symptoms to an extent necessitating operative treatment from those whose clinical course does not indicate intervention under the age of one year. All the infants exhibited major obstruction at the level of the infundibulum, but it is not possible to define differences in severity from the angiogram. This study did, however, show that infundibulum is a mobile structure in this age group and may contribute more to the overall obstruction than narrowing of the pulmonary valve.

Reference
1. Simril, W. A. and Thurston, D. (1955). Normal interpediculate space in spines of children. *Radiology,* **64,** 340–347

10
The present indications of palliation in Fallot's tetralogy

D. Waterston

Two years ago at this Conference we had an interesting session on the treatment of Fallot's Tetralogy and at that time I spoke for our Unit at Great Ormond Street and made out what we thought was a good case for palliative procedures in certain infants with Fallot's tetralogy. These were the ones under six months of age who were in severe trouble and would not survive under the best medical care. We showed what we thought was a good case with a low mortality rate for shunt procedures in this very selected group of babies. At that time, two years ago, we produced our figures going back to 1953. We showed an overall mortality rate of 16% in a total of 401 shunts of various kinds in children with Fallot's tetralogy. I then gave the more up to date figures which are relevant and our shunts for Fallot's tetralogy in infants from 1970 to 1972 showed that our mortality rate had improved enormously. It was difficult to be sure whether this was due to better postoperative care, or better surgical technique but from a total of 54 shunts in this period we only had three deaths and they were probably explainable for other reasons than the cardiac lesion.

We were happy with this approach until recently with satisfactory figures for early correction of transposition of the great vessels during the first six months of life, we thought it wise to go more carefully into our figures for Fallot's tetralogy. Dr James Taylor who you have heard previously in this Symposium looked more critically into this special group of infants under six months of age with Fallot's tetralogy on a more long term follow-up, that is to say, not the immediate or short term hospital follow up. Of 40 infants who came for investigation and treatment because of bad trouble, from Fallot's tetralogy, by far the greatest number were under three months of age so you must realise that the figures we are dealing with now are a specialised group who need urgent treatment for Fallot's tetralogy under three months of age.

Our figures in this group show that we had an overall total mortality rate of 27%, but you must realise that this was not altogether an operative mortality because this included the children who had no surgery but died from other causes. That is to say, cerebral thrombosis, gastro-intestinal haemorrhage or thrombosis and other complications of their high haemoglobin and tendency to thrombosis. It seems therefore that if we can produce a mortality rate of less than 25% for total correction under bypass in this age group, and I would remind you that the group I am talking about are under six months of age, then there should be no indication for palliating these children. It is, I think, a little more complicated than these figures show, because there will always be the difficult complicated infant coming in perhaps moribund and who needs urgent investigation. I talk especially about those ones who have complications such as cerebral thrombosis and in whom there might be an abnormally high risk on putting on to bypass for total correction.

We obviously have not come to any final decision about the definitive care in these infants under six months of age. There are many factors to be taken into consideration. That is to say, the type of outflow tract from the right ventricle, the condition of the pulmonary valve, the size of the main pulmonary artery, and the main branches, and also of course the age of the child. What I have brought out in this short paper is not only the surgical skill required for total correction, but also the overwhelming need for perfect investigation in these sick infants, urgent bypass surgery being available throughout the 24 hours, expert anaesthesia and, of course, the all important after-care of these babies.

11
Total correction after previous Blalock-Taussig shunt

M. F. Sturridge

A very large number of Blalock–Taussig operations were very satisfactorily performed by Sir Thomas Holmes Sellors at the Middlesex Hospital predominantly in the late 1940s and early 1950s. Sir Thomas' policy at that time was to perform a pulmonary valvotomy in infants with Fallot's tetralogy that were in need of some immediate help and a Blalock–Taussig-type shunt in the older child. Most of these Blalock operations were done in patients over the age of four years and some of them quite late in life. At the present time palliative procedures of this type would not be considered. It is therefore interesting to realise that patients can live to become adults with Fallot's tetralogy.

At the London Chest Hospital and the Middlesex Hospital a group of 32 adults with Fallot's tetralogy were operated on. Thirty-one of these patients were aged between 21 and 40 years, with a mean of 28 years, and one patient was 54 years of age. Of the 32 patients, nine had had no previous operative treatment; their mean age was 31 years and their haemoglobins, which is perhaps a measure of severity, range between normal up to 25·7 g % with a mean of 19. Therefore most of these were in fact deeply cyanosed and were incapacitated although some of them who had had no previous surgical treatment often denied that they were very symptomatic and they were leading lives which later on they admitted were very restricted. One of these patients in addition to having a total correction had his aortic valve replaced, the valve in this case being a prolapsing cusp-type valve, and had severe aortic regurgitation. Also in this group, there were two deaths which will be discussed later.

The remaining 23 patients had had some previous operative procedure, two of these had had a closed pulmonary valvotomy; again these were performed not in infancy but at about the ages of four or five, one had had a total correction and 20 had had a left Blalock operation. One of these 20 had had bilateral Blalock operation and one had also had an attempted total correction. This patient who had had an attempted total correction was 28 years of age with a very large patch in the outflow tract, a VSD that was still open and florid tricuspid regurgitation. She was also in ventricular failure with a large liver, ascites and oedema. The patient's tricuspid valve was therefore replaced, a patch was used to cover the VSD and a homograft was inserted in the outflow tract. There was also a single right pulmonary artery which had a stenosis on it and had to be resected and although the operation was successful the patient did not survive.

Therefore the 20 patients who had already had the left Blalock operation, now had total corrections and in all but two of them, the Blalock anastomosis was dissected out and ligated. In one of them the Blalock anastomosis was not demonstrable before operation; it was not audible and has not appeared since. In the other, the dissection appeared to be introducing great hazards to the procedure and was abandoned. This patient has since been investigated and does not have any significant shunt. A further two of these 20 patients had pulmonary atresia when they presented in adult life and were severely incapacitated, very cyanosed and were found to have pulmonary hypertension with a pressure in their pulmonary arteries at systemic level; they were not correctable. There were three hospital deaths and two late deaths. Of these late deaths, one patient, who had apparently a very satisfactory total correction, went out of hospital and three months later suffered cardiac arrest. His VSD was sewn up and everything seemed intact but this is one of the problems that occur with people who have massive ventricles. The other late death was a patient who had an outflow tract reconstruction. This patient had a large patch in his outflow tract, but after about a year he had a fairly florid tricuspid regurgitation and it was found that he had bilateral branch stenosis. He died on reoperation. There were also two patients who had a homograft outflow tract created and another two had patches in their outflow tract. These operations were successful.

Thirteen of the 20 patients are alive. Therefore, taking the series as a whole of the 32 patients, only 22 are alive and well. Two were inoperable and there were six hospital or operative deaths. Among the hospital deaths were the first three operated on and three of the last 27 which shows an improvement in operative technique. Two of the hospital deaths were late deaths and occurred at one year and a year and three months after the total correction.

Therefore the Blalock operations were successful, probably because they were done in older children. If you believe that in Fallot's tetralogy there is a need to develop the left atrium and left ventricle, then it is possible that this shunt helps these patients. But if you believe it is helped in any other way by developing the pulmonary valve or the outflow tract or by alleviating any of the coagulation problems associated with it then it is not that this shunt has failed to do this, but that these are added complications to an otherwise already complex condition.

12
Total correction after the Brock procedure
S. C. Lennox

In 1968, Lord Brock retired from the staff of the Brompton Hospital. Attending the out-patient clinic at that time were a number of patients all of whom, having been born with tetralogy of Fallot, had subsequently had an infundibular resection. In many ways these patients were similar. The first thing was that they were all alive and this of course was due to the brilliant pioneering surgery of Lord Brock in the early 1950s. Secondly, they were probably the products of parents who refused to accept the inevitable for their children at that time and who brought them from all over the country to Brock for operation. Probably because of that background, these patients, having been at least partially corrected, went on to have a good education, some going to university. Most of them had good jobs and some of them were married and had family responsibilities. The problem then was what to do with these patients attending out-patients. Did they require a fuller correction and if so when should this be done? Most, in fact, were expecting a further operation at some stage and they were naturally worried about when this should be because of their family and work responsibilities. Clearly the main problem was that with a large ventricular septal defect their right ventricle was at systemic pressure. The question was, 'Could this be tolerated?' Those who had a less than optimal correction were still cyanosed and they were presumably also at risk from cerebral embolism and cerebral abscess. Those who had more than an optimal correction were left with a large left-to-right shunt and they were at risk from pulmonary hypertension. In deciding which patients should be advised to have an operation there was also concern about the operative mortality and morbidity. As it happened, sufficient patients attended with severe enough symptoms to advise operation. At present 15 patients have had a further operation. Of these eight were female, seven were male and they were aged between eight and 46 years. The two youngest aged eight and 11 were from other surgeons, referred subsequently. The mean age was 24 years (Table 12.1).

Thirteen of these patients had one previous operation which was an infundibular resection plus or minus a pulmonary valvotomy and they had their operation from six to 22 years previously. Two had, in addition to their infundibular resection, a Blalock–Taussig shunt at a separate operation. These were six and 16 years previously (Table 12.2). All patients were symptomatic, the most important symptoms being breathlessness on exertion and tiredness (Table 12.3). In four there was

Table 12.1 The number of patients with tetralogy of Fallot who have had a further operation after the Brock procedure

15 patients
8 female
7 male
Ages: 8 years – 46 years
(Mean 24 years)

Table 12.2 Patients with tetralogy of Fallot who were further operated on after the Brock procedure but had had previous operations

One previous operation (13)
Infundibular resection ± pulmonary valvotomy; 6–22 years previously
Two previous operations (2)
Infundibular resection ± Blalock–Taussig; 6–16 years previously

Table 12.3 Symptoms of patients born with tetralogy of Fallot who had subsequently had an infundibular reaction

Breathless on exertion	15
Tiredness	15
Increasing cyanosis	4
Orthopnoea	1
Acute episodes of breathlessness	1

increasing cyanosis, one patient deteriorated rapidly over 18 months and ended up in severe heart failure and another had an interesting symptom of episodes of acute breathlessness which she had had at irregular intervals over the three previous years.

At operation there were a number of problems. There were usually dense adhesions from their previous operations and these adhesions were mainly over the left side. This meant that when operating through a median sternotomy incision the further one dissected away from the midline the more dense the adhesions. Early on in some patients oozing from behind the heart was experienced which was difficult to control and so it was soon decided to free only as much of the heart as was necessary to do the operation. As a result most patients did not have a

Table 12.4 Results of total correction performed after the Brock procedure in 15 patients

Hospital deaths (1)
Complications
   Renal failure (1)
   Wound dehiscence (1)
   Gastro-intestinal (1)

left ventricular vent inserted. Secondly the adhesions obscured the anatomy of the coronary arteries making the ventricular incision more hazardous. The intracardiac anatomy was often distorted. This distortion might have occurred not only from the previous closed surgical manipulation, but also from the effect of growth on a tethered heart. It was interesting that in the intracardiac anatomy often apparently very little had been done to resect the infundibulum and despite this the patients had a left-to-right shunt. This poses the question, 'Just how much of a resection is necessary in order to relieve obstruction?' The operation was performed in the standard way; the remaining infundibulum was resected and the ventricular septal defect closed with a Dacron patch. When necessary a pulmonary valvotomy was performed. Of the 15 patients operated on there was one hospital death (Table 12.4). While resecting the infundibulum of this patient a cusp of the aortic valve was separated from its anulus. This was repaired, but after coming off bypass the heart behaved poorly, the left ventricle appeared distended and it seemed that the probable cause was aortic regurgitation. The aortic valve, which was in fact quite abnormal, was replaced and the patient eventually came off bypass, but unfortunately died some hours later. It was interesting that this was the only patient who had an obvious early diastolic murmur before operation. This had been thought to be due to pulmonary regurgitation, but subsequent events suggest that it was in fact due to aortic regurgitation.. One patient came off bypass poorly, was obviously desaturated and in this patient the atrial septal defect had not been successfully closed. After closing the defect he came off bypass well.

Eleven patients had an uneventful recovery, one developed renal failure which responded to treatment after two weeks, another dehisced his wound and this had to be resutured and the third had a considerable amount of nausea and vomiting, but this cleared after ten days.

Unfortunately there have been two late deaths (Table 12.5). One of these

Table 12.5 Late deaths after total correction of tetralogy of Fallot following the Brock procedure

Follow-up: 2 months – 51 months	
Late deaths	(2)
Well	(12)

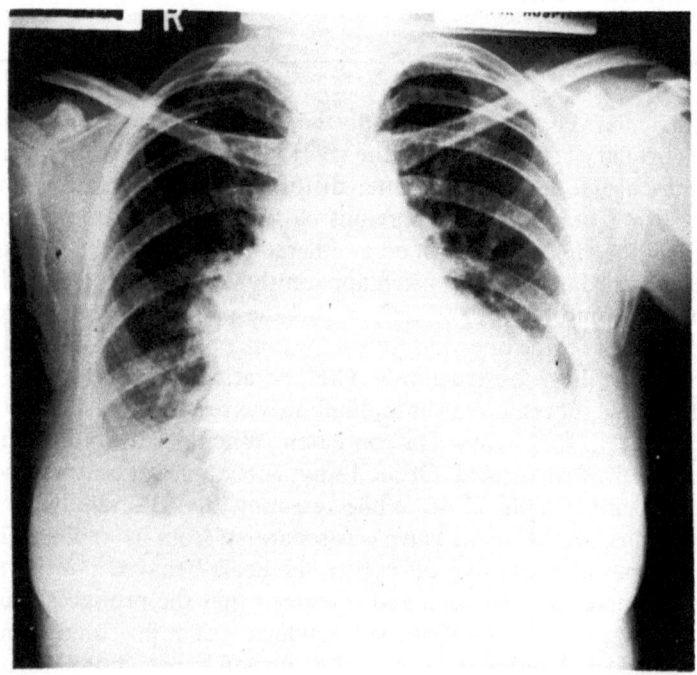

Figure 12.1 Preoperative X-ray showing a large heart in a totally disabled patient in severe failure.

was in the patient who had the attacks of acute breathlessness. She had made a perfectly good recovery following operation, but several months later suddenly had another of these attacks and died. Presumably the attacks were due to bouts of dysrhythmia. The second patient left hospital well, but some weeks later developed a large left-to-right shunt due to reopening of her ventricular septal defect. On admission to hospital she was found to have potassium of only 2 mEq/l and while this was being treated she arrested and could not be resuscitated.

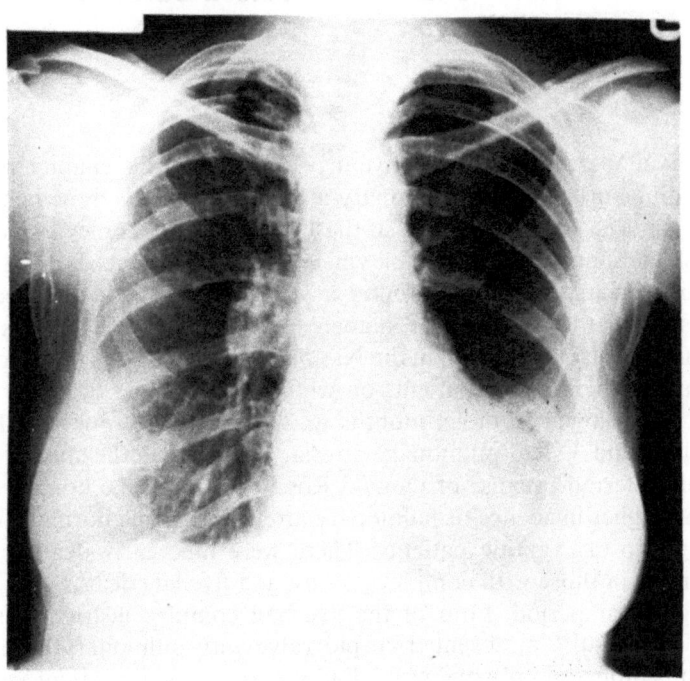

Figure 12.2 Postoperative X-ray showing a large reduction in heart size.

The remaining 12 patients have progressed well and are now leading normal lives. The longest follow-up is 51 months. The most spectacular radiological change was in the oldest patient who presented in severe heart failure (Figure 12.1). This patient was totally disabled and in severe failure and the preoperative X-ray shows a large heart. She has now returned to a very active life travelling around the world and her latest X-ray shows a large reduction in heart size (Figure 12.2).

13
Radical corrective surgery after Waterston shunts
Jane Somerville and Rosa Barbosa

Of David Waterston's many inventive operations this chapter refers to ascending aorta to right pulmonary artery anastomosis done behind the superior vena cava and called in the United States, Cooley's operation. At the National Heart Hospital, where this has been the shunt of choice for eight years, it has been found a very good palliative procedure in terms of what it was done for, namely to maintain relief of hypoxia.

The patients operated on in the National Heart Hospital were not small infants. In the first 100 patients on whom this operation was performed their ages ranged from six months to 29 years; forty-one had Fallot's tetralogy and 39 had pulmonary atresia. This reflects the special type of patient referred because of Donald Ross' work with the homograft and is a far higher incidence of pulmonary atretics than one normally expects in a group of cyanotic patients. There were nine early deaths, mainly occurring in those with complex lesions, and five late deaths over a three to eight year period. Four of the five had complex heart disease such as tricuspid atresia, absent tricuspid valve with pulmonary atresia and transposition and only one was a Fallot with a too large shunt who died in congestive failure. Two patients had spontaneous closure of the shunt and in the others, the shunt remained open and adequate. However, it became clear in the last three years that at the National Heart Hospital mortality for total correction in Fallot's tetralogy and pulmonary atresia was rising. Naturally the hospital was concerned, and as the patients were not different from earlier cases and the problems of postoperative care and surgical technique had improved, it was wondered whether it was anything to do with this shunt. Therefore, the group of 45 patients who had correction two to eight years after Waterston's anastomosis were studied in detail. They were aged four to 27 years at the time of total correction. In 28 Fallot's nine were lost; they were a bad group of Fallot's but no different from anybody else's and in 17 pulmonary atresias with homograft correction eight were lost. In a parallel series of patients with pulmonary atresia who had not had this shunt there were 16 patients who had either Blalock, Potts' or bilateral shunts or lived on a natural duct, which, of course, is the easiest thing to deal with; only two of these patients were lost. Therefore, clearly something was wrong, accepting that perhaps the group in whom the aorta–right pulmonary artery anastomosis had been performed was a little worse and could account for this devastating mortality.

The first thing to do was to examine the mode of death in detail.

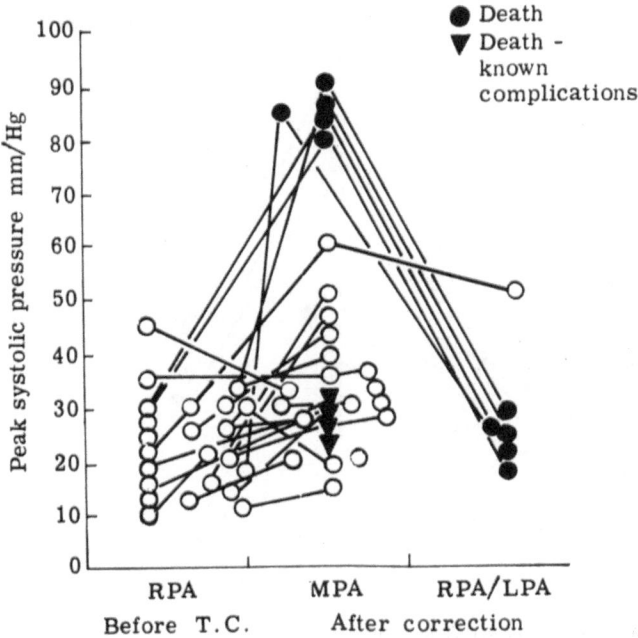

Figure 13.1 (a) Pulmonary artery pressures in a group of patients with Fallot's tetralogy who had total correction after a Waterston anastomosis

Figure 13.1a shows the group of patients with Fallot's tetralogy who had total correction after a Waterston anastomosis. Four patients died with normal central pulmonary artery pressures but there were surgical factors to account for these such as haemorrhage, coronary obstruction, etc. There were four patients with a high central main pulmonary artery pressure and none of the other surgical factors. They came off bypass with a low or falling P_{O_2}. The distal left pulmonary artery pressure was sometimes low and sometimes the right was lower distal to the anastomosis, but even after reconstruction of Waterston and opening the left pulmonary artery out as far as possible the central pulmonary artery pressures out into the hila remained high. This group of patients died within 24 h of operation or on the table with low cardiac output, falling

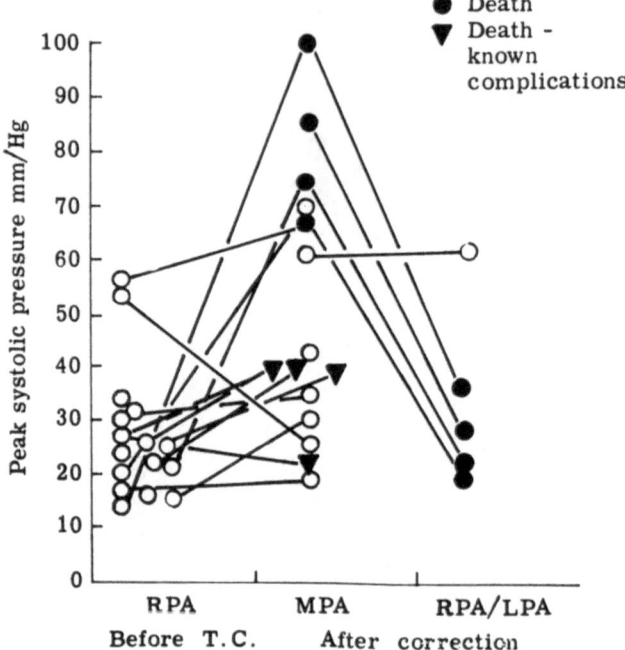

Pulmonary artery pressures -
pulmonary atresia T.C.
at operation

Figure 13.1 (b) Pulmonary artery pressures in a pulmonary atretic group of patients with Fallot's tetralogy who had total correction after a Waterston anastomosis.

P_{O_2} and increasing acidosis despite various attempts to reduce this central pressure.

Looking at the pulmonary atretic group the story is the same, only worse (Figure 13.1b). In two patients the right pulmonary artery pressure was slightly elevated before total correction and the same situation occurred as in Fallot but was more serious. Therefore, the first obvious question to be answered is – was this due to actual pulmonary arteriolar damage and disease, such as occurs when a large shunt is left for a long time? A preliminary summary of Eckhardt Olsen's work in the examination of both lungs in 13 patients who died showed that only one had serious hyptertensive changes (grade III) in the right lung and this was a boy whose shunt had been working for six years. In five patients there were mild hypertensive changes in the right lung and nothing unusual in the left; none of the 13 really had changes to suggest arteriolar damage in the left lung. Thus it would appear from this that in only one patient might the shunt have caused peripheral pulmonary arteriolar disease in the right lung which was obvious from the angiocardiogram done beforehand (Figure 13.2) and that these particular problems are not simply related to the production of irreversible pulmonary vascular disease or damage.

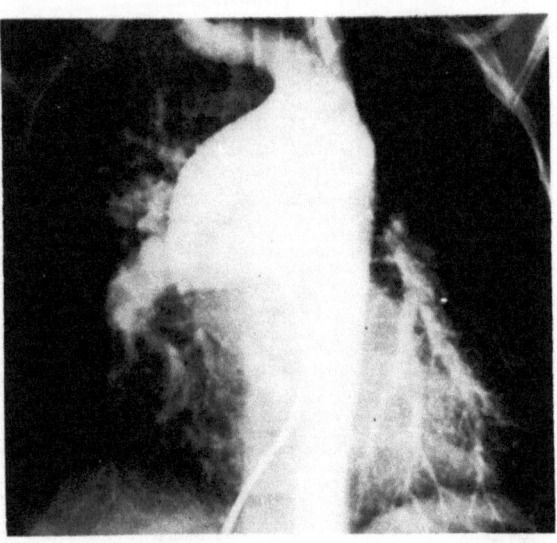

Figure 13.2 Preoperative angiocardiogram showing peripheral pulmonary arteriolar disease in the right lung

Other factors were then examined. Kinking of the right pulmonary artery so that only that lung is perfused is quite common after this operation (Figure 13.3) both in those who do well after correction and those who die. It is accepted that it is in part due to technical problems and also, particularly in those with an anterior or right aortic arch as is common in pulmonary atresia, that it may be difficult to avoid. When kinking and lone perfusion of the right lung occurs in Fallot, everything may be all right if the right ventricular outflow remains open and the rest of the pulmonary circulation and left lung is perfused. But if the right ventricular outflow becomes atretic, as is common after a good shunt in a severe Fallot, there may be little or no flow out into the left lung or stimulus to the growth and development of the rest of the pulmonary arteries. In pulmonary atresia the problem is more serious because if there is no duct or man-made left-sided shunt, there is nothing to stimulate growth of pulmonary arteries proximal to the Waterston anastomosis and intrapulmonary thrombosis may occur. There was one such patient at the National Heart Hospital who had type 1 pulmonary atresia and had an ascending aorta–right pulmonary artery shunt at the age of five months. Now, seven years later the shunt is still patent but there is no perfusion of his central pulmonary arteries or left lung – it is known that in infancy he had central pulmonary arteries perfused by a duct. This patient developed the central pulmonary hypertension and died with the described syndrome.

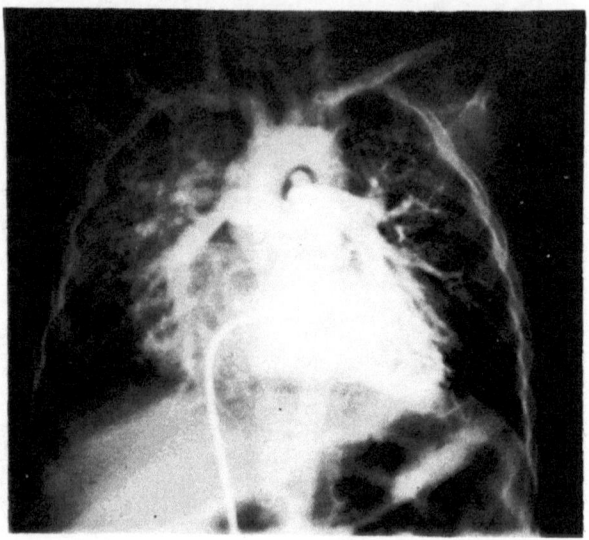

Figure 13.3 Postoperative angiocardiogram showing kinking of the right pulmonary artery so that only that lung is perfused

Thus, looking at the total group it would appear that the problem might be related to a combination of kinking of the right pulmonary with lone perfusion of the lung and leaving the shunt for a number of years. A Fallot under particular circumstances shunted young, i.e. below the age of three and left uncorrected for several years, who has a kinked right pulmonary artery is at risk, particularly if the perfusion from the rest of the lung is poor. Patients with pulmonary atresia, shunted under seven years and left uncorrected for three to four years will inevitably have the problem if there is no perfusion of the left lung from a duct or previous shunt. To put the other side of the story, results of total correction after Waterston operation are very good if one does not encounter this problem. It is common to have a minor stenosis in the right pulmonary artery where the shunt was closed and in only one patient was it severe. Formal repair and reconstruction of this area is required and closure of the stoma inside the ascending aorta is usually not adequate, particularly if preoperative aortography has demonstrated kinking.

In summary, the National Heart Hospital has encountered a problem which has increased mortality at total correction of Fallot and pulmonary atresia after Waterston's anastomosis. It manifests as a high central pulmonary artery pressure after bypass, with falling cardiac output and P_{O_2} and death. It does not appear to be due to peripheral pulmonary arteriolar disease although there are minor changes in the right lung. It is possibly related to deflection of blood into the once poorly perfused left lung which cannot cope, but it is not related to the production of severe pulmonary arteriolar disease which may appear after Potts anastomosis and other large shunts left *in situ* for many years. The problem appears to be related to hypoplasia and hypoperfusion of the central pulmonary arteries and left lung with subsequent unbalance of ventilation/perfusion.

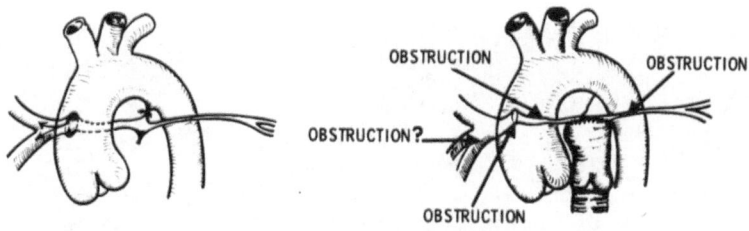

Figure 13.4 Hypoplasia and hyperperfusion of the central pulmonary arteries and left lung with subsequent unbalance of ventilation/perfusion

Those patients who are at special risk of this complication are those young Fallot's with kinked right pulmonary artery (Figure 13.4) left over three years and any pulmonary atresia left in this state for over two years. The Fallot problem is now solved by early correction but where primary correction is inadvisable owing to anatomy, local problems, strikes and politics some Fallots and patients with pulmonary atresia may require a shunt. Therefore if an aorta to right pulmonary artery shunt is done, patients must be investigated early and electively, irrespective of clinical results in order to see whether there is kinking so that internal renal pulmonary artery is being developed or not; this is particularly important in pulmonary atresia. If kinking is present, early correction is mandatory or a shunt on the left side in the case of some atretics may be needed before the ideal time for total correction is reached. If faced with this problem of kinking, the surgeon must formally take down the shunt and repair the pulmonary artery, but this alone will not solve the problem. However, this an extremely successful palliative shunt.

14
Current concepts in the management of Fallot's tetralogy

A. Starr

Perhaps as a result of inexperience, early in the 1960s the author began to explore total corrective operations applied early in life in the tetralogy of Fallot.

Figure 14.1 shows a typical angiogram in a patient with a good size of pulmonary artery who was selected for operation at about 10 months of

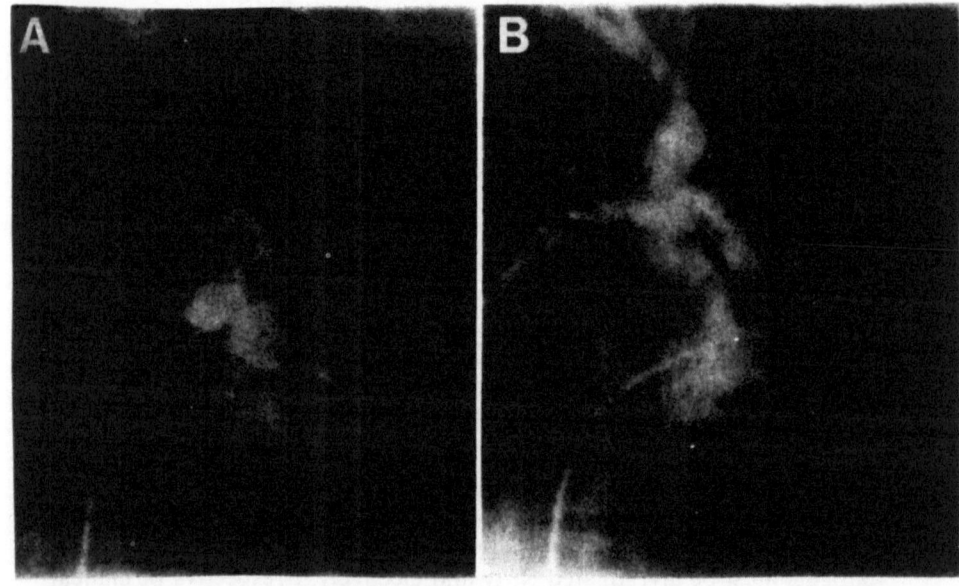

Figure 14.1 Right ventricular angiogram in the anteroposterior projection from a representative infant in Group 1. Severe muscular infundibular hypertrophy is evident. The pulmonary artery is of adequate size. On the first systole following contrast injection, dye enters the pulmonary artery (A) and does not enter the aorta until the next systole (B). This is a valuable sign and indicates the dynamic nature of the outflow tract obstruction in this group of patients.

age. The first systole after injection of contrast medium is actually filling the pulmonary artery before the aorta. The oblique view shows a very tight infundibular stenosis. On the other hand, it is still possible to see some infants who have a marked discrepancy between the aorta and the pulmonary artery. In this type of case the author continues to use a Waterston shunt. Whether the shunt should be abandoned or not is an open question. This must be analysed not only in terms of the summation of various mortalities, but also in terms of trying to base the operation of tetralogy of Fallot on an understanding of the basic pathology, and the basic anatomy and the way in which this disease progresses. The concepts of the development of this condition should govern the techniques that are applied surgically. If the surgery is related in this way to the basic disease mechanism rather than solely to operative mortality, it should then be possible to arrive at a method of treatment which would ultimately have the minimal operative mortality.

In 1964 the author began to explore the possibility of early total correction. At that time, a philosophy that the age and the weight of the child was of secondary importance , was adopted. Patients were therefore selected from the younger age groups on the basis of the size of their pulmonary artery on angiocardiography. In an analysis of experience from 1964 with 59 patients who presented themselves under the age of two for the care of tetralogy it was found that 25% were not sufficiently symptomatic to warrant any consideration of surgery in this age group. These were all angiographically proven tetralogy of Fallot. Sixteen patients (27%) had a shunting procedure, mostly Waterston shunt and almost half the group had total correction. The age distribution of these cases shows considerable overlap. This indicates that the primary consideration, except in those infants under the age of two months, was based upon consideration of the surgical anatomy rather than on the age of the patient. Some of the total corrections were performed in very sick infants under the age of six months; the youngest total correction was performed in an infant of 10 weeks of age. On the other hand, some shunt operations were performed in the second year of life in patients with very severe malformations of the pulmonary artery and marked hypoplasia or pulmonary atresia. There is also overlapping in the weights of these infants, but, in general, the shunt procedures were performed on the very small babies—less than four kilos— although some shunts were performed in the larger children based upon an evaluation of the surgical anatomy. The smallest sized patient who had a total correction was a five kilo infant. The mean size at the time of shunt, was 4.9 kilos and somewhat higher for the totally corrected group. Therefore both forms of therapy are still used; the total correction in young infants who have favourable anatomy and a shunt procedure in those infants who have highly unfavourable anatomy.

Table 14.1 shows the results in this series of patients. By 1972, 28 total corrections had been performed, with two operative deaths – a mortality of

7%. During the same period, 16 shunting procedures were carried out, most of them on infants under the age of 3 months and the mortality was 31%.

It seemed reasonable to divide these patients up into various groups depending upon their degree of cyanosis. There was a large group of patients who had relatively normal haematocrits or only slight elevation in

Table 14.1 Comparative operative and late mortality rates

| *Treatment* | *No. of patients* | Deaths | |
		Operative	*Late*
Total correction	25	2 (8%)	0
Shunt	16	5 (31%)	0
No surgery	13	–	6
Totals	54	10 (18.5%)	6

haematocrit (group 1). These patients had little or no cyanosis at rest but had apnoeic episodes and constituted a large proportion of the patients on whom total correction was performed. Eight of them were under one year of age. Another group of patients (group 2) with more severe pulmonic stenosis who were cyanosed at rest but who also had spells of infundibular spasm were also recognised. A third group of patients had more severe cyanosis at rest but did not have a muscular element to their symptoms; they had higher haematocrits than the other patients. Finally there was a fourth group. These patients had persistent severe cyanosis and were found on angiocardiography to have atresia, or severe hyperplasia of the pulmonary artery. It is primarily in this group that the shunt procedures were performed.

An interesting insight into the natural history of the tetralogy of Fallot as it had been observed in a group of 40 patients followed in the author's clinic from early life to the time of operation. All the 40 patients were asymptomatic at birth. By the time the first hospital visit was made, which was at a mean age of 5.8 months, 21 of these 40 patients were still asymptomatic, but increasing numbers developed symptoms which are related to these groups and sub-groups, so that 15 of them were only slightly cyanotic at rest but had apnoeaic episodes. Three were moderately cyanosed and one was quite severely cyanosed at rest. By the time cardiac catheterisation was performed at a mean age of 12.7 months, these patients were beginning to shift into the more advanced disease groups, so that by the time of operation—in these 40 patients at a mean age of 17.7 months—the majority of the patients were in the group 2 and group 3 categories. These observations reinforced what has always been known, i.e. tetralogy of Fallot, even in early life, is a progressive disease. With close follow-up even during the first year of life, this progression can readily be demonstrated.

Categorising of patients according to the degree of cyanosis is of some surgical consequence with regard to the use of outflow tract patching. For example, in the group 1 patients, who had total correction, who were only slightly cyanotic at rest and whose primary symptom was spells, outflow tract patches were used in only 41% of the patients. In those patients with more severe disease who were moderately cyanosed at rest, outflow tract patches were used more commonly—in 73% of the patients. In the group 3 patients who were severely cyanosed at rest, all required outflow tract patches. Therefore, in the total number of cases, there was a 64% incidence of outflow tract patches and nine of these 28 patients had a patch placed across the pulmonary annulus. This is a very radical treatment to apply to a very young infant in whom the use of artificial materials may have to be discussed further. The anatomical findings at surgery also correlate very well with the degree of cyanosis prior to surgery. For example, of 23 patients in groups 1 and 2, infundibular obstruction was found alone in 83% of the patients. In those in group 3, without spells, infundibular obstruction was commonly associated with pulmonary valvular obstruction.

The technique of surgery in correcting tetralogy has always been to use a vertical ventriculotomy with cardiopulmonary bypass. The infundibular hypertrophy is resected and then the ventricular septal defect is exposed during the period of cardiac anoxia with aorta cross-clamping. The author does not use the left ventricular vent but instead uses the ventricular septal defect to vent the left side of the heart. A sucker tip is placed through the ventricular septal defect and with traction to the left, as the heart relaxes, the defect gradually comes into view. Simple interrupted sutures are used with a Teflon felt patch to close the defect. No attempt is made to stray far from the margin of the defect. On the contrary, if the margin of the defect is free of conducting tissue it is then possible to place the sutures directly in the margin of the defect without creating heart block.

Rather a large patch was used in the ventricular septal defect, the size of the patch approximating to the size of the aortic diameter rather than the the size of the defect itself. The ventricular septal defect may be left open until the heart has been resuscitated. Air is expelled from the left ventricle and then finally the sutures are tied on what used to be called the crista but is now called the conus septum.

One patient who was closed without a right ventricular outflow tract patch and was the only patient in the series to require reoperation for continued infundibular obstruction. However, despite that continued obstruction of a

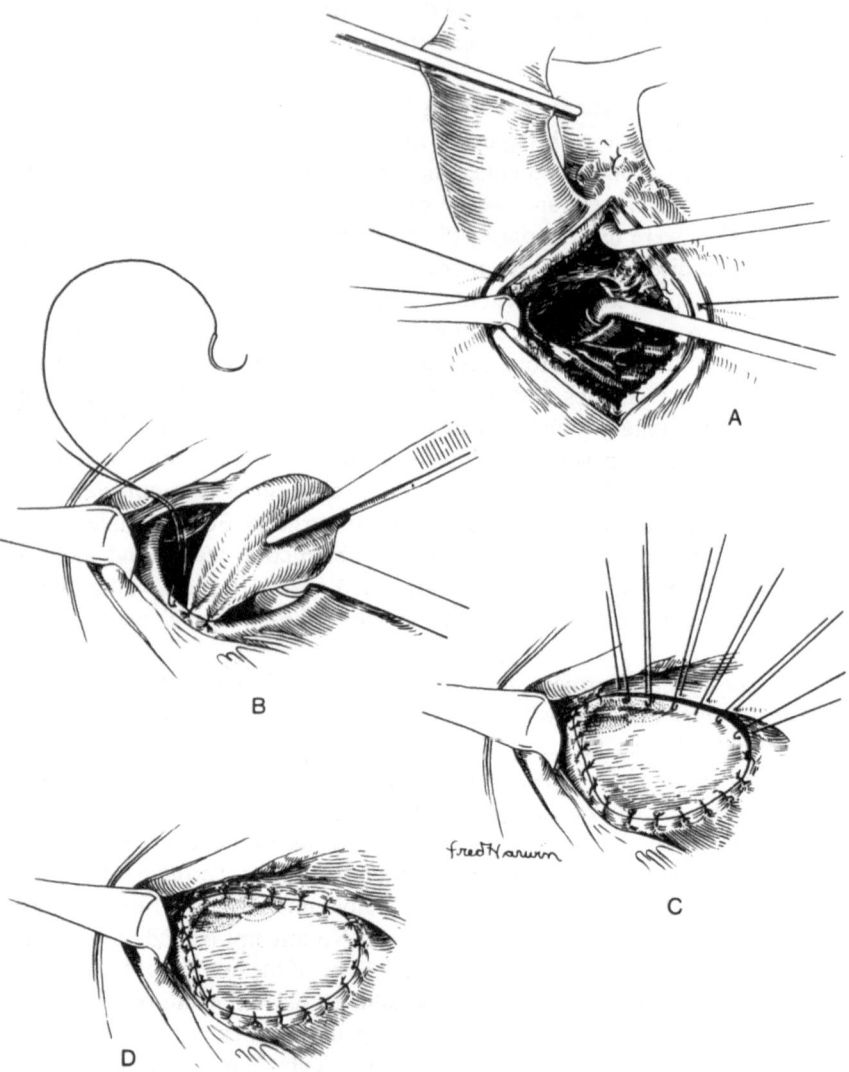

Figure 14.2 A, Aortic cross-clamping is required for exposure of the ventricular septal defect. An intracardiac sucker is placed through the defect and retracted to the left to facilitate exposure. B, Suturing begins in the midportion of the caudal rim of the defect and proceeds clockwise to the crista supraventricularis. Compressible Teflon felt is always used. Each suture is tied immediately after placement, and traction on the patch by the assistant facilitates exposure for the next suture. C, Sutures are then placed counterclockwise beginning again at the caudal margin. The last few sutures are left untied and the aortic clamp is removed. Air is evacuated through the ventricular septal defect as the heart resumes beating. D, The last few sutures are tied in the beating heart, thus completing closure of the ventricular septal defect. A left ventricular vent in unnecessary.

moderate degree, the child did very well. Figure 14.2 illustrates another operative view of the defect in tetralogy of Fallot showing the sucker tip in the defect with traction to the left, the aorta cross-clamped and the heart quite relaxed. Sutures were placed through the margin of the defect with impunity. At the point of the tricuspid annulus the suture line leaves the

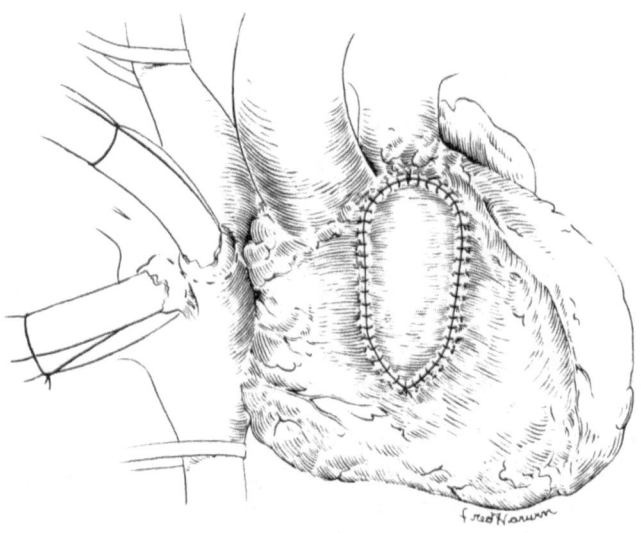

Figure 14.3 If the outflow tract is inadequate, a woven Teflon patch is inserted with a running suture. If the pulmonary annulus is inadequate, the patch is placed across the annulus and even into the left pulmonary artery (see text).

margin of the defect and sutures were placed in the area leading up to the conus septum. The conus septum was used in the repair. The outflow tract patches used tend to be quite large (Figure 14.3).

There has been no instance of heart block. In the author's experience it has been difficult to produce even transient block in patients with tetralogy of Fallot. Only one patient required a tracheotomy for prolonged artificial ventilation. Incidence of right ventricular failure in the immediate postoperative period was relatively low—one patient had a cerebrovascular accident with complete recovery. The possible key to the performance of total correction at an early age is the ability to avoid heart block since the production of this complication in a small infant would be a very difficult problem to manage. There were no late deaths in this group of patients. In this unit the author is fortunate in having an excellent follow-up system which relates to the relative geographic isolation of Portland, Oregon and the fact that most of these patients reside in an area which is serviced by the unit and for whom the follow-up programme is an excellent one. All the corrected patients were completely asymptomatic and all

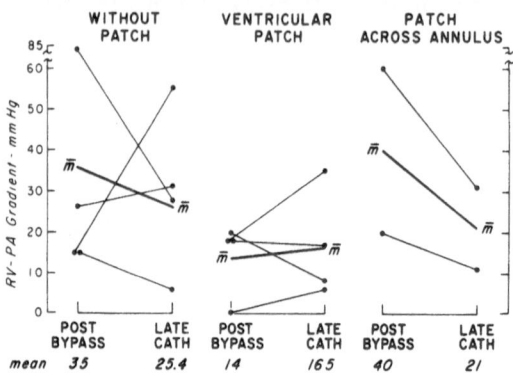

Figure 14.4 A comparison of gradients across the outflow tract at operation and at late cardiac catheterization in patients with and without outflow tract prostheses.

showed normal growth and development which was quite different from the results that have been seen with palliative operations in terms of this most important parameter. The ability to relieve pulmonic stenosis in this age group is shown in Figure 14.4. This illustrates a group of patients whose right ventricular to pulmonary gradient without a patch was 35 mm Hg. The highest gradient was in the child requiring reoperation—84 mmHg. On late catheterisation, the mean gradient was 25 mmHg and the highest gradient found was 55 mmHg in a patient who was reoperated. Therefore there is some decrease in the gradient across the outflow tract with time even in patients in whom a patch is not used. In those patients who had a ventricular patch, the mean gradient was 14 mmHg and the late gradient was 16.5 mmHg. None of the patients who had a ventricular patch had a significant gradient on the cardiac catheterisation. In the two patients who had postoperative studies, who had a patch across the annulus, the mean gradient, immediately after surgery was 40 mmHg and this fell to 21 mm Hg after operation. One patient had a gradient of 60 mmHg that fell to 31 mmHg following operation. Others have also demonstrated that when a patch is placed in the right ventricular outflow tract there is a tendency for moderate gradients measured at the time of operation to become less at the time of late cardiac catheterisation.

Table 14.2 compares the right ventricular to the aortic pressure ratio as measured immediately after surgery and at the time of late catheterisation.

It can be seen that in a group that had no patch, the mean ratio at the time of operation was 0.6 dropping to 0.44. In those with a patch across the outflow tract, the mean ratio was 0.47 dropping to 0.36, and in those with a patch across the annulus, the mean ratio was 0.6 dropping to 0.37. This again shows that a patch across the outflow tract can produce a very profound fall in the right ventricle to aortic pressure ratio when measured after late cardiac catheterisation. The highest ratio in the entire series was seen in an infant with a ratio of 0.89 without an outflow tract prosthesis. A result at this level would be accepted, but it would be preferable to have a maximum ratio of 0.75.

Table 14.2 Relief of pulmonic stenosis—immediate and late results (11 patients)

Treatment	No. of patients	RV: aorta pressure ratio (mm Hg)			
		Immediately postop.		Late catheterization	
		Mean	Range	Mean	Range
Without patch	5	0.60	0.32-0.89	0.44	0.26-0.82
Ventricular patch	4	0.47	0.35-0.75	0.36	0.23-0.55
Patch across annulus	2	0.61	0.40-0.82	0.37	0.25-0.48

Patients were also studied after operation in terms of various parameters. These patients were grouped into those who had an outflow tract prosthesis on the ventricle only, those who had a patch through the annulus and those that had no outflow tract patch at all. In this group of patients, 35% had some mild dilatation of the right ventricle, 53% were considered to have some residual constriction of the outflow tract on angiocardiography and 29% had a mild bulging of the outflow tract. Those patients that had a patch across the annulus, had a very high incidence of right ventricular dilatation compared to those that had no outflow tract patch at all. It must be emphasised again, however, that all these patients were completely asymptomatic.

The cardiac index in the left ventricular ejection fraction in the two groups of patients have been measured late after total correction in infancy. When those patients without an outflow tract prosthesis are compared with those with an outflow tract patch the cardiac index is very much the same in both groups of patients. The A-V oxygen difference is very much the same and the left ventricular ejection fraction is a mean of 0.64 in the group without an outflow tract patch and a mean of 0.66 in patients with an outflow tract patch. This is of some significance because late cardiac catheterisation in unoperated tetralogy of Fallot, or in patients operated upon late in life, shows significant decrease in left ventricular performance.

So at least in terms of left ventricular ejection fraction, it can be said that total correction in infancy, in addition to its other advantages, would tend to preserve left ventricular function when compared to total correction later on in childhood.

The author was also very interested in the size of the pulmonary artery and in the demonstration that the total corrective operation performed early in life enhances growth of the right ventricular outflow tract. This was done by making a ratio between the pulmonary artery and the aorta in terms of their diameters as measured at postoperative cineangiocardiography. The results after surgery were compared with results before operation in terms both of the diameters and of the ratio of the areas. There was a highly significant difference in these measurements with a significant increase in the ratio of pulmonary artery to aorta in the postoperative period as compared to before correction of tetralogy. So it would appear that the application of early correction, in addition to preserving left ventricular function, also enhances the growth of the pulmonary artery in relation to the size of the aorta.

What about the problem of pulmonary insufficiency? In 17 patients studied after total correction in infancy, the right ventricular end-diastolic and pulmonary artery pressures were equal in five (29%) of the patients. This shows that a significant pulmonary insufficiency has been created in this group of patients operated upon early in life. Of course those patients with a patch through the annulus all had pulmonary insufficiency whilst of those patients without an outflow tract prosthesis, only three had evidence of severe pulmonary insufficiency. Despite this relationship, the author will continue to use outflow tract patches in patients in whom there is fear of leaving residual significant obstruction, since an early postoperative obstruction is of much more serious consequence to the patient than a pulmonary regurgitation discovered on late cardiac catheterisation in a patient who otherwise had no symptoms.

Another very important area for evaluation in patients who have early total correction is measurements of their mentation. We have basically two alternative techniques for the total correction of tetralogy in early life; either total cardiopulmonary bypass or the use of hypothermia with core cooling. As has been demonstrated in adults' the use of circulatory arrest may be damaging to mentation and so the author has been interested in establishing relatively normal psychometric data in patients who have had total correction of tetralogy of Fallot using cardiopulmonary bypass. Insofar as the intelligence quotient and the development quotient is concerned, the patients in this group of postoperative tetralogies fall into the normal range with a score of 104 in intelligence quotient, somewhat above the average in the US compared to a standard group. The development quotient is very similar and the same order of magnitude as a group of patients who had cardiac catheterisation but who did not have heart disease of the tetralogy type.

We have compared the late results on cardiac catheterisation in three groups of patients. One group was obtained from the literature, giving figures for patients operated on between the ages of three and 20 years a second group of patients were aged between four and six years and were operated on at the University of Oregon and a third group of patients were aged between 10 weeks and 23 months and were operated on at the author's institution. Comparison was made in terms of the right ventricular systolic pressure on late cardiac catheterisation, i.e. the mean values in a large group of patients. There was very little difference in the mean right ventricular pressure of patients operated upon early in life and then studied later compared to patients operated upon in the older age groups. Therefore, the application of total correction in this age group does not compromise the late haemodynamic result in terms of right ventricular systolic pressure, in terms of right ventricular to pulmonary artery systolic gradient and in terms of right ventricular end-diastolic pressure. The mean right atrial pressure was within normal limits in all of the patients studied late after total correction in infancy showing relatively satisfactory right ventricular function.

In conclusion, the author currently feels that total correction should be applied early in life if the anatomy is favourable. When there is a pulmonary artery to aortic ratio of above 0.3 and when the operation is applied in this manner, one can expect a low operative mortality, and excellent late haemodynamic results. The growth of the pulmonary annulus can be documented, there is normal left ventricular function and there is normal growth and development of the child. Of equal importance is the lack of anxiety on the part of the parent who has to take care of a child undergoing multiple operative procedures, if a course is one of initial palliation followed by total correction. Summarising the current status of the treatment of tetralogy of Fallot is a difficult task and this may change with time, but, for the present, it seems prudent to apply total correction as early in life as possible. This has many advantages in terms of economics, in terms of a child's physical and mental development and in terms of avoiding all other complications of tetralogy of Fallot such as brain abscess and continued cyanosis. Despite this, it seems reasonable to apply shunt procedures to patients who present themselves within the first month or two with very severe anatomic deformities, such as severe hypoplasia of the pulmonary artery and complete atresia of the pulmonary artery. These are patients in whom total correction must be considered as an experimental approach. The application of total correction to more favourable anatomic situations is not at the present time an experimental approach. It has been established as providing a low operative risk and takes its cue from knowledge of the progressive course of tetralogy of Fallot. Many patients operated on in the first year of life had only mild cyanosis and the main symptom was spells. These patients would either die in infancy without operation or would progress to more severe forms of tetralogy with more difficulty and a greater risk for surgery later on. The application of total correction to this group of unfavourable cases with atresia and its proper place remains to be determined but for the present at least, early application seems to be the trend and it is certainly one that will be followed in Oregon.

15
Primary total correction of Fallot's tetralogy under the age of two years
M. H. Yacoub

Since January 1972 it has been our policy to perform total correction in all infants and children with Fallot's tetralogy who require surgical treatment. This has been stimulated by the disadvantages of the two stage procedures which include:
1. Subjecting the child to two operations.
2. Continued subnormal growth after the first stage.
3. Risk of development of progressive pulmonary vascular disease.
4. Risk of cerebral complications.

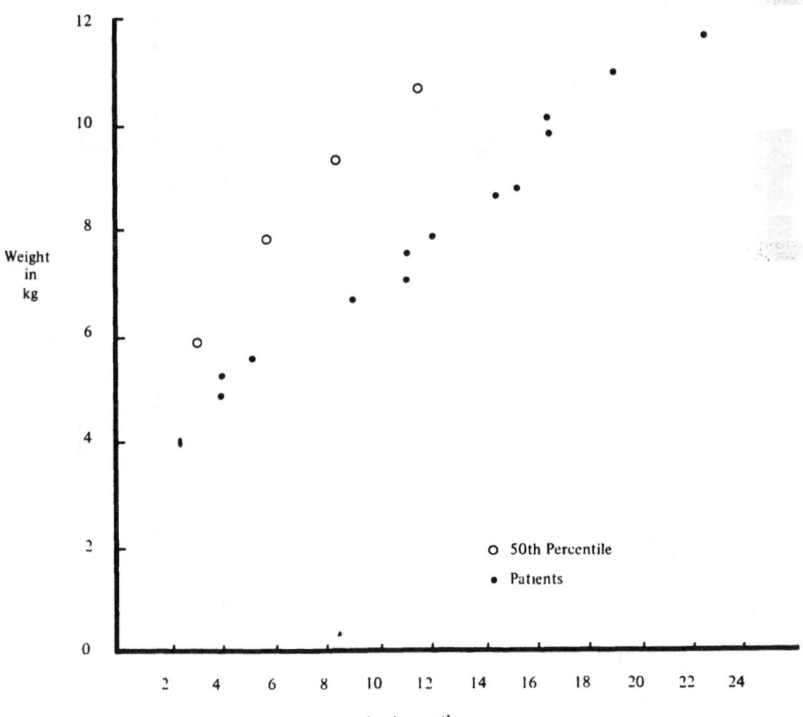

Figure 15.1 Age-weight relationship at time of operation

95

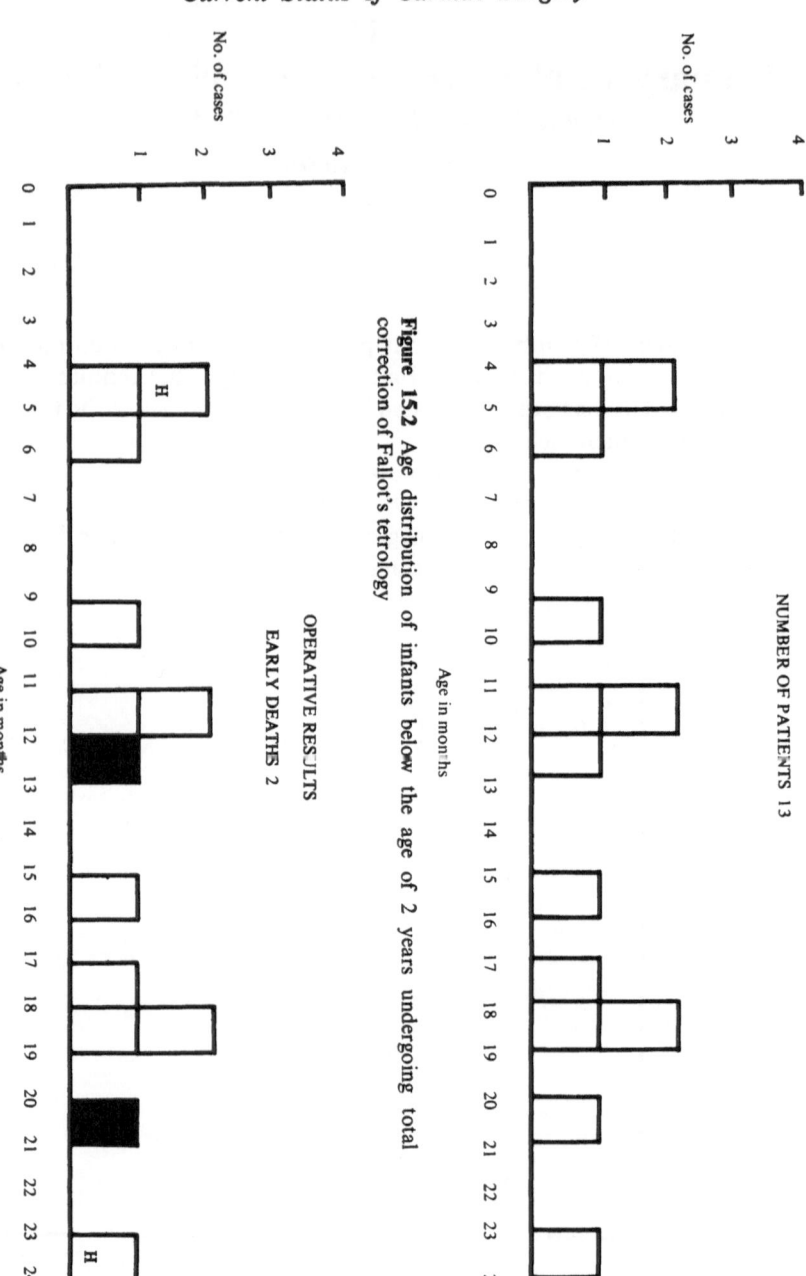

Figure 15.2 Age distribution of infants below the age of 2 years undergoing total correction of Fallot's tetrology

Figure 15.3 As Figure 15.1 showing deaths. H = homograft reconstruction

NUMBER OF PATIENTS 13

OPERATIVE RESULTS

EARLY DEATHS 2

5. High combined mortality of the first stage, the waiting period and the second stage.

During this period 13 patients below the age of two years underwent total correction. Their ages varied from four to 23 months and six were below the age of one year (Figure 15.2). Their weights, at the time of operation, ranged from 3.5 to 11 kg and were below the 50th percentile in all cases (Figure 15.1). The indication for operation (Table 15.2) was retarded growth and progressive cyanosis in eight, cyanotic attacks

Table 15.1 Total correction of Fallots tetralogy below the age of 2 years. Indications for surgery

Retarded growth and progressive cyanosis	8
Cyanotic spells	2
Both	3

in two and both in three patients. In patients with cyanotic attacks operation was performed as soon as possible without the effect of beta-blockers. The diagnosis was confirmed by cardiac catheterisation and angiography in all patients. The angiographic findings included infundibular stenosis alone in two patients, infundibular and pulmonary valve stenosis in seven and hypoplastic pulmonary valve ring in four. Underdevelopment of the pulmonary valve ring or vessels was not regarded as contraindication to early correction. Patients with pulmonary atresia or absent pulmonary valve are not included in this series.

Surface induced profound hypothermia with rapid rewarming using cardiopulmonary bypass was used in all patients. This method was similar to the Koyoto–Barratt–Boyes technique. In our patients surface cooling to a nasopharangeal temperature of 24 °C was followed by further cooling using cardiopulmonary bypass. The repair was performed during a period of circulatory arrest varying from 40–55 min. Aortic homograft reconstruction of the outflow tract was performed in two patients (aged four and 23 months). For this purpose the non-coronary cusp of a fresh adult-sized homograft with the attached aortic leaflet of the mitral valve was used. This technique has the advantage of preserving the patient's own outflow tract and valve cusps thus allowing continued growth. No outflow patches were used in any of the remaining patients.

There were two postoperative deaths (Figure 15.3). One occurred early in our experience in a patient with a hypoplastic pulmonary valve ring who was left with a large gradient across the outflow tract and developed low cardiac output state 24 h after operation. The second death occurred in a child who developed a cerebrovascular accident 24 h after operation. The remaining infants and children made smooth recovery and continued to be clinically well during the period of follow-up. The growth pattern reverted back to normal in all patients as illustrated in Figure 15.4,

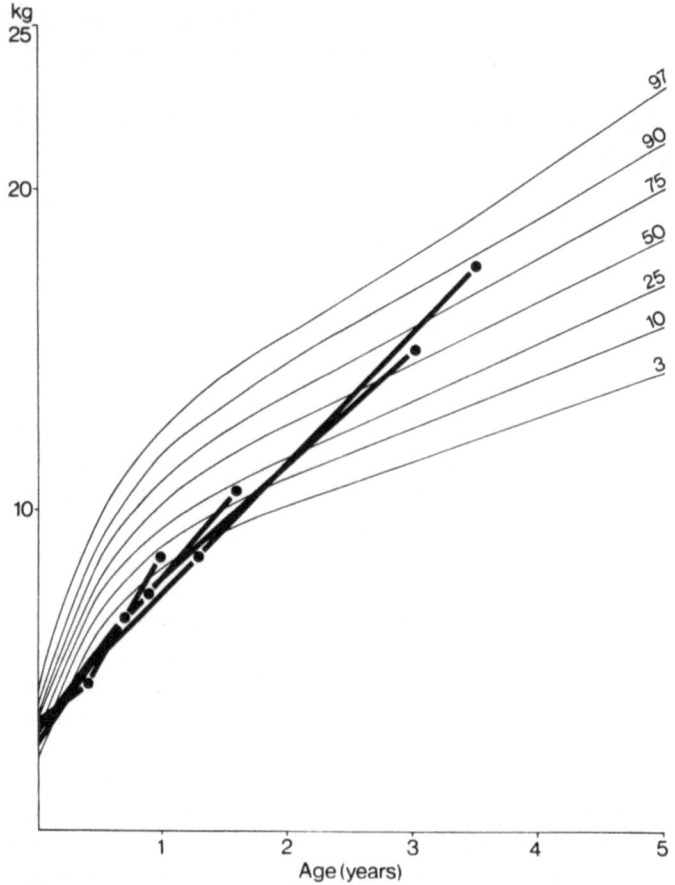

Figure 15.4 The growth pattern after operation

which shows the weights at birth, at the time of operation and later. Pulmonary diastolic murmurs were not observed in any of the patients including those who underwent homograft reconstruction of the outflow tract.

The haemodynamic response, both immediately after repair and at late

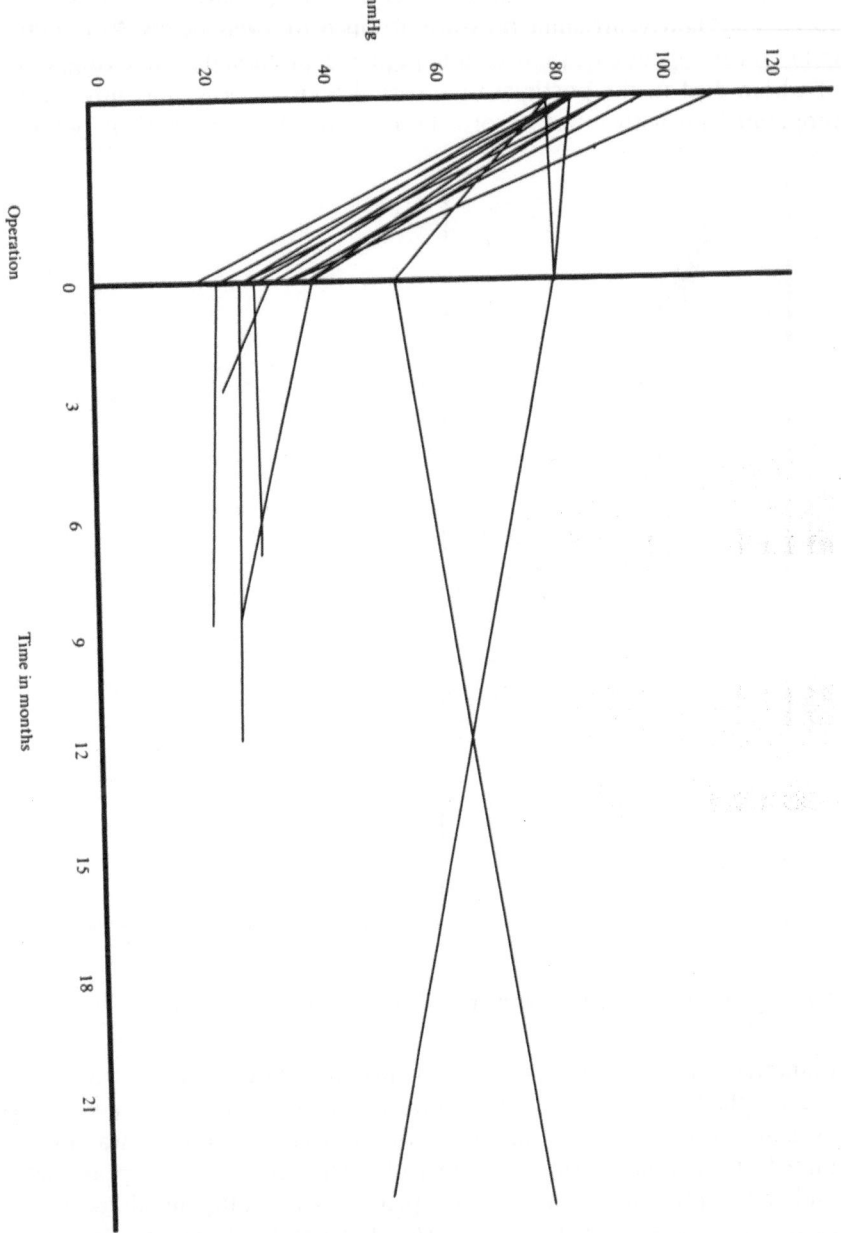

Figure 15.5 Right ventricular pressure after recatheterisation.

catheterisation was good in all but three patients (Figures 15.5, 15.6 and 15.7). The right ventricular pressure dropped to levels below 40 mmHg in all but three patients (two with hypoplastic pulmonary valve ring, one of whom died in the postoperative period and the other has now been reoperated on with insertion of a homograft; the third patient, whose

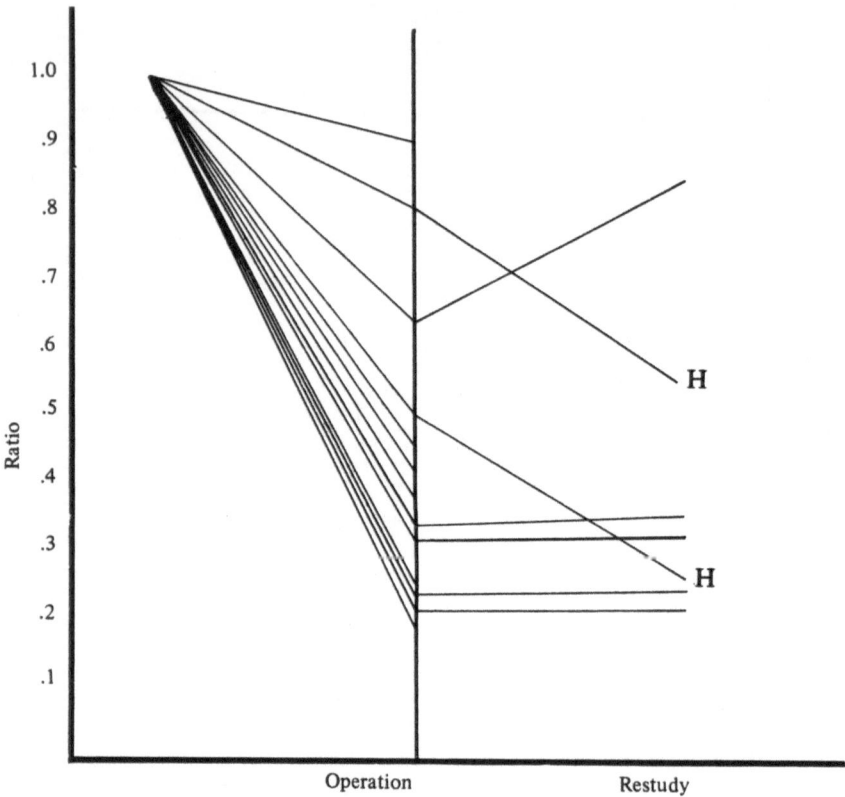

Figure 15.6 RV:LV ratio after operation. H = homograft reconstruction

pulmonary valve ring was of adequate size showed further drop to acceptable levels at recatheterisation). The drop in right ventricular pressure observed at the time of operation, following repair, was maintained at recatheterisation (Figure 15.5). The ratio between peak right and left ventricular pressures dropped to below 50% in all patients, apart from the three mentioned earlier (Figure 15.6) and the drop was marked in the patients with homograft reconstruction of the outflow (H in Figure 15.6). At recatheterisation the gradient across the right ventricular outflow tract (Figure 15.7) was 10 mmHg or less in four, 30 mmHg in one and 55 mmHg in another (the latter patient has been reoperated on with insertion of a homograft resulting in drop of the gradient to 5 mmHg). None of the patients had any degree of postoperative pulmonary hypertension which is observed in some of the older patients.

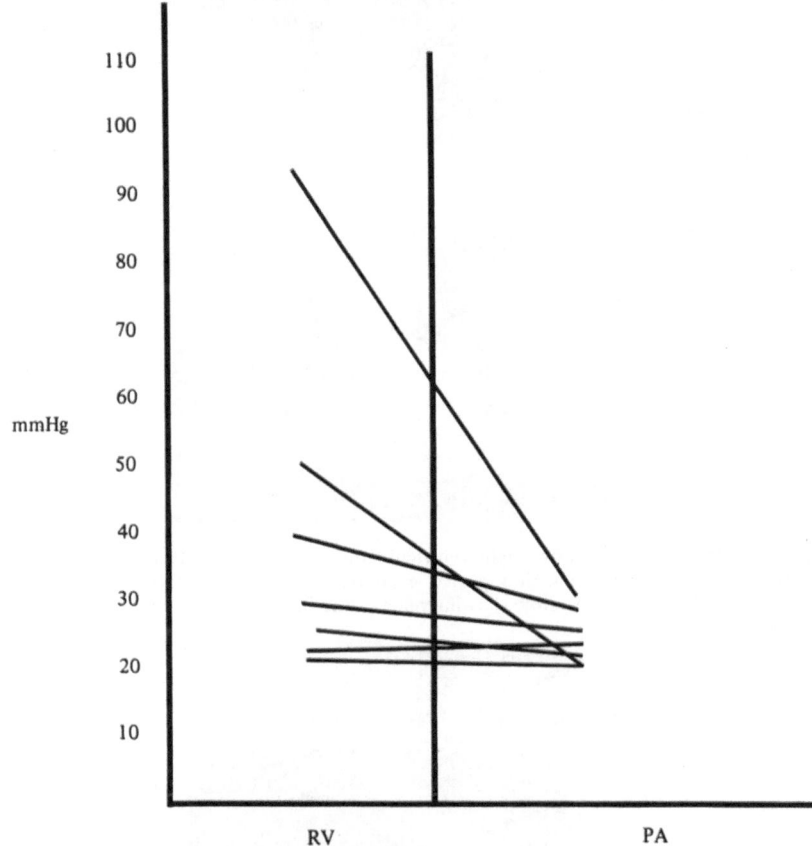

Figure 15.7 RV/PA gradient at late catheterisation

There were no residual shunts detected in any of the patients re-investigated. Figures 15.8a and 15.8b show pre and postoperative right ventriculograms in a patient with isolated infundibular stenosis who presented with repeated cyanotic attacks. Relief of the stenosis is seen in the postoperative film taken during systole. Figure 15.9 is a post-operative right ventriculogram after aortic homograft reconstruction of the outflow tract showing the large size of the outflow tract and reconstructed main pulmonary artery. The homograft valve cusp can also be seen.

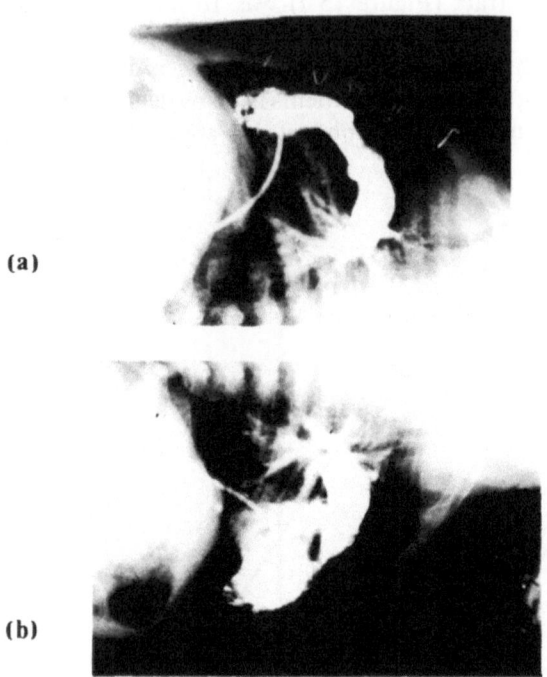

(a)

(b)

Figure 15.8 (a) Preoperative right ventriculogram in a patient with isolated infundibular stenosis who presented with repeated cyanotic attacks (b) Postoperative right ventriculogram taken during systole showing relief of the stenosis

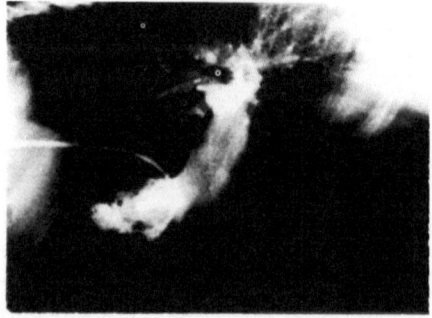

Figure 15.9 Postoperative right ventriculogram after aortic homograft reconstruction of the outflow tract

This experience has encouraged us to continue the policy of performing total correction in all symptomatic infants and children who require surgical treatment regardless of the severity of the anatomical lesion.

16
Correction of tetralogy of Fallot
W. Klinner

Total correction of tetralogy of Fallot which was first performed by Lillehei in 1954, exactly 20 years ago, seems today to be a routine procedure, which can be carried out with low risk.

However, there is no congenital disease which shows more difference in its anatomical appearance than tetralogy of Fallot. Although the always huge VSD is rather uniform, there is extreme variance in respect to location and degree of pulmonary stenosis, the pattern of coronary arteries, overriding of the aorta, the size of the pulmonary artery and its branches or even of the left ventricular outflow tract. Tetralogy of Fallot originates from malformation of the conus and is present from birth. It most probably does not progress in its anatomical appearance itself. Only secondary malformation such as right ventricular hypertrophy or the extent of infundibular stenosis might progress with age as does clinical cyanosis.

Many hazards always accompany the course of a surgical intervention. These are (1) possible severing of major branches of coronary arteries, with successive myocardial infarction of part of the right ventricle or even the septum (2) inability to reduce the right ventricular pressure to an acceptable two-thirds of the left ventricular pressure (3) persistant complete heart block (4) left heart failure due to narrowing of the left ventricular outflow tract as a result of closing the VSD with a small patch and (5) there is always the danger of recurrence or reopening of the VSD.

INDICATIONS, TECHNIQUE AND PROBLEMS OF POSTOPERATIVE CARE

Although every case of tetralogy should be considered correctible, there are cases, predominantly those with pure valvular stenosis and a very small pulmonary artery, in which, despite extensive outflow tract reconstruction, the pressure in the right ventricle remains high, i.e. equal to systemic pressure.

In such patients with pure valvular stenosis and narrow pulmonary artery we rely on doing a closed valvotomy first, postponing total correction of the malformation for two to four years, until the pulmonary vascular bed has become wider. A modified and small version of the Tubbs dilator is sometimes useful in this procedure.

In severely ill cases a Blalock anastomosis during infancy might still have its place. The author prefers it to the Waterston shunt, at least after the age of three months because of the many complications that have been seen with the shunt, particularly if it is not adequately done when either pulmonary hypertension or stenosis of the right pulmonary artery results. After three months of age an adequate Blalock shunt always can be achieved. There is no chance of pulmonary hypertension and should further correction be necessary at a later date, the anastomosis is quite easy to take down, whether it is on the right or left side.

Patients who do not need a palliative procedure or shunt in infancy probably will not need one before the age of three or four years when anatomical correction of the cardiac disease is more conveniently carried out. As soon as the diagnosis is established and favourable anatomical conditions revealed, correction of the malformation should be performed before the child starts school. In cases with an extremely unfavourable anatomical condition a palliative procedure should be considered, leaving the final decision until the heart is fully exposed at the time of surgery.

At this stage the author would like to point out that the proper classification of tetralogy of Fallot seems to be very difficult. Classification makes sense only if it is done according to anatomical conditions and not from a clinical point of view. A clinically very ill child with severe cyanosis can be at operation, a technically low-risk case. On the other hand, patients with only mild cyanosis without history of fainting or squatting can be very difficult to correct. This is easily explained insofar as children with fainting spells and squatting usually have an infundibular stenosis, which can be resected, whereas cases with pure valve stenosis quite often have a very narrow valve ring and pulmonary artery. A previous Brock or shunt procedure *per se* does not increase the operative risk, but these cases are usually the ones with unfavourable anatomical conditions, since otherwise the palliative procedure would not have been done before.

Since 1959 to the end of 1973, 652 corrective procedures have been performed at the Department of Cardiac Surgery in Munich. There has been a hospital mortality of 17.3% and a late mortality of 3% (Figure 16.1). This statistic also includes the cases that were operated on during a time in which inexperience accounted for a good many deaths. During the last 10 to 12 years, there has been an annual mortality of about 10–15%. In 1971 and 1972 there were 111 cases with a hospital mortality

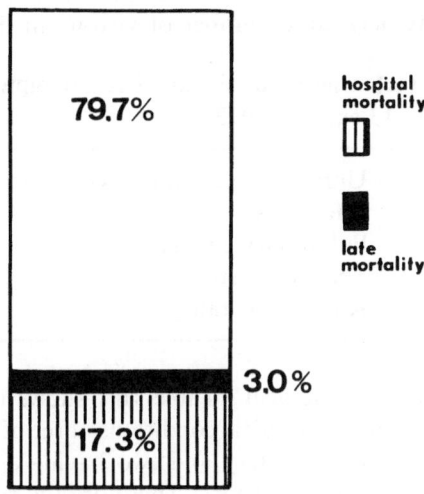

Figure 16.1 Correction of tetralogy of Fallot

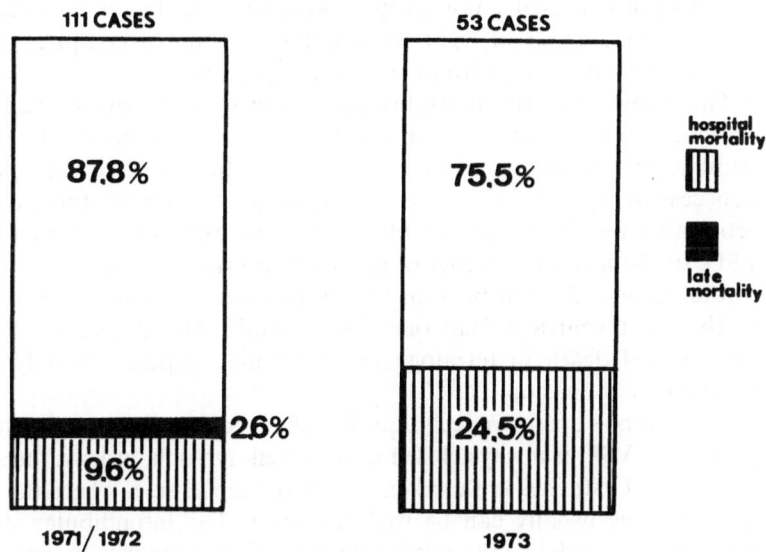

Figure 16.2 Correction of tetralogy of Fallot

of about 10% and a late mortality of 2.6% (Figure 16.2). From May to December 1972 36 consecutive cases were operated on without any hospital mortality. Starting the new year, three consecutive cases died because of infection. All three patients were operated on on days with an extremely large number of visitors in the theatre. Why did another

Table 16.1 Causes of death after attempted correction of tetralogy of Fallot in 13 cases in 1973

Unfavourable anatomical conditions	7
Infections	3
Pulmonary edema	1
Technical error	1
Right heart failure	1

10 die during the year? Table 16.1 shows that seven of them had very unfavourable anatomical conditions, three of them having only one branch of the pulmonary artery and two having a relationship of 5 or 6 : 1 of aorta to pulmonary artery. Therefore the reason for these deaths lies in the fact that correction was attempted in cases in which the risk apparently was very high, with the result that there were more deaths than would normally be expected – not on the operating table, but three to 20 days after surgery, either of right heart failure or due to complications of prolonged ventilation, with pneumonia, sepsis, etc.

This shows that the mortality figure can be kept low, if cases with extremely unfavourable anatomic conditions are eliminated. The second point is to consider what else can happen during surgery to prevent a successful outcome, e.g. excessive bleeding after a preceding palliative procedure, the danger of AV block, the possibility of reopening of the VSD, or damage to branches of coronary arteries with subsequent myo-cardial failure. As can be seen reoperation can often do more damage to the right ventricle than one would think. The difference between success and death in tetralogy of Fallot may depend on only a few millimeters of incision.

The author's operative technique has changed very little during the past years. The VSD is always closed using a Teflon patch, at least the size of the defect. U-stitches are used except on the septal side, where the endo-cardial tissue usually can be well-preserved. The infundibular stenosis is resected as widely as possible and the valvular stenosis is opened by splitting the two commissures from the ventricular level. The decision for an outflow tract patch should be made before opening the heart in order to avoid a T-shaped incision. The outflow tract patch which should always extend to the bifurcation is sutured in with continuous 4-O Prolene sutures. The better the haemodynamic correction, the less the postoperative worry. Bleeding in severe cyanotic cases can be almost always completely controlled by careful haemostasis and right heart failure can usually be overcome by proper digitalisation. Severe and prolonged right heart failure is quite often evidence for a partially reopened VSD. This, as everybody will agree, is a reducable but not completely preventable complication. In the author's cases there were 66 reopenings (10.1%). Most cases occurred when direct sutures were used; least when Teflon patches were used (Figure 16.3). 3.7% cases with reopened defects had to be operated on again; two cases twice. In some cases the operation had to be done as an emergency in the early postoperative days. Thirteen (32.4%) patients died during or as a result of the procedure. Judging from the high mortality figures in the first 10 years, it is probably better to operate as soon as a large left to right shunt is established, and not wait until there is definitive right heart failure or until pulmonary hypertension is imminent. In the author's experience a major reopening of the VSD – sometimes combined with residual stenosis – has been the only reason for reoperation. Restenosis alone has never led to re-operation. The late results in cases who left the hospital with at least reasonable haemodynamic conditions are excellent. A review of cases showed that 90% of the surviving patients are able to carry out a

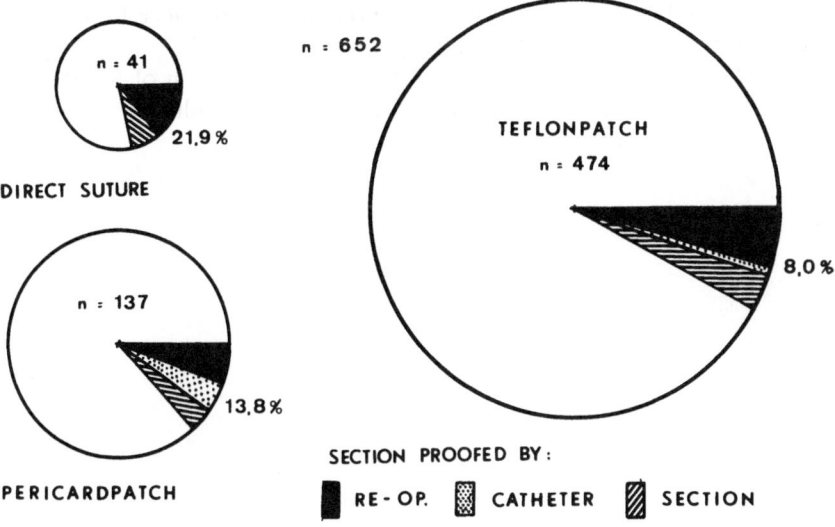

Figure 16.3 VSD – frequency of recurrence

normal pattern of life, more than 50% engage in sports and all go to school or work.

SUMMARY

1. Tetralogy of Fallot is in the majority of cases a correctable congenital malformation.
2. There are cases which due to very unfavourable anatomy cannot be operated on with the expectation of obtaining acceptable haemodynamic conditions and therefore carry a large operative risk. In these patients a two stage operation should be considered.
3. Correction in infancy most probably will not lower the risk involved in a two stage operation.
4. Only children with fainting, always originating in infundibular stenosis might be an indication for corrective procedure during the first or second year of life.
5. Cause for reoperation is (almost exclusively) a reopened VSD. Residual stenosis as well as mild to moderate pulmonary incompetence is usually well tolerated.
6. Late results in haemodynamically well-corrected cases are excellent and guarantee these patients a normal life, probably also a life expectancy close to normal. How far this concerns the patients with residual abnormalities which in the author's present opinion do not require reoperation, as there are small recurrent VSDs, residual stenosis with a pressure gradient of not more than 40 and pulmonary incompetence, has yet to be evaluated.
7. Altogether after 20 years experience, the correction of tetralogy of Fallot continues to be one of the most difficult but also most gratifying procedures.

17
Revaluation after total correction of Fallot's tetralogy

F. Fontan and A. Choussat

In cases of total correction of Fallot's tetralogy, if a purely clinical evaluation is made based on the absence of any functional symptomatology and the staturoponderal development, the results may be considered good or very good in 91% of the cases, average in 6% and poor in only 3%. However, this clinical evaluation is insufficient and must be compared with objective data obtained from a more complete check-up including radiology, electrocardiography, ergometry and haemodynamics. Therefore for two years, a programme of systematic revaluation of patients, on an average six months after correction of Fallot's tetralogy has been undertaken.

During this period – March 1972 – among 73 patients operated on with three deaths (4% mortality) 65 patients were revaluated, four of them twice, to give a total of 69 revaluations. Most of the patients operated on were between four and 10 years old, with an average age of seven – although the present tendency is to operate earlier (Figure 17.1).

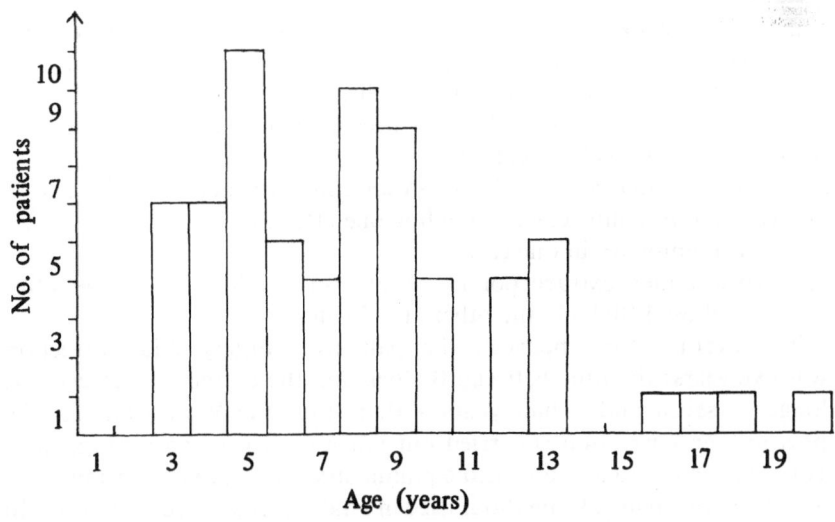

Figure 17.1 The age of 65 patients undergoing total correction of Fallot's tetralogy

Types of stenosis. The anatomical types of obstacles in the outflow tract of the right ventricle are shown in Figure 17.2: isolated infundibular pulmonary stenosis in 16 cases, associated with a pulmonary valvular stenosis in 23 cases or an association of both with hypoplasia of the ring

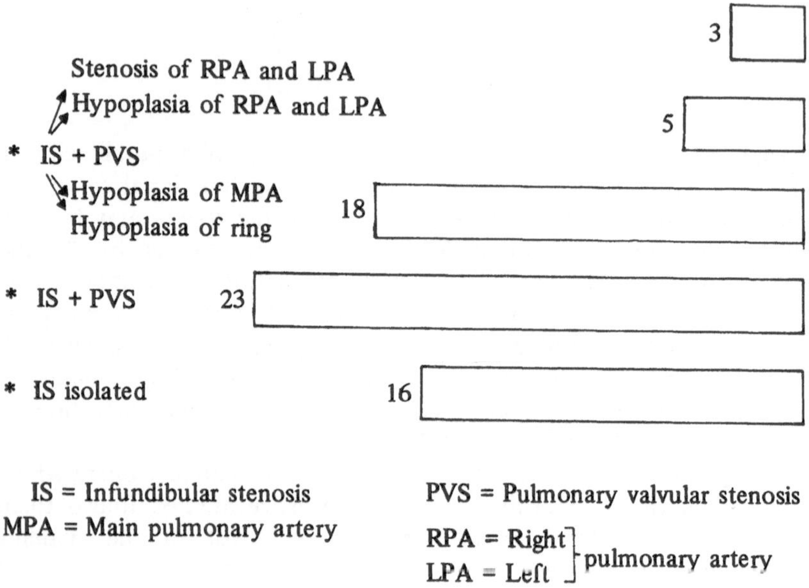

Stenosis of RPA and LPA
Hypoplasia of RPA and LPA

* IS + PVS

Hypoplasia of MPA
Hypoplasia of ring

* IS + PVS   23

* IS isolated   16

IS = Infundibular stenosis   PVS = Pulmonary valvular stenosis
MPA = Main pulmonary artery   RPA = Right ⎤
                                     LPA = Left ⎦ pulmonary artery

Figure 17.2 Anatomical localisations of obstruction to right ventricular outflow

and of the trunk in 18 cases, hypoplasia of the branches of the pulmonary artery in five cases and finally, in three cases, absence of stenosis of the pulmonary arterial branches.

Previous palliative surgery. Twenty-three patients had one or several palliative operations beforehand:
 – Blalock in 15 cases, of which 13 were still permeable
 – Waterston in nine cases, including one after Blalock
 – Cavopulmonary in one case
 – Brock under extracorporeal circulation in two cases; one after thrombosed Blalock, the other after Waterston.

The average time between the palliative surgery and correction was five years; the time between Blalock and the corrective surgery was longer – seven and a half years – than after the Waterston. At the present time correction is carried out much earlier, on an average after two years so as to avoid possible pulmonary arterial hypertension.

Technique of repair. The methods used in total correction are as follows: In all cases, an infundibulolysis with infundibulectomy has been carried out;

in 47 cases, a pulmonary commissurotomy. On the other hand, what is important and this should be noted, is that in this series of 65 patients, only seven patients had an enlargement patch, five at the level of the ring and the trunk of the pulmonary artery and two at the level of the infundibulum.

This is a policy which is voluntarily restrictive and which favours a residual gradient to a pulmonary insufficiency, i.e. a gradient between the right ventricle and the trunk of the pulmonary artery.

RESULTS OF THE REVALUATION

Cardiac volume. The cardiac volume has been estimated using a simplified method which likens the heart to an ellipsoid with a certain enlargement (0.4).

The possibility of reproducing these measurements, particularly in infants is questionable. Nevertheless, even in unfavourable circumstances, the variations in cardiac volume are below 10% and there is a reasonable reproductibility, particularly in the same subject. The normal values defined by Harris have been adopted. He showed that there was a closer relationship between the cardiac volume and the weight than between the cardiac volume and the overall body surface.

It was thought necessary to split up this series of patients according to whether a previous palliative operation had been carried out or not.

In the 42 patients who underwent a complete correction right away, the cardiac volume was normal in 29 patients before the correction. After the correction, the cardiac volume was normal in only one third of the cases, i.e. 14 out of 42. In the 23 patients who underwent a complete correction after previous palliative surgery, the cardiac volume was normal before correction in 14 out of the 23 patients. After corrective surgery it was normal in only 5 out of 23 patients. What are the elements responsible for this increase in the cardiac volume? Angiographic images suggest that pericardiac participation cannot be considered. A dilation of the right atrium, or more important of the infundibular zone and of the ventriculotomy zone may be considered. Perhaps this almost constant increase in the cardiac volume can also be explained by the increase in the volume of the left cavities.

It is important to underline that there are no close relationships between the variations in the cardiac volume and the favourable or unfavourable haemodynamic results.

Electrocardiography. Study of the electrocardiogram shows that the disorders in the auriculo-ventricular conduction are practically nil. These disorders include an auriculo-ventricular block of first degree and an in-

termittent nodal rhythm which is replaced, at effort, by a sinus rhythm. On the other hand, in this series, the disorders in the intraventricular conduction were constant, as they are in most series:
- incomplete block of the right branch in one-fifth of the cases
- complete block of the right branch in 61% of the cases
- in 18% of the cases, there was a complete block of the right branch associated with a left anterior hemiblock with QRS axis at −30°.

The interpretation of such an electrocardiographic image is still questioned; some writers, notably Wolf, Rowland and Ellison, have come to pessimistic conclusions. They compared a series of patients operated on for Fallot's tetralogy and who presented such an electrocardiographic image with a series of control patients operated on for Fallot's tetralogy who only presented a complete or incomplete block of the right branch. For the writers, the number of sudden deaths from serious ventricular arrhythmias and auriculo-ventricular block was much more frequent when this electrocardiographic image existed. In fact, these pessimistic observations would seem to have resulted from patients who presented a transitory phase of auriculo-ventricular block after the operation. Other writers, on the other hand, do not attach any particular significance to these troubles in the intraventricular conduction and this is the author's attitude as there has been no phase of auriculo-ventricular block.

Ergometry. Fourteen asymptomatic patients have been submitted to an ergometric evaluation, with study of their oxygen consumption. The following observations were made:
- most of them had a tolerance to effort lower than normal
- there was an unchanged gradient of pressure between right ventricle and pulmonary artery during an isometric effort
- there was no relationship between the importance of the gradient and the level of tolerance to effort.

Epstein, in six asymptomatic patients operated on for Fallot, noticed that the gradient which before effort fluctuated between two and 20 mmHg could increase and reach 75–100 mmHg during effort.

Haemodynamics. The haemodynamic explorations were aimed at estimating different elements:
- and on the other hand, the quality of the outflow tract of the right ventricle, both at rest and when making an effort, on the haemodynamic data and on the angiographic data; the existence of a pulmonary insufficiency was estimated by studying the dilution curves of ascorbic acid and the angiographic data.

In searching for a possible residual ventricular septal defect, different means have been used. Oxymetry was tried in all the cases, but this was not effective, particularly in cases with small residual shunts. The left side was studied in all cases after injection of the contrast product into the right ventricle or into the trunk of the pulmonary artery. Selective angiography of the left ventricle was carried out thanks to a Botal hole which was voluntarily resected during the operation. Finally, in 47 cases, the curves of cardiogram dilution were examined.

These different means of exploration suggest that there were no further cases of residual VSD apart from those already observed, i.e. there was only a low percentage occurrence – 4.5% – when using this technique for closing of the VSD.

In studying pressure relationships, only one case of pulmonary arterial hypertension was observed, in a two-year-old child who, at the age of one, underwent a Waterston aorto-pulmonary anastomosis and complete correction sixteen months later. Six months after complete correction of the malformation, a control evaluation was made and pressures of 90 mmHg both in the right ventricle and in the trunk of the pulmonary artery were found, with a 77% arterial desaturation. However there was no residual shunt and the angiography in the left ventricle affirmed that there was no residual VSD, but that this child clearly had a pulmonary vascular illness. It was not possible before the Waterston operation and before the complete correction, to measure the pulmonary arterial pressures. Was this pulmonary arterial hypertension due to the Waterston operation or were there other causes? A recent article by Macgoon, Danielson, Wallace and Mair (J. Thorac. Cardiovasc. Surg., January 1974, page 70), reports 61 cases of pulmonary arterial hypertension among 1400 patients who had been operated on for Fallot's tetralogy. A certain number of these patients had undergone an aorto-pulmonary anastomosis beforehand, notably a Potts' anastomosis, but some of them had undergone complete correction with no previous operations.

The study of the pressure gradient between the right ventricle and the pulmonary artery, has shown that in 10 cases, there was no gradient (Figure 17.3). In a certain number of cases on the other hand, there was a gradient of variable importance with, in four cases, a gradient of more than 75 mmHg. The great majority of these residual gradients are located at the level of the pulmonary ring and, much more rarely, at the infundibular level. This results from the voluntarily restrictive policy with regard to the placing of a transannular patch so as to avoid pulmonary insufficiencies since the choice was finally between the existence of a residual gradient or of a pulmonary insufficiency.

If the right ventricular pressures at the end of the operation and on an average six months later at the time of the control are compared, it can be seen that the great majority of these pressures have remained stable or have dropped particularly when they are below 60–70 mmHg. In three cases, however, the pressures have increased in a completely abnormal manner to 90–100 mmHg. Consequently, it would seem that when during the operation, the right ventricular pressure is below or equal to 60 mmHg, there is a good chance that afterwards, the pressures will remain within satisfactory limits. On the other hand, when the pressure is above 75 mmHg, it rarely drops and remains quite stable or has a tendency to increase. However, these pressure measurements take place,

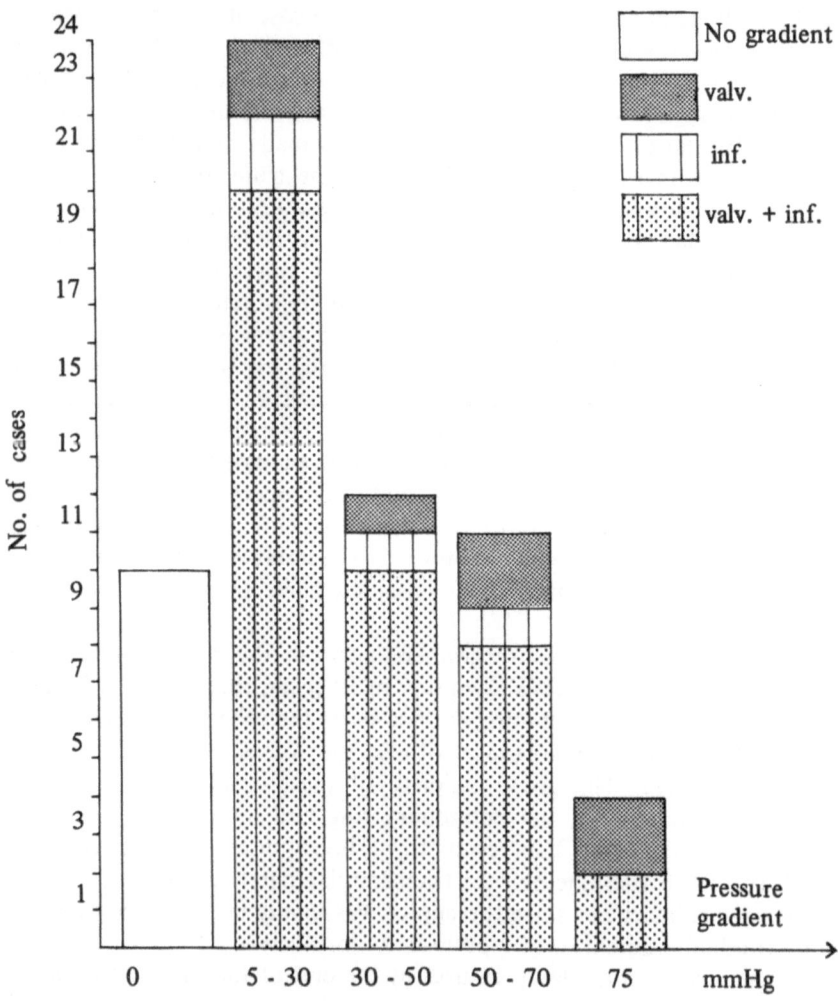

Figure 17.3 RV/PA pressure gradients in 65 patients undergoing total correction of Fallot's tetralogy. Mean delay between correction and evaluation = 6 months

on average, six months after the correction and therefore they may be sensitive to later modifications.

The study of the relationship between the right ventricle pressure and the aorta pressure shows that, when it is below 0·6, it remains stable or tends to drop in the great majority of cases. When, on the other hand, it is above 0·7, it tends to increase and when in the intermediary zone of

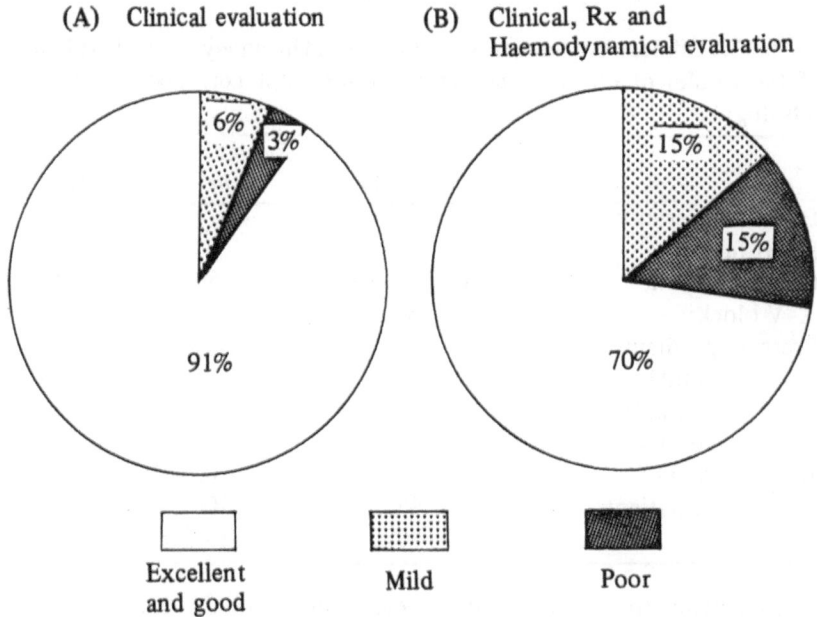

(A) Clinical evaluation

(B) Clinical, Rx and
     Haemodynamical evaluation

Excellent and good   Mild   Poor

Figure 17.4 Follow-up studies in 65 patients undergoing total correction of Fallot's tetralogy

uncertainty, between 0·6 and 0·7 it leads to the discussion of whether or not a patch should be put in place, notably at the level of the pulmonary ring.

In summary, some important residual gradients are observed but we have for corollary a small number of noticeable pulmonary insufficiencies, estimated with dilution of ascorbic acid and angiographies in the main pulmonary artery. In these rare cases, other than in the immediate postoperative period, a higher death rate after correction has not been observed as in other series, nor has there been any special difference in the late follow-up (Figure 17.4).

CONCLUSIONS

On the basis of objective classification together with clinical data, an evaluation of the cardiac volume, a cardiometric evaluation and evaluation of the haemodynamic and angiographic results, 70% of the patients have a result which is good and 15% have an average result – either they have a cardiac volume 30% above normal or they have a higher gradient ranging between 50 and 75 mmHg. The remaining 15% either show a very great increase in the cardiac volume, or a gradient higher than 75 mmHg, or residual VSD (Table 17.1).

Table 17.1 Clinical, ergometric, radiological and haemodynamical evaluation of the results of 65 cases operated on for total correction of Fallot's tetralogy

	Results		
	Excellent and good	*Mild*	*Poor*
Exercise tolerance	+ +	+ +	+
Heart failure	0	0	+
Cardiac volume	N or < 30%	< 50%	> 50%
A–V block	0	0	+
Pressure gradient			
– < 50 mmHg	+		
– 50–75 mmHg		+	
– > 75 mmHg			+
Residual VSD	0	0(+ ?)	+
Number of patients	45	10	10
%	70%	15%	15%

Comparing the isolated clinical evaluation and the evaluation and bearing in mind other factors, it can be seen that if the result was good or very good in 91% of the cases, it remains good or very good in only 70% of the cases (Figure 17.4).

Therefore, this study shows up different factors for which it may be possible to improve the result, i.e. capacity of effort, cardiac insufficiency and increase in the cardiac volume which depend on other factors, the most important being the residual VSD which must be avoided. In so far as the haemodynamic conditions are concerned, a right ventricle – left ventricle pressure relationship lower than or equal to 0·6 is accompanied by a good postoperative condition in all cases; a pressure relationship higher than 0·75, calls for an enlargement of the outflow tract of the right ventricle. Between 0·6 and 0·75 it is a matter of choice, either a high residual pressure or the risk of pulmonary insufficiency later on, the development of which is not very well known. Obviously a long-term study on two groups of patients, one having a residual gradient and the other having a pulmonary insufficiency, would be informative.

18

The need for homograft reconstruction of the right ventricular outflow in Fallot's tetralogy

D. N. Ross

It would be difficult to get uniformity of opinion as to whether a homograft should be used in the right outflow tract in Fallot's tetralogy. The best approach in the first instance is to consider whether there is a need for a major outflow tract reconstruction at all. Secondly, having decided on reconstruction, when would a homograft conduit be the ideal method? In the author's opinion the decision to do an outflow tract relieving operation must be based upon the well-known and accepted criteria of the pressure gradients across the outflow and the residual right ventricular pressure. In fact the final determinant of whether one does a major outflow tract reconstruction is dependent upon whether the residual obstruction lies at or about the valve ring level. The difficulties of a hypoplastic valve ring are well-known. The easiest method of assessing this, depending upon the size of the child, is to pass one's index or little finger up through the outflow tract. The soft muscle will be pushed aside but the fibrous valve ring will act as a barrier. Under these conditions one will generally divide the valve ring and reconstitute with some form of patch reconstruction.

Even more common, and perhaps more difficult to evaluate, is the sphincter-like smooth outflow tract which constricts and acts as a tight constricting ring right up to the valve ring. Thinning this muscle by sharp dissection right up to the valve ring is often unsuccessful as a means of relieving the obstruction and usually requires a vertical incision through the sphincter and the valve ring.

There are two other important related points. The first is that to assess this type of residual outflow obstruction it is essential to have the coronaries perfused and the heart in normal tone and beating. Secondly, the ventricular incision would be better as a vertical incision, if not in all cases, at least in all those in which is anticipated some outflow tract difficulty. The vertical ventriculotomy has a great deal to commend it, particularly where difficulty is anticipated, as it offers the chance of extending the incision downwards and upwards right into the pulmonary artery.

Having decided upon a form of reconstruction, what sort of material should be used? Pericardium had a great vogue and has many attractions for it is biological material. Unfortunately aneurysm or some degree of dilatation is an increasingly common finding and now so frequently described that Dacron – occasionally covered with pericardium if bleeding through the patch occurs – is favoured as a form of patch recon-

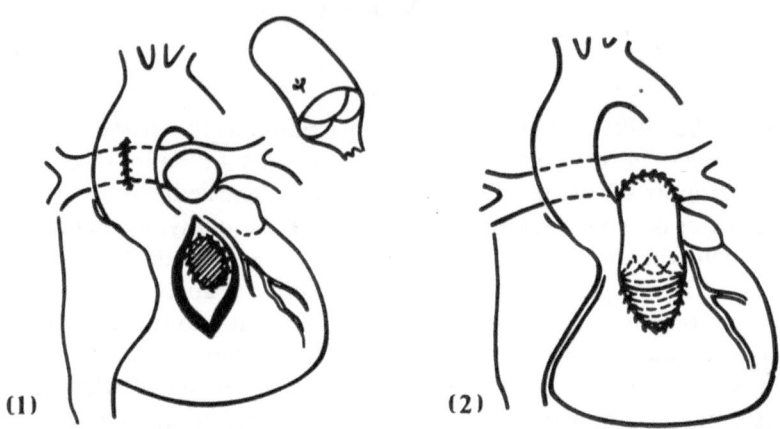

(1)   (2)

Figure 18.1 Reconstruction of right ventricular outflow tract. The VSD has been closed and the homograft conduit is ready for insertion.
Figure 18.2 Reconstruction of the right ventricular outflow. The homograft conduit in place.

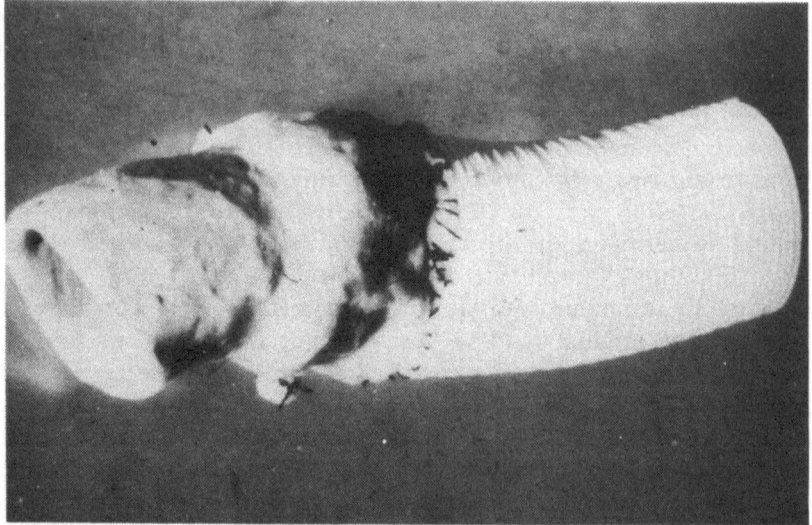

Figure 18.3 Dacron conduit with a homograft incorporated.

struction. Having decided upon a major reconstruction through the valve ring, when is a homograft conduit necessary? At the one end of the spectrum there is the type 1 pulmonary atresia with a small main pulmonary artery and a long narrow muscular infundibular sphincter. This anatomical configuration favours a homograft reconstruction (Figures 18.1 and 18.2). At the other end of the spectrum is the syndrome of ventricular septal defect with absent pulmonary valves, again not a typically Fallot type condition but one in which there would be no difficulty in deciding to put in a homograft valve. In between these extremes, a homograft should be used when there is no residual *functional* pulmonary valve tissue remaining after opening through the valve ring. Often just remnants of thickened valve tissue with platelet adherences are found. Under these circumstances it is better to excise the cusp remnants completely and fix a homograft conduit in place. Currently homograft valves collected within 24–48 h after death are used. These are trimmed of excess fat and contaminated tissues and a good length of ascending aorta is retained as a conduit. The specimen is then immersed in antibiotic tissue culture solution (Jenabi) and kept in an ordinary domestic refrigerator. Viability testing shows that these valves retain a significant proportion of their cells in a viable state for up to eight weeks (Jenabi) and this is an indication that the culture has not been denatured. At the time of surgery the coronary vessels are tied off and the aorta is trimmed to the required length and degree of obliquity. It is convenient to add a segment of Dacron conduit to the lower end for incorporation in the ventriculotomy incision. In the United States it is popular to use Dacron conduits with a homograft incorporated (Figure 18.3). No real difficulties have been found apart from calcification in the aortic wall of the homograft. There have been no known complications relating to the valve cusps which remain flexible and functional. The advanced degenerative changes described by McGoon have not been seen and perhaps it is the type of preparation of his conduits with irradiation which has caused some of the marked changes.

The author's longest functioning right ventricular homograft reconstruction has been in place since 1966 (eight years). This patient, who has recently been re-studied, still has a functional valve mechanism. John Kirklin has also just reported an 18-year-old patient who was killed in a motor car accident who had a homograft in place for two and one-half years, which at the time of death showed 'perfect preservation of the original elastic tissue of the graft and no calcification'. In cases of Fallot, a right ventricular reconstruction – not necessarily a homograft – has been used in almost 50% of cases, which is a high proportion and corroborates Jane Somerville's reports that many patients had in fact rather crooked outflow tracts and near atresia. Also most of them have had previous shunts. Of the patients requiring an outflow tract reconstruction (about 50%) approximately half of these so far have been done with a patch and the other half with a homograft.

The mortality in patients using the patch has been 15·5% whereas the mortality using the homograft has been 42%. The big discrepancy in mortality may not encourage use of homografts but the unacceptably high mortality can be accounted for on the basis that the cases have had difficult hypoplastic outflows and the programme in the past has been first to try and avoid a patch altogether, then to reconstruct with a patch of pericardium or Dacron and then finally when these measures had been proved to be unsatisfactory, and after a prolonged bypass, to use a homograft. In future once a clear need for an outflow tract reconstruction is seen a homograft will be used immediately.

Table 18.1 Applications of right ventricular outflow reconstruction with a valved conduit

1. Aortic valve replacement with pulmonary autograft
2. Pulmonary atresia
3. Severe Fallot's tetralogy
4. Truncus arteriosus
5. Transposition with ventricular septal defect
6. Tricuspid atresia
7. Common ventricle

Table 18.2 Right ventricular reconstruction with homograft valved conduit for pulmonary atresia and severe Fallot's tetralogy

48 patients	24 pulmonary atresia
	24 severe Fallot
21 hospital deaths	12 with unrelieved RV hypertension RV ⟩ LV pressure
	9 with residual hypertension RV > ½LV pressure

Part 3

Prosthetic Valves

19
The design characteristics of heart valves
K. Reid

The status of cardiac valve replacement still remains an ambivalent one. On the one hand are surgeons prompted possibly by earlier bitter experience who now advocate mechanical prosthetic valve replacement. They uphold essentially the ball-valve principle or its simple variants and urge that valve research be directed to solving such problems as tissue ingrowth on artificial fabrics to avoid embolic phenomena or to developing materials or coatings which will resist wear and corrosion in the blood stream. They are not principally concerned with modification of the basic design principles of their valve.

Simple mechanical valves of this type have a wealth of clinical experience behind them and despite constant modifications there is the certain knowledge that such valves are reasonably reliable. On the other hand are surgeons whose instincts and empirical judgements find offensive the crude solution provided by mechanical prosthesis differing so fundamentally from nature's valves. Since Durran and Gunning in Oxford in the early '60s first demonstrated in animals the feasibility of long-term homograft replacement, devotees of biological valves have used in clinical practice a wide variety of processed tissues as valve cusp substitute materials. Often regrettably these have been used without an adequate experimental basis. It would not I think be unfair to say that the case for biological valves currently rests on the supposition that live cells transplanted either from a recently dead person, often weeks later, or freshly as autologous tissue, are likely to survive as a valve substitute. While the use of fresh nutrient homograft valves would appear to have prolonged homograft survival, the weight of evidence clinically and experimentally indicates that they too may have a limited lifespan.

A third approach, and the one I am advocating here, is the development of man-made leaflet valves.

In order to understand normal aortic valve mechanics, a perspex aortic root was made incorporating nylon-reinforced silastic cusps; the cusps were mounted so that they were fully open in their relaxed position without any elastic recoil tending to close them. The model was placed in a pulsatile water tunnel, the valve being presented with a laminar uniform stream, dynamically identical with that measured in the outflow tract of animals and man.

Our conclusions were that normal aortic valve action is a vortex-dependent mechanism of high efficiency. The geometry of the sinuses of Valsalva being crucial in effectively regulating the fluid dynamic forces responsible for efficient closure and for ensuring coronary artery flow in systole.

Using dye studies, we showed that high velocity vortexes form near the sinus ridge. It was observed that fluid enters the sinus over the free-cusp margin, leaving at the corners.

There is considerable variation of pressure within a sinus so that a coronary ostium positioned near the ridge, a stagnation point in fluid dynamic terms, would be fed at a higher pressure than one lower in the sinus and systolic coronary blood flow would be correspondingly enhanced.

Pulsatile flow was studied by filming simultaneously cusp position and aortic velocity. Frame-by-frame analysis enables aortic velocity and valve opening to be demonstrated graphically as functions of time.

This technique showed that the valve mechanism comprises four distinct phases – opening, fully open (the quasi-steady phase), deceleration and reversed flow. The opening phase occupies 15%, the fully open 55% and the deceleration phase 30% of total systolic time. The cusps are thus three-quarters of the way shut before forward flow ceases.

Gregg has demonstrated that the essential adaptive response to exercise is a marked increase in systolic coronary blood flow, so that it often exceeds diastolic coronary flow. In exercise, when systolic peak velocity and pressure at the sinus ridge rises, systolic coronary flow will be correspondingly increased. The sinus of Valsalva and the position of the coronary ostea have an important architectural role in enabling these functional changes to occur. The results indicate that the ideal aortic valve replacement should produce no impedence to aortic-systolic flow, should close with less than 2% reverse flow and should not cause turbulence.

A separate study was undertaken to define more precisely the design criteria for a prosthetic mitral valve by considering the flow pattern and end-diastolic ventricular silhouette in normal hearts and in subjects in whom the mitral valve had been replaced by either a disc valve or a homograft. The geometric configuration of the mitral valve, is such as to allow a vortex to be trapped in the retro valvular zones, in a manner analogous with the fluid motion of the sinus of Valsalva. Cine studies indicate opaque medium entering the ventricle as a broad slug which quickly expands as the valve opens to its full extent with the whole of the ventricular surface distal to the cusp tip receiving the impact of entering fluid. The mitral valve remains fully open for the major part of diastole, closing after the onset of atrial contraction. When the mechanical valve is in the mitral position, the normal filling pattern is exactly reversed. The proximal heart cavity fills first and the more distal major portion of the ventricle never fully dilates. The distal heart wall appears to be drawn inward paradoxically and the heart assumes a turnip-shaped appearance. Given an appreciation of the normal ventricular filling pattern that achieves an optimum distension of the heart muscle for a given volume flow in unit time, it is obvious that in the circumstances of the disc valve the ventricle labours at a very great mechanical disadvantage. In the case of the homograft valve, a central jet of fluid rapidly reaches the internal apex of the heart and causes the distal portion of the cavity to dilate. The proximal heart cavity is unaffected by the thrust of fluid entering the chamber and the heart assumes a pear-shaped appearance. The duration of diastole and the flatness of the ventricular filling curve after the early filling phase, suggests that it is vortex decay that is especially critical to mitral valve closure, and atrial contraction should be seen as the means of imparting additional energy to a dying vortex in late diastole. As diastole shortens, and the atrial filling curve moves to the left, as the heart speeds up, so the need for atrial contraction in valve closure diminishes.

The configuration of the atrium and ventricle makes it comparable in fluid dynamic terms with a diffuser except that in the heart the mouth of the diffuser is guarded by a valve. A standard method in fluid dynamics for estimating the quantity of fluid flowing through a pipe is to utilise a diffuser or venturimeter. This comprises a short length of pipe tapering to a throat and then re-expanding to its original diameter. By measuring the pressure differences at the inflow of the taper and at the narrowest portion, it is possible to calculate the quantity of liquid flowing at a given time. It is found that as the fluid velocity increases as it reaches the narrowest throat, so the pressure declines. If, however, the throat diameter is small compared with the outflow diameter, there is too rapid a rate of expansion of the tube for the fluid cone to run full. This causes a loss of pressure. If lateral suction is applied by a series of small tubes beyond the constriction, or in the case of the heart, there is elastic recoil or a vortex mechanism, the fluid cone is allowed to run full. As a result, pressure recovery is much enhanced. Using a similar system, Akaret, a German engineer, has shown that pressure recovery may be nearly doubled since the jet can be fully expanded. In a similar way, the mitral valve presents a boundery-layer control situation, in which initially elastic recoil and later a vortex both pay a part. In this way, pressure recovery for full ventricular dilation is enhanced by promoting full expansion of the jet. The effect being to spread and direct the streamlines towards the ventricle walls which therefore behave as a pressure-recovery surface.

While it is convenient to consider the non-valvular functions of the aortic valve as relating principally to systolic coronary blood flow, it is clear that the non-valvular functions of the mitral valve are concerned with ventricular filling. Thus, it is not sufficient to state that the ventricle fills merely because of an atrioventricular pressure difference. It must be added that the ventricle fills in a highly characteristic manner. And any device which interferes with the normal ventricular filling pattern seriously compromises cardiac function, particularly when there is a reduction in the duration of diastole.

The realisation of a man-made aortic valve or mitral valve prosthesis which reproduces the normal valve mechanisms, remains the most desirable but elusive goal. In the short term the stumbling block has proved to be not a design but a materials problem. The valve is made from silastic and Dacron – the principal feature is that the valve lies in a fully-open position, and though the orifice looks triangular in this particular view, in fact it conforms to a cylinder.

20
Echocardiographic studies following mitral valve replacement
D. G. Gibson

This chapter describes the application of echocardiography to studying alterations in the pattern of left ventricular filling due to mitral valve replacement, and so differs from previous investigations in which echoes have been recorded from the homograft[1] or prosthesis[2] itself. The method depends on recording echoes simultaneously from the interventricular septum and the endocardial surface of the posterior wall of the left ventricle. The distance between the two represents the transverse dimension of the left ventricle and is derived from an echocardiogram using a simple digitising technique that has been described elsewhere. This dimension is plotted, together with its rate of change, continuously throughout the cardiac cycle and a typical example from a normal subject can be seen in Figure 20.1. In normal subjects, the peak rate of increase of dimension of the left ventricle during the rapid phase of filling has a mean value of 10 cm s^{-1}, but is only maintained for a short period at the start of diastole. In the presence of rheumatic mitral stenosis, the filling pattern is significantly modified and in 10 patients who required valvotomy, had a mean value of 4 cm s^{-1}. In addition, the rapid early phase was lost, but lower levels were maintained throughout the period of ventricular filling.

The effects of three types of mitral valve replacement on the pattern of left ventricular filling are shown in Figure 20.2. These are derived from patients in whom Starr–Edwards prostheses (composite seat), Björk–Shiley (pyrolite disc) or cuff-mounted, inverted aortic homografts had been inserted in the mitral position. It is apparent that in all three groups of patients, the peak rate of diastolic wall movement was reduced, although not to the low levels seen in those with critical mitral stenosis. Although there was considerable overlap between the three groups, the lowest values of peak rates of wall movement were recorded in patients with Starr–Edwards prostheses. These patients included not only those with small (size 2) prostheses, but also those in whom a larger prosthesis had been inserted into a small left ventricular cavity to replace a mitral valve that was previously stenotic.

A number of factors may be involved in this reduction in peak filling rate. A direct relation between stroke volume and peak filling rate has previously been demonstrated[3] and it is well-established that after mitral valve replacement, cardiac output, and therefore stroke volume, may not return to normal.[4] A second abnormality may be the presence

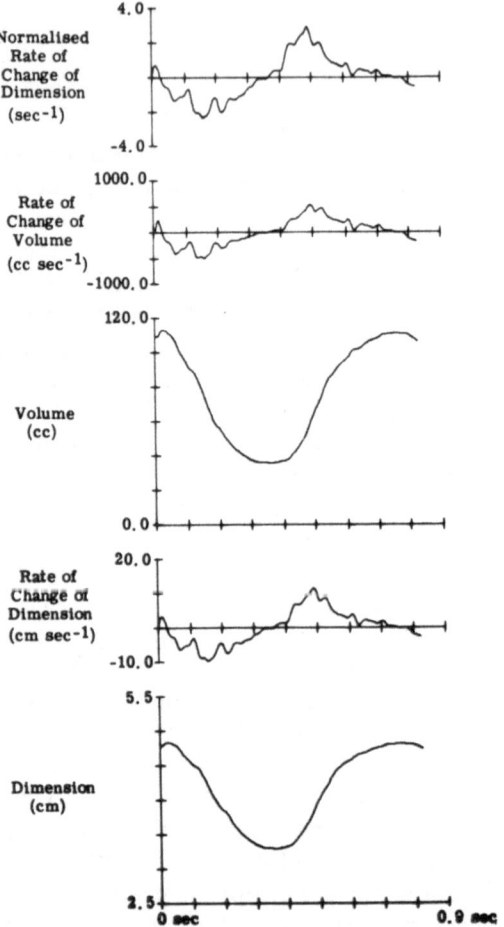

Figure 20.1 Computer plot of left ventricular dimension and its rate of change throughout a single cardiac cycle from a normal subject. Values of left ventricular volume are derived as the cube of the dimension. Zero time corresponds to the Q wave of the ECG

of pulmonary hypertension and associated disturbance of septal movement although this is probably unimportant, since filling rates may become normal in the presence of a mitral paraprosthetic leak, although severe pulmonary hypertension may be present. The most likely mechanism for reduced filling rate, however, is that the prosthesis itself is obstructive, as has been documented haemodynamically by a pressure difference across the valve during diastole.[4] The importance of assessing the function of prostheses *in situ* in the left ventricle is illustrated in Figure 20.3. This is the echocardiogram of a patient with a No. 3 Starr–Edwards prosthesis in the mitral position, who developed a low

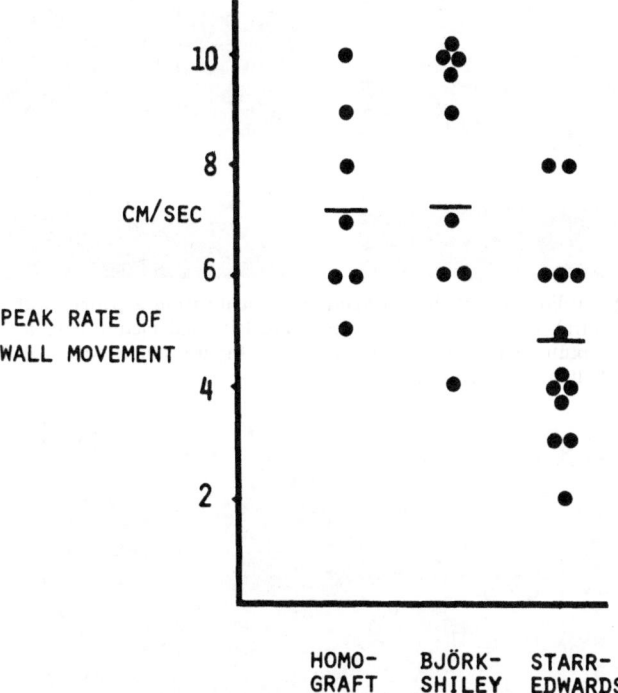

Figure 20.2 Peak rate of increase of left ventricular dimensions during diastole in three groups of patients after mitral valve replacement.

cardiac output in the postoperative period. The motion of posterior wall and septum are virtually parallel to one another and the apex of the cage impinges on the septum, while the ball of the prosthesis can be seen to take up a position half-way down the cage during diastole, thus explaining the very abnormal filling pattern seen in this patient.

Figure 20.2 illustrates peak left ventricular rates of diastolic wall movement in 3 groups of patients following mitral valve replacement with an inverted aortic homograft, a Bjork-Shiley prosthesis or a Starr-Edwards prosthesis. Comparison suggests that on haemodynamic grounds, there is little difference between a Björk–Shiley prosthesis and an inverted aortic homograft. In some patients, particularly those in

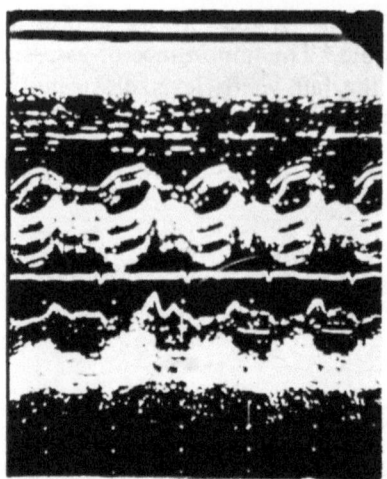
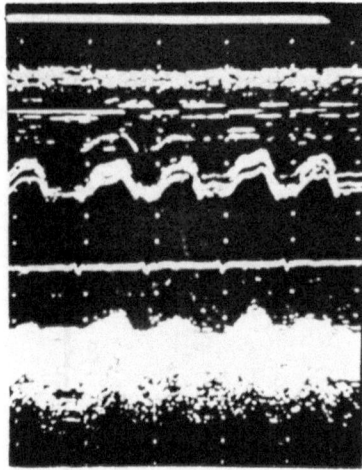

Figure 20.3 Echocardiograms of the left ventricular cavity from a patient with a No. 3 composite seat mitral Starr–Edwards prosthesis. The left hand picture demonstrates the interventricular septum and the posterior wall. When the transducer was angled a little, echoes from the ball and cage also become apparent

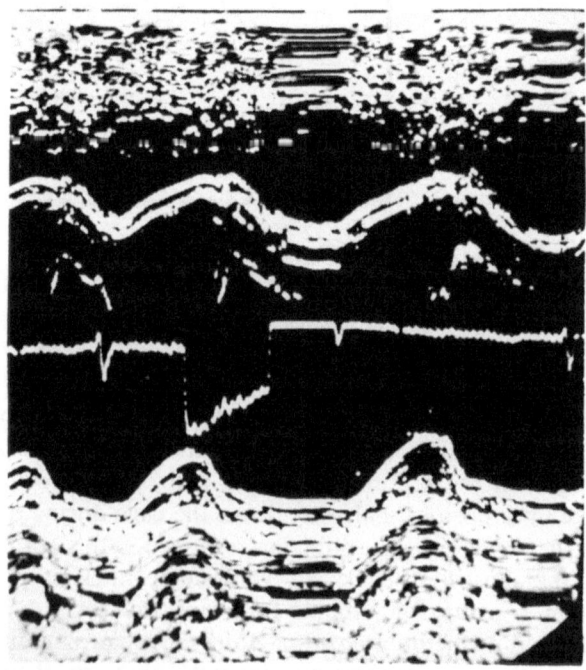

Figure 20.4 Echocardiogram of the left ventricular cavity from a patient with a normally functioning mitral Starr–Edwards prosthesis. Septal motion is reversed, with a dominant anterior movement during systole

whom the left ventricular cavity is small, however, a Starr–Edwards prosthesis may be associated with low rates of wall movement, comparable to those seen in patients with mitral stenosis.

Echocardiography has also proved of value in the assessment of patients suspected of having a mitral paraprosthetic leak. This is a

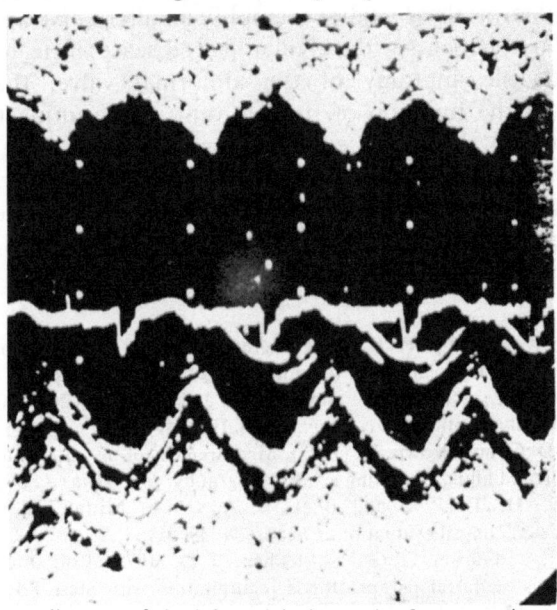

Figure 20.5 Echocardiogram of the left ventricular cavity from a patient with a severe mitral paraprosthetic leak. Septal motion is normal and the calculated stroke volume is 130 ml

difficult diagnosis to make clinically, since a pan-systolic murmur is usually absent, or when present, originates from the tricuspid valve. The patient deteriorates, or fails to improve after mitral valve replacement, the venous pressure is elevated and the chest radiograph shows cardiac enlargement and pulmonary congestion, so that the clinical picture is indistinguishable from left ventricular dysfunction. In the presence of a normally functioning mitral Starr–Edwards prosthesis, septal movement is reversed, the dominant movement during systole being in an anterior rather than in a posterior direction (Figure 20.4). In 9 patients out of 11 with mitral regurgitation due to a paraprosthetic leak, septal movement had returned to a normal pattern (Figure 20.5), and in the tenth, the site of regurgitation at operation was found to be dominantly through the ring, rather than round it.[5] Reversion to a normal pattern of septal movement also occurred in two patients with a normally functioning mitral prosthesis but who had, in addition, unsuspected aortic regurgitation, and was present in spite of severe pulmonary hypertension and increased right ventricular stroke volume due to tricuspid regurgitation. Its absence in patients with left ventricular dysfunction or obstructed protheses suggested that normal septal movement reflected abnormal early diastolic filling of the left ventricle, the normally functioning prosthesis being to some extent obstructive.[4]

In general terms these studies exemplify an alternative approach to the investigation of patients with valvular heart disease: instead of being concerned with the anatomy of the abnormal valve, they document alterations in the function of the left ventricle resulting from stenosis or regurgitation. When taken in association with those designed to delineate abnormal anatomy, they allow a very full description of the overall disturbance and in many cases allow cardiac catheterisation to be dispensed with.

References

1. Gianelly, R. E., Popp, R. L. and Hultgren, H. N. (1970). Heart sounds in patients with homograft replacement of the mitral valve. *Circulation,* **42,** 309
2. Johnson, M. L., Paton B. C. and Holmes, J. H. (1970). Ultrasonic evaluation of prosthetic valve motion. *Circulation,* **Suppl. II, 3,** 41
3. Gibson, D. G. and Brown, D. (1973). Measurement of instantaneous left ventricular dimension and filling rate using echocardiography. *Brit. Heart J.,* **35,** 1141
4. Kezdi, P., Head, L. R. and Buck, B. A. (1964). Mitral ball valve prosthesis. Dynamic and clinical evaluation. *Circulation,* **30,** 55
5. Miller, H. C., Gibson, D. G. and Stephens, J. D. (1973). Role of echocardiography in diagnosis of mitral paraprosthetic regurgitation with Starr–Edwards prostheses. *Brit. Heart J.,* **35,** 1217

21
Myocardial preservation during aortic valve replacement

R. N. Sapsford

Myocardial preservation has been, and still is, a major problem in aortic valve surgery. In order to determine the safety of coronary perfusion as compared to profound hypothermic non-perfusion arrest, one technique of coronary perfusion with moderate hypothermia and one technique of profound hypothermic non-perfusion arrest using cardiac cooling by the perfusate in patients undergoing elective aortic valve replacement were studied in a prospective and randomised manner. Special study techniques were necesary since simple hospital mortality and morbidity rates for this operation are low. Operation and cardiopulmonary bypass times were significantly reduced when profound hypothermic non-perfusion arrest was used. In the early postoperative period no statistical differences were observed between the two groups of patients with respect to haemodynamic performance, myocardial metabolism, isoenzyme release and the electrocardiogram. However, present data indicates that the majority of the patients studied incurred myocardial cell necrosis.

Table 21.1 A randomised study of the safety of coronary perfusion as compared to profound hypothermic non-perfusion arrest

	No. of patients	per cent
Randomised in pairs per surgeon	78	
Randomisation adhered to	64	82.1
Coronary perfusion (C.P.) used	31	48.4
Hypothermic non-perfusion arrest (H.N.P.A.) used	33	51.6

A process of randomisation was applied to all patients in the Department of Surgery at the University of Alabama undergoing primary elective isolated aortic valve replacement between the 1st February and 4th July 1973. This yielded 64 patients (Table 21.1). One patient in the study died in the operating theatre of intractable left ventricular fibrillation; coronary perfusion had been employed to replace his valve. There were 31 patients in the coronary perfusion group: both coronaries were perfused in all but one patient, the perfusate temperature was 32 °C and during the perfusion the heart was not allowed to fibrillate. There were 33 patients in the profound hypothermic non-perfusion arrest group and they were placed on bypass at 25 °C after four minutes. In this group the perfusate temperature was lowered to 15 °C for two minutes and the aorta was cross-clamped.

Table 21.2 Operation and temperature times in a group of 64 patients undergoing primary elective isolated aortic valve replacement

	TEMPERATURES AND OPERATION TIMES		
	Coronary perfusion Mean + S.E. (n)	*Hypothermic non-perfusion arrest* mean ± S.E. (n)	
Myocardial temp. (°C) (at aortic cross clamp)	31.0 ± 0.4620 (25)	22.4 ± 0.6439 (26)	*p*<.001
Myocardial temp. (°C) (at aortic release)	29.6 ± 0.4637 (24)	24.6 ± 0.7121 (26)	*p*<.001
Operation time (mins.) (aortic cross clamp to release)	68.3 ± 2.544 (31)	49.7 ± 1.576 (33)	$p < .0001$
Total cardio-pulmonary bypass time (mins.)	82.4 ± 2.712 (30)	65.1 ± 2.135 (33)	p< .0001

The perfusate temperature was then raised to 28 °C and the heart was vented in all the patients via the left atrium. Myocardial temperatures were recorded when the aorta was cross-clamped and when it was released. Studies were performed at six periods in the first 56 hours postoperatively when cardiac output, heart rate, arterial, left and right atrial and left ventricular pressures were measured. Coronary sinus and arterial plasma were analysed for lactate and pyruvate levels, coronary sinus or right atrial plasma was analysed for the isoenzyme creatine phosphokinase (CPK). The MB isoenzyme of CPK is specific for myocardial necrosis yet the method is of sufficiently low sensitivity to avoid elevations with atriotomies, needle puncture of myocardium or multiple defibrillation attempts. Lactatedehydrogenase isoenzyme fractionation was also performed on these samples since haemolysis was low enough to give valid

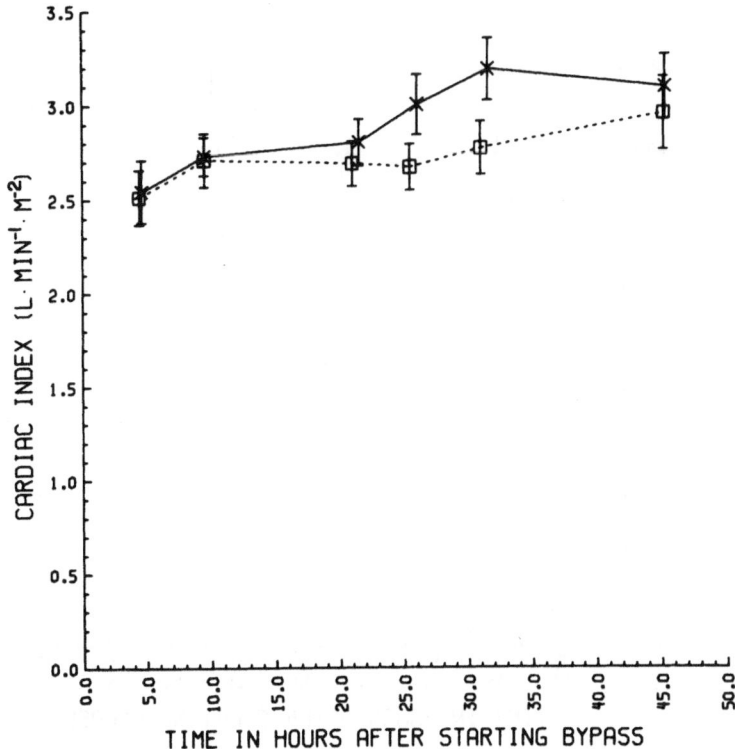

Figure 21.1 Cardiac index plotted against time for two groups undergoing primary elective isolated aortic valve replacement. × = coronary perfusion group; ☐ = profound hypothermic non-perfusion group

results. The data set was analysed by a variety of statistical techniques, including appropriate data transformations, when departures from a normal distribution were encountered.

Seventy-seven items were tested for significant differences between the two study groups. These included vital statistics such as age and sex; symptoms; stenosis or incompetence at the aortic valve, findings on X-ray, the elctrocardiogram and at cardiac catheterisation, together with observations and measurements at operation, such as the left ventricular wall thickness and diameter. Of these, only two were found to be different. This demonstrates the success of the randomisation procedure since the theory of chance predicts at least two such occurrences.

Table 21.2 depicts certain operative measurements. The myocardial temperatures at both aortic cross-clamping and release times were significantly different for the two groups as expected. Cross-clamp time

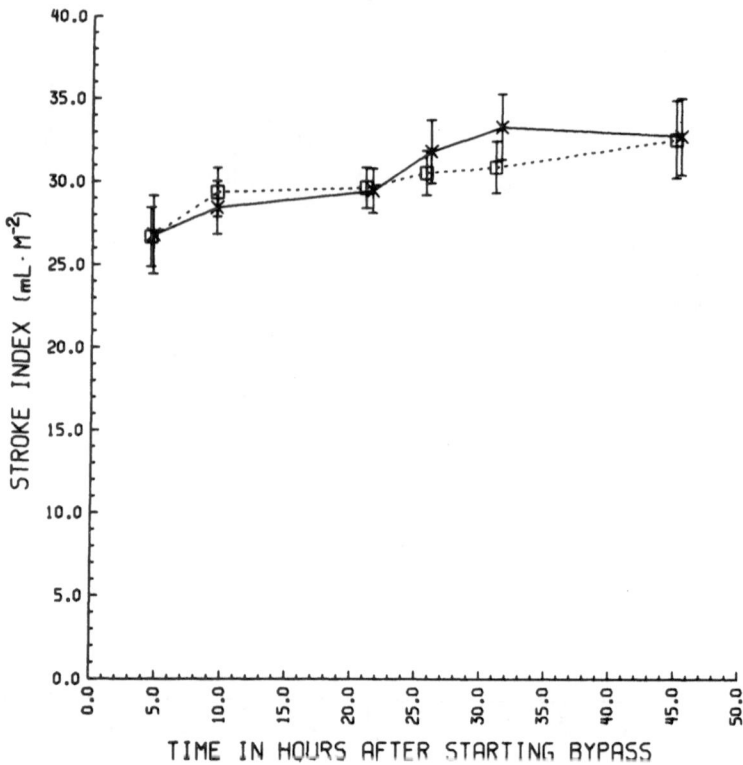

Figure 21.2 Stroke index plotted against time for two groups undergoing primary elective isolated aortic valve replacement. × = coronary perfusion group; □ = profound hypothermic non-perfusion group

using profound hypothermic non-perfusion arrest was 27% less than when using coronary perfusion and total cardiopulmonary bypass time was 21% less.

The haemodynamic data was analysed against time. Figure 21.1 shows the time in hours after bypass on the horizontal axis and the variable to be examined, i.e. the cardiac index, on the vertical axis. The mean values at the six study periods for the coronary perfusion group are indicated by the crosses with one standard error of the mean, joined by the solid line. The profound hypothermic non-perfusion arrest group are indicated by the open squares joined by the dotted line. The cardiac arrest was not significantly different for the two groups. The stroke index shown on Figure 21.2 indicates that there was no difference between the groups. Figure 21.3 shows the stroke-work index and again there was no difference between the groups.

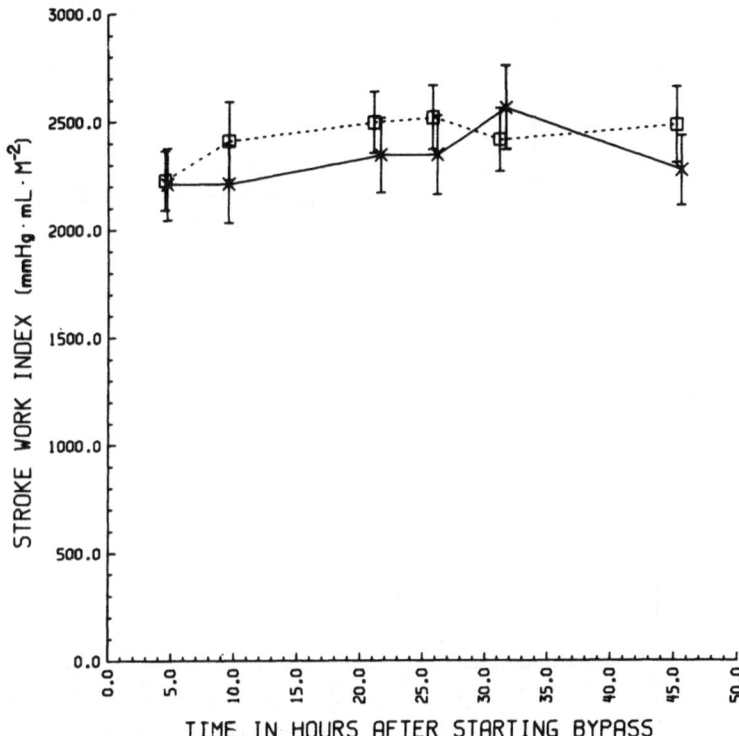

Figure 21.3 Stroke-work index plotted against time for two groups undergoing primary elective isolated aortic valve replacement. × = coronary perfusion group; □ = profound hypothermic non-perfusion group

The left ventricular peak pressure derivative or DP/DT was normalised by dividing it by the pressure developed during isovolumetric contraction. There was no difference between the groups (Figure 21.4). The ratio of the tension time index (TTI) and diastolic pressure time index (DPTI) as an index of coronary blood flow is shown in Figure 21.5. Once more, no difference between the groups was observed.

Figure 21.6 shows the percentage transmyocardial lactate extraction, which was low at first then rising to normal levels at about six to ten hours. Once again no differences could be demonstrated. The arterial to coronary sinus excess lactate was high early postoperatively, falling quickly to near zero. No difference between the groups was observed (Figure 21.7).

With the method used, any detectable CPK(MB) is an indication of myocardial cell necrosis in humans. In both groups, this preoperative level was zero, but at four to nine hours postbypass peak levels of MB were detected, although these disappeared over the next 40 h when

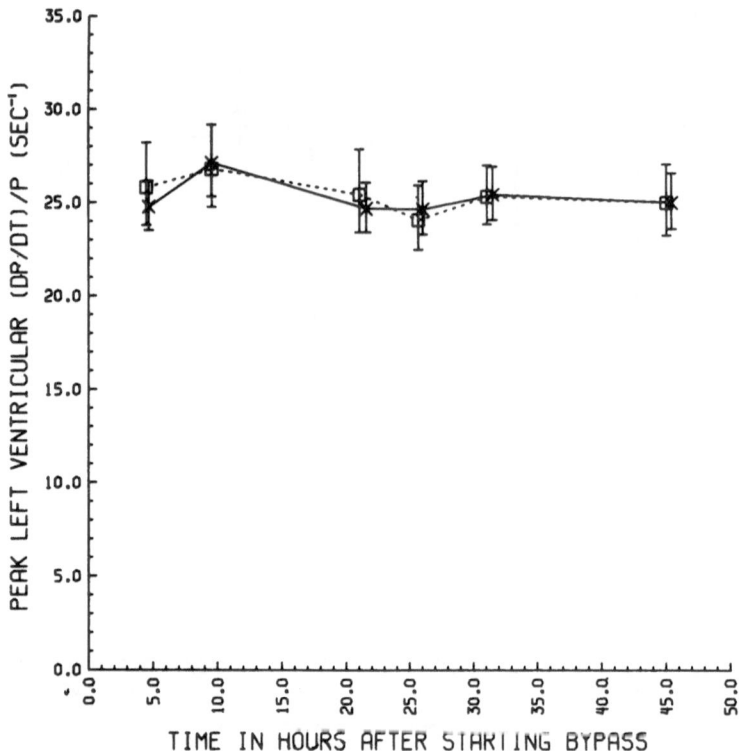

Figure 21.4 The left ventricular peak pressure derivative plotted against time for two groups undergoing primary elective isolated aortic valve replacement. × = coronary perfusion group; □ = profound hypothermic non-perfusion group

the levels and the time course of the isoenzymes were similar in both groups (Figure 21.8). An excess of LDH isoenzyme 1 over LDH isoenzyme 2 is presumptive evidence of myocardial necrosis. When this occurs the ratio of LDH1: LDH2 becomes greater than 1. This occurred on the average about 16 h postbypass in both groups, but again both groups were nearly identical (Figure 21.9).

Table 21.3 is an analysis of individual patient isoenzyme response – this information was available in 48 patients. An absence of CPK and LDH1 less than LDH2 indicates no necrosis. This occurred in only two patients. The detection of CPK (MB) and an excess of LDH1 over LDH2 is diagnostic of necrosis. This occurred in 33 or 69% of these patients. An additional six patients had an LDH1: LDH2 reversal without detectable CPK (MB). This is presumptive evidence of necrosis and ongoing work indicates that there may have been an early and transient appearance of

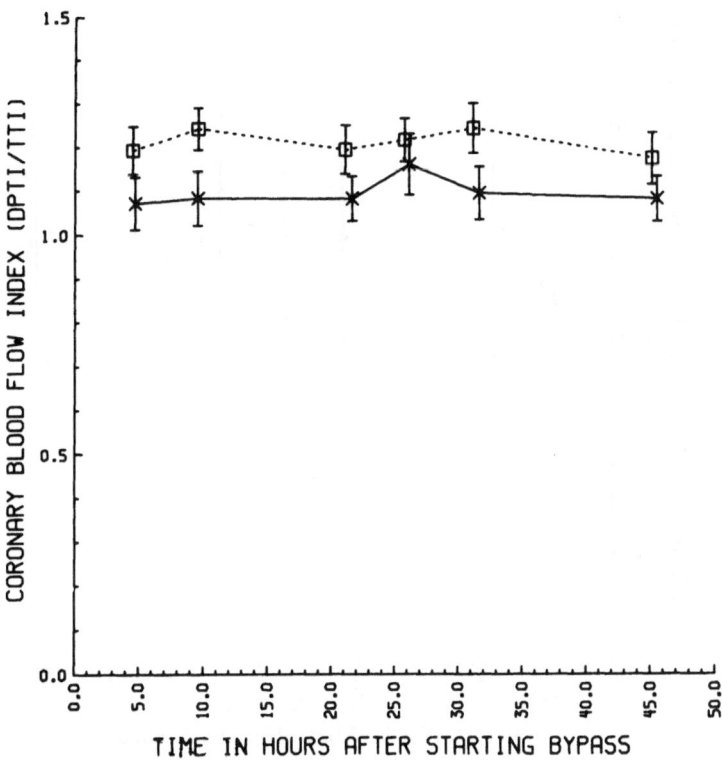

Figure 21.5 Coronary blood flow index plotted against time for two groups undergoing primary elective isolated aortic valve replacement. × = coronary perfusion group; □ = profound hypothermic non-perfusion group

Table 21.3 Analysis of individual patient isoenzyme response to assess myocardial necrosis

	No CPK-MB LKH1<LDH2	CPK-MB and LDHI⋝LDH2	No CPK-MB LDHI>LDH2	CPK-MB and LDHI<LDH2	Total
Coronary perfusion	1	14	4	3	22
Ischaemic arrest	1	19	2	4	26
Totals	2 (4.2%)	33 (68·7%)	6 (12.5%)	7 (14.6%)	48
Interpretation	None	Diagnostic	Presumptive	Indeterminate	

p for table by χ^2 test is not significant

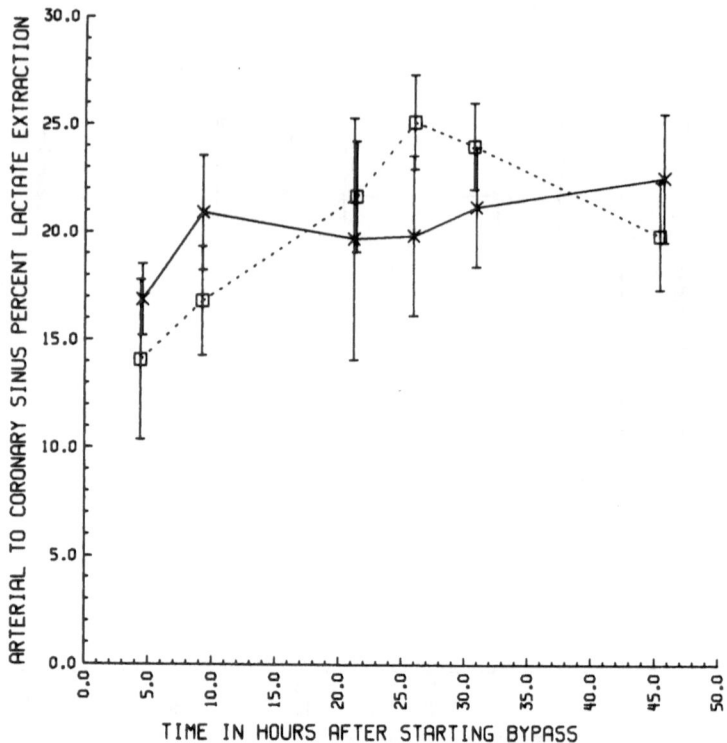

Figure 21.6 The percentage transmyocardial lactate extraction plotted against time for two groups undergoing primary elective isolated aortic valve replacement. × = coronary perfusion group; ☐ = profound hypothermic non-perfusion group

CPK (MB) missed by our sampling in this group. At the present time it is not possible to interpret the presence of CPK (MB) with a normal LDH1 : LDH2 ratio which occurred in seven patients, but it is becoming apparent that this is also diagnostic of myocardial cell necrosis. Thus, viewed conservatively, 39 or 81% of these patients had diagnostic or presumptive evidence of myocardial cell necrosis. As regards the proportion of patients in each of the four categories shown, there was no significant difference between the groups.

Significant changes occurred in the electrocardiogram for both groups postoperatively. These were interpreted as either new ischaemic changes, or when quite characteristic as indicative of myocardial infarction. The two groups are clearly mutually exclusive and these changes occurred in 27% of all the patients. Half of these were interpreted as ischaemic changes and the other half as infarction. There was no statistical difference

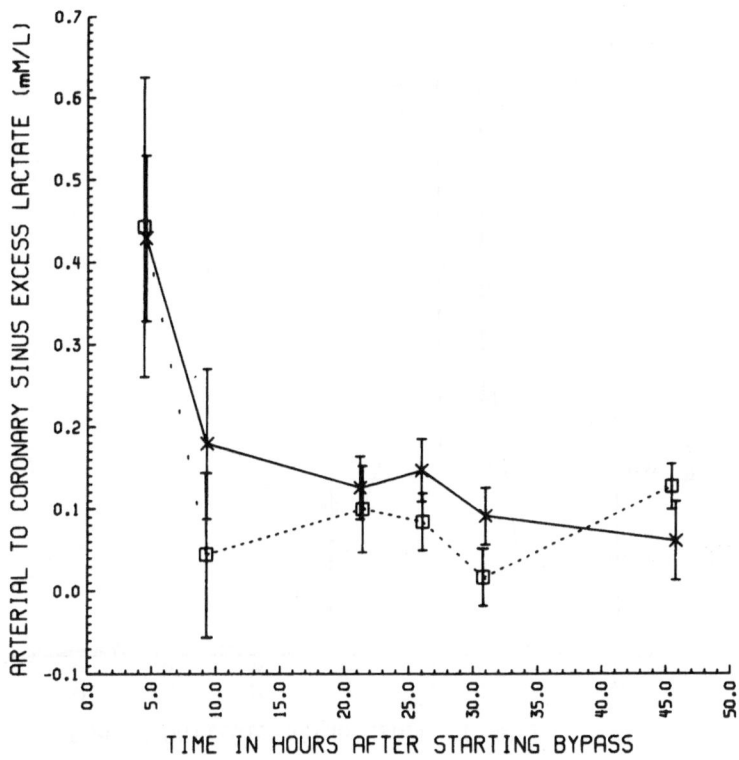

Figure 21.7 Arterial to coronary sinus excess lactate plotted against time for two groups undergoing primary elective isolated aortic valve replacement. × = coronary perfusion group; □ = profound hypothermic non-perfusion group

Table 21.4 Electrocardiographic evidence of myocardial injury (7–10 days postoperatively)

	Coronary perfusion	*Ischaemic arrest*	*Total*
New ischaemic changes	2	5	7 (13.5%)
New myocardial infarctions	5	2	7 (13.5%)
No changes	20	18	38 (73.0%)
Total	27	25	52

p for table by χ^2 test is not significant

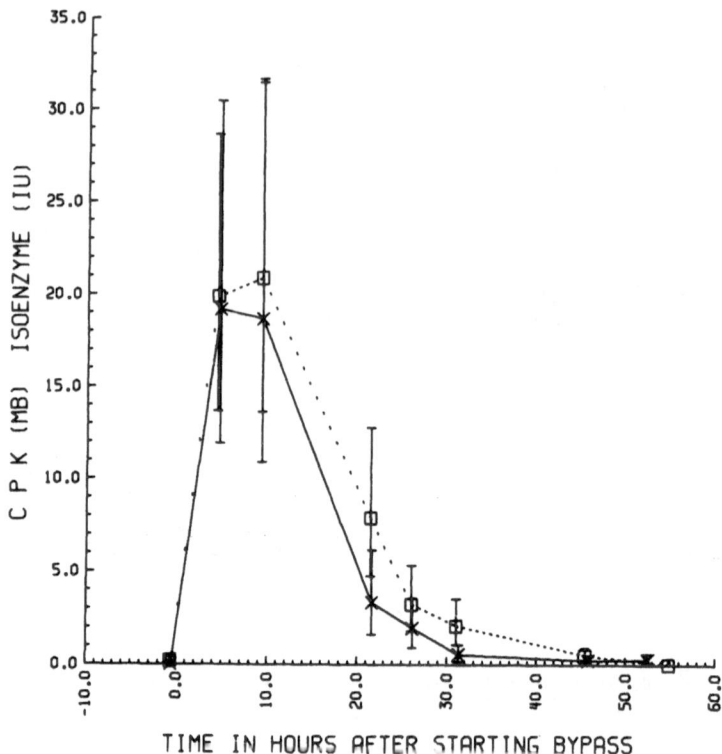

Figure 21.8 Levels of CPK (MB) isoenzyme plotted against time for two groups undergoing primary elective isolated aortic valve replacement. × = coronary perfusion group; □ = profound hypothermic non-perfusion group

in the incidence of these changes between the two groups. All patients with these changes, who had isoenzyme studies done showed isoenzyme patterns diagnostic of necrosis (Table 21.4).

In summary, we have demonstrated that the profound hypothermic non-perfusion arrest technique used significantly shortens the aortic cross-clamp time and cardiopulmonary bypass time. There was no difference between the two techniques in terms of early postoperative cardiac performance, metabolism, isoenzyme release or the electrocardiogram and the majority of patients sustained myocardial injury irrespective of the method of myocardial preservation used. It is evident that a lot of further work is necessary to elucidate what causes this cell necrosis. The only factors common to the two methods in this study were the first and the last 10 minutes of cardiopulmonary bypass. Recent work on denatured protein microaggregates which form early in the course of cardiopulmonary

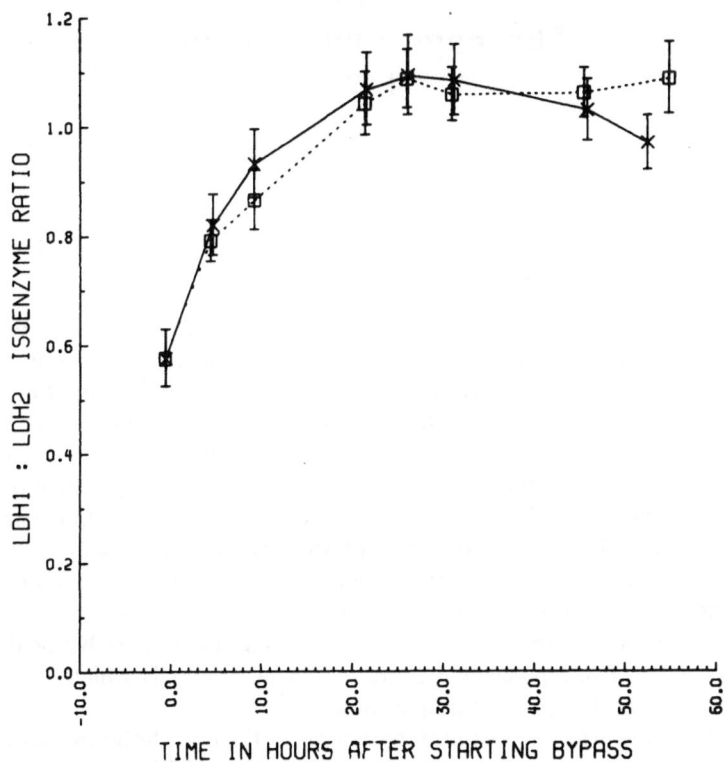

Figure 21.9 LDH1:LDH2 isoenzyme ratio plotted against time for two groups undergoing primary elective isolated aortic valve replacement. × = coronary perfusion group; □ = profound hypothermic non-perfusion group

bypass may be an important cause of this cell necrosis and this can really only be assessed by further randomised trials of this sort eliminating one factor at a time.

22
The cage ball prosthesis

A. Starr

Discussions about the theoretical aspects of valve design are always very interesting. If we turned the engineers loᴄ se, completely, they would design many exotic prostheses which would be highly imaginative and they would function very well. Unfortunately, we are limited by the problem of thrombosis. The design of an artificial valve must take into account the environment in which the valve will be used. The approach to the problem of valve replacement has really been to free ourselves of as many of these engineering considerations as is possible and see how prostheses can be used to solve a clinical problem rather than to try to achieve the ultimate in duplicating the beautiful design of the natural living valve.

The author will review his experience during the past twelve or thirteen years with valve replacement using prosthetic materials which are almost always in the ball-valve configuration.

The Model 6120 is the mitral prosthesis of the non-cloth-covered variety which is currently used, and the Model 6310 or 6320 series is the cloth-covered variety used (Figure 22.1). Figure 22.2 shows the results to date in an actuarial display with the Model 6120 valve or the non-cloth-covered standard mitral prosthesis. In this group of patients whose follow-up has extended to nine years, there have been no patients who required a replacement of this valve. In addition, the problem of infection during this period is quite small so that the chance for a patient to have an infection by the end of eight years' follow-up is about 2 or 3%. Also, the chance for a patient to live to the eighth or ninth year after operation, after isolated mitral valve replacement with this type of prosthesis, is 70%. A disturbing feature with this valve, however, is the continued incidence of thromboembolic complications occurring throughout most of the period of follow-up, so that by the time the patient reaches eight or nine years after operation, the chance for a thromboembolic episode is about 30%. This valve is still in rather widespread current use possibly because most of these emboli are transient ischaemic attacks with no neurological sequelae—many of them are missed entirely by the clinician. This is especially so if the patient is not seen frequently at the hospital that performed the operation. And so while the incidence of emboli is disturbing, it is really not as bad as it may appear from an actuarial display.

Because of this continued incidence of emboli, which is characteristic of probably all non-cloth-covered valves and maybe all prosthetic valves, the author was interested in evaluating those prostheses which are capable of

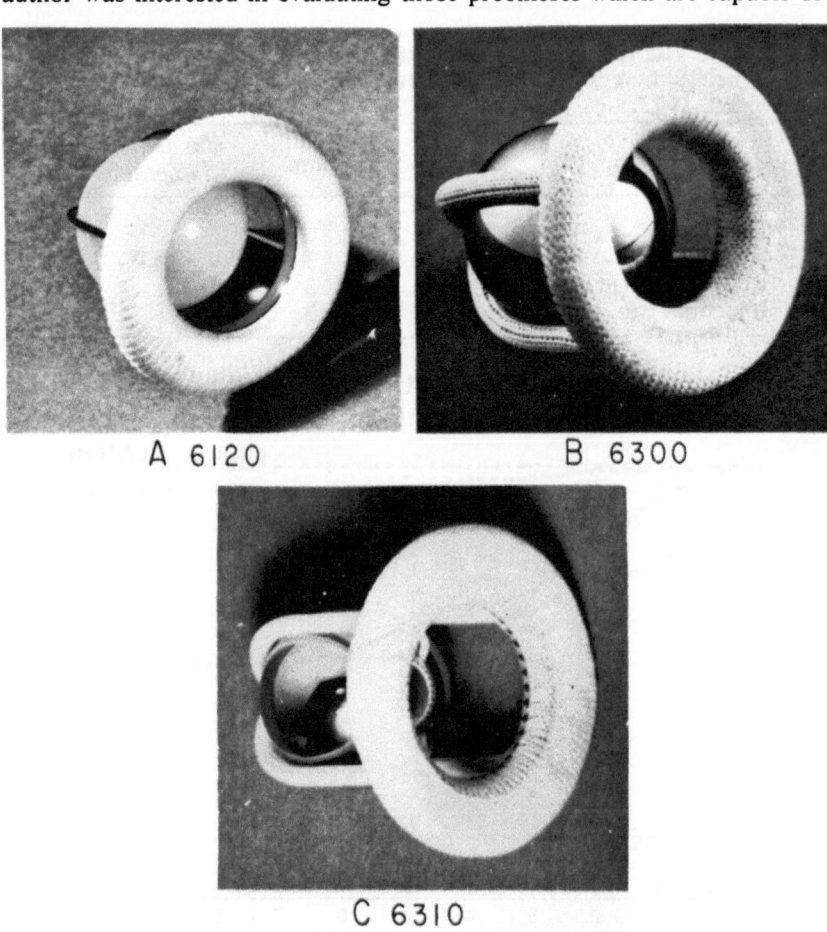

Figure 22.1 (a) Model 6120—the mitral prosthesis of the non-cloth-covered variety (b) Model 6300—cloth-covered mitral prosthesis (c) Model 6310—cloth-covered mitral prosthesis

being covered with autogenous material. In 1967, after a period in the experimental laboratory, use of a completely cloth-covered prosthesis was initiated. Then, in 1968 the author began to use the composite seat prosthesis. The results obtained with this prosthesis, the composite seat mitral valve completely cloth-covered (as of September 1973), are shown in Table 22.1

as ordinary percentages. The operative mortality, for example, throughout this period which is now in excess of five years, was 2% and the actual late mortality was 10%, i.e. a total mortality of 12% using this prosthesis. The total incidence of emboli has been 5%. There has been need for replacement in 3% of the patients, either from perivalvular leak or thrombosis

Table 22.1 The results for isolated mitral valve replacement (in percentages) using a completely cloth-covered composite seat prosthesis. September 1973.

Model 6310–6320	Early	Late	206 patients Total
Mortality	2	10	12
Emboli	2	3	5
Re-replacement	0	3	3
Infection	0	3	3

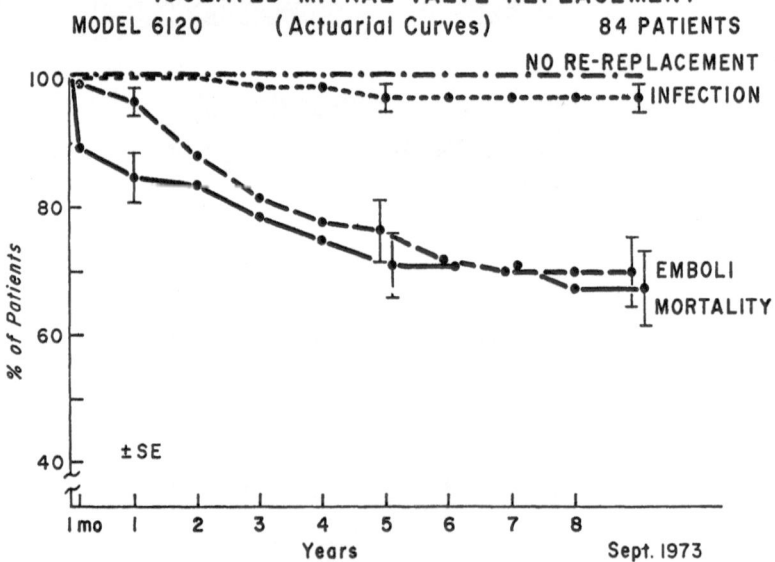

Figure 22.2 The results of mitral valve replacement (in an actuarial display) using the Model 6120 valve of the non-cloth-covered standard mitral prosthesis

of the prosthesis. Infection occurred in 3% of the patients. These figures are somewhat misleading because in actuarial display it can be seen that the chance for a patient surviving five years is 80% (Figure 22.3). The actual figures show that 88% of the patients are alive, but an actuarial display indicates not what has happened in the past but what one can expect in the future from one's past experience. This is a very good way of displaying surgical information. The chance for patients surviving five years with this prosthesis is therefore 80%. The operative mortality which of course occurs over a very short period, is almost the same on an actuarial display as it would be in actual percentage—quite small. Most important, the incidence of

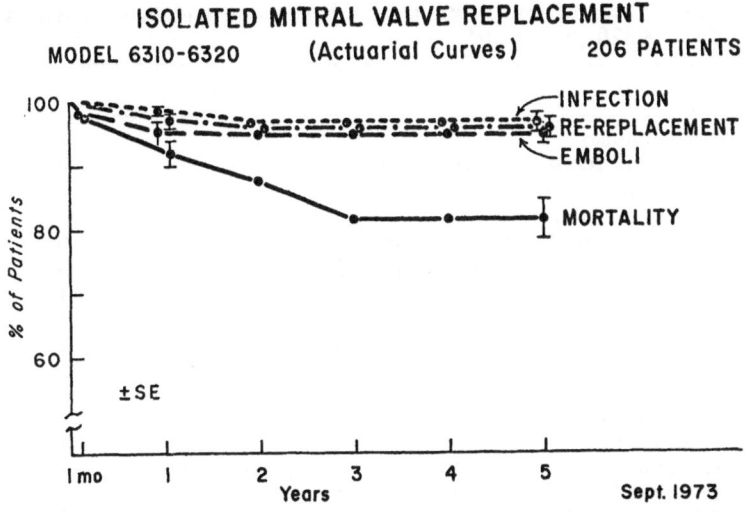

Figure 22.3 The results of mitral valve replacement (in an actuarial display) using completely cloth-covered prostheses.

emboli with a cloth-covered mitral prosthesis is enormously changed from the incidence with non-cloth-covered mitral replacement. Figure 22.3 shows that there is an early incidence during the first year and then the curve remains completely stable. Transient ischaemic attacks are virtually unknown in patients following cloth-covered mitral valve replacement so that by the end of five years, the chance for a patient to have an embolus is about 5%. All these patients had far-advanced mitral valve disease and the majority had atrial fibrillation. When patients with mitral stenosis following commissurotomy or unoperated mitral disease are followed-up, it is possible to recognise the extremely small percentage of embolic episodes which occurs with this type of prosthesis, when compared with the naturally-occurring emboli. The replacement rate is quite small—about 3% at the end of five years. The chance for infection with a cloth-covered valve is no greater than the chance for infection with a non-cloth-covered valve. However, infection can occur as late as the second or third year after implantation.

Table 22.2 shows the causes of late death in the first 150 patients with the composite seat mitral prosthesis. Most of these deaths were related to cardiac causes but only three of the deaths in this entire series were related to the prosthesis itself. Two were due to endocarditis, one occurred at five months and another at 17 months following operation. One patient died from an unrecognised massive leak which was actually a dehiscence of the suture line occurring about six weeks after operation.

Table 22.2 Causes of late death after mitral valve replacement with the Model 6310–6320 prosthesis*

Causes of Death	
1. Cardiac causes	9
(a) Deaths related to prosthesis	3
Endocarditis (5,17)	2
Leak (14)	1
(b) Deaths unrelated to prosthesis	6
Myocardial failure (4, 13, 33)	3
Coronary artery disease (26)	1
Arrhythmia (31)	1
Quinidine intoxication (11)	1
2. Non-cardiac causes	5
Intestinal obstruction (irradiation) (27)	1
Ashtma (1)	1
Chronic obstructive pulmonary emphysema (3)	1
Pyelonephritis with septicemia (34)	1
Chronic renal disease (20)	1
3. Unknown	1
Total	15 (10%)

*Figures in parentheses indicate months after operation

There were many cardiac deaths which were not related to the prosthesis. Many deaths were due to myocardial failure, coronary artery disease, arrhythmias and so on. In only one patient was there a failure to have an autopsy in this series of mitral valve replacement. Thus, this is very accurate information concerning late causes of death following mitral valve replacement with a cloth-covered mitral valve.

Prosthetic-related Complications
Haemolysis is unknown with mitral replacement in the author's series of patients. In the presence of a small leak, of course, haemolysis can occur with any valve. No patients were observed with haemolysis, nor was it necessary to reoperate or transfuse any patients with haemolytic anaemia. There was, of course, no evidence of ball wear in any of the patients; the poppet of the hollow stellite is virtually indestructible. There was evidence of cloth tear in the orifice of one patient and this has indeed been a

problem in other series, perhaps occurring more frequently than in this series.

There is no incidence of strut cloth tear on the mitral valve prosthesis as there is in the aortic position. Only one patient required reoperation (in February 1973) for thrombotic stenosis of the prosthesis but since then one

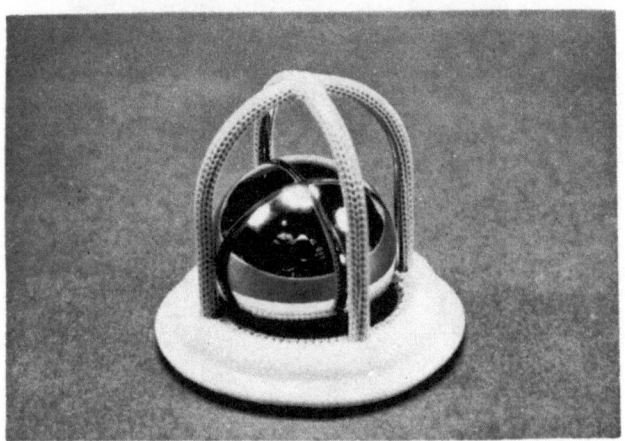

Figure 22.4 Cloth-covered mitral valve prothesis—Model 6400

or two additional patients have been seen. One patient was explored thinking there was a thrombosis in the orifice of the valve but the findings at operation showed a normal valve. It was simply a very small prosthesis and a very small ventricle.

Because of the problem of orifice cloth tear, the orifice was redesigned to increase the height of the studs and change the nature of the cloth. At the same time, an inner track on each strut was built into the prosthesis not because there was any evidence of cloth tear in the mitral position of any clinical significance, but because there was evidence, in examining prostheses at the time of late death, of some flattening of the fibres at the base of the strut suggesting that perhaps with many years or decades of use there may be wearing of the cloth in those areas. This valve has now been used for 23 months but not exclusively—only when it has been available, since it is quite a difficult prosthesis to make (Figure 22.4). The results with it are identical to the results achieved with the previous composite seat valve and both prostheses are probably, at least over the first decade, easily interchangeable in terms of results.

The problem with aortic valve replacement is that it has had a very similar evolution. Time does not permit a complete evaluation of this valve which has been in widespread use from 1961 to 1965 (Figure 22.5). Dr Björk remembers putting that prosthesis in as one of the earliest in Europe.

The current prostheses which are in use are the non-cloth-covered standard type of aortic prosthesis and the composite seat aortic prosthesis. The time span very similar to the mitral prosthesis. Model 1200-60 has been in use since 1966, and model 2310-20 since 1968 (Figure 22.6).

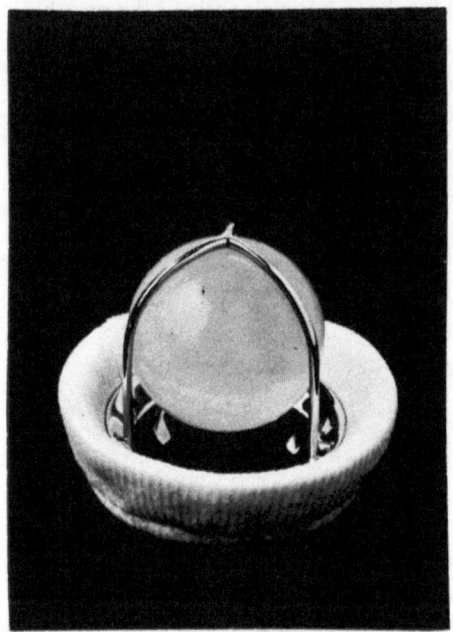

Figure 22.5 Non-cloth-covered aortic valve prosthesis—Model 1000

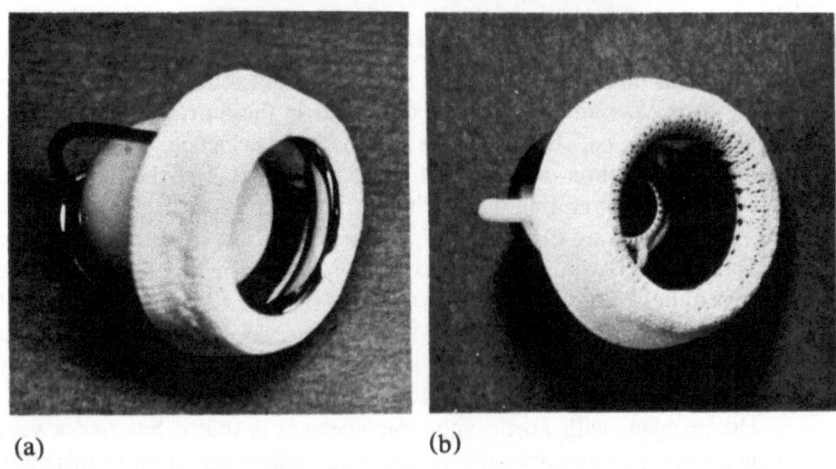

(a)   (b)

Figure 22.6 Aortic valve prostheses (a) Model 1200—non-cloth-covered valve (b) Model 2310—composite seat valve

The results obtained with these currently-used prostheses are shown in Figure 22.7. Again, the problem of infection is a small one–about a 2 or 3% chance at the end of eight years. There have been two instances of re-replacement of the Model 1200 valve, but never for valve failure and never for ball variance. Fatty infiltration of the silicone-rubber poppet in this

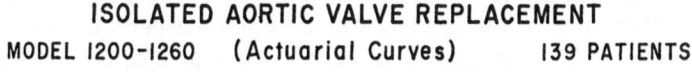

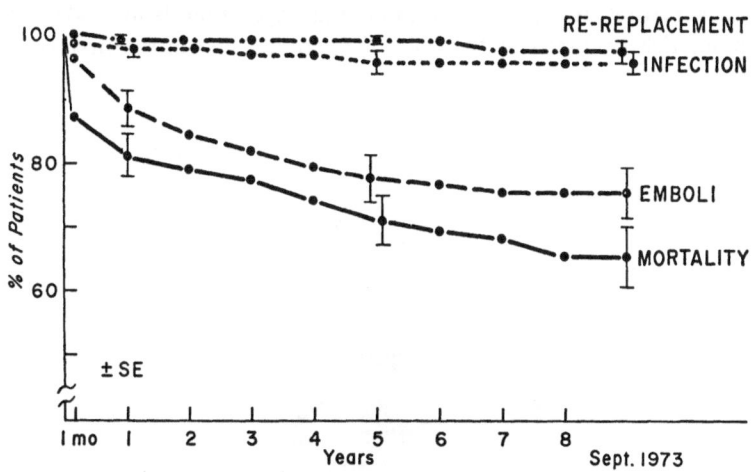

Figure 22.7 The results of aortic valve replacement (in an actuarial display) using Model 1200 —1260.

group of patients has not occurred with this design despite the fact that its use extends back to 1966. These re-replacements were performed for infection. The chance for a patient surviving to nine years after operation is 70%. However, like other non-cloth-covered prostheses, there is a continued incidence of thromboembolic problems with this prosthesis so that at the end of eight years the chance for an embolic episode is approximately 20%. Again, these episodes are primarily transient ischaemic attacks and so, despite this incidence of emboli, this valve remains in rather widespread use. It is a very reliable valve and the results with it are quite predictable. It avoids many of the problems that may be associated with cloth-covered aortic valve replacement. This is the valve that the author's Unit has used since 1968–the composite seat prosthesis. Many of the patients with this prosthesis also had coronary artery surgery, since the development of this valve occurred during the era of coronary artery surgery (Figure 22.8). Table 22.3 shows that at the time the curves were made, 49 such patients were included and the operative mortality was only 6% in this group of combined operations.

Figure 22.9 shows the results obtained thus far with the composite seat aortic prosthesis. Twenty-seven patients who had close clearance or intermediate clearance valves were excluded from consideration. These were a modified prosthesis used during a period of six months which led to a very high incidence of thrombosis with sticking of the ball in the open position. Excluding those cases, the results in 258 patients can be seen. Again, there was a low incidence of infection, despite the cloth-covered configuration. The operative mortality was about 8%, the chance for a patient surviving for six years after this operation being 80%. The maximum risk occurred at the time of operation and in the first year of

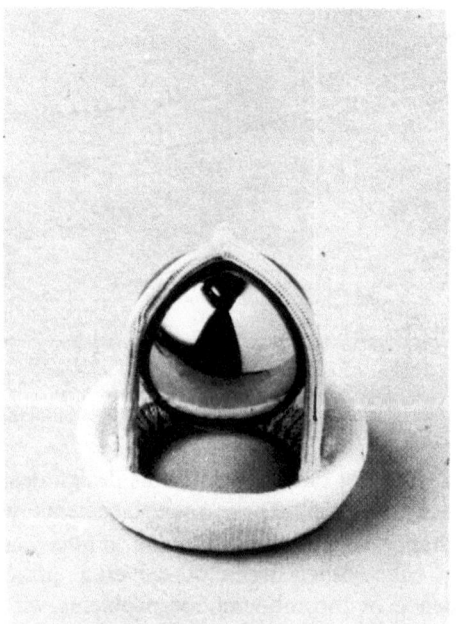

Figure 22.8 Composite seat aortic prosthesis—Model 2320

Table 22.3 The operative mortality for patients with composite seat aortic prosthesis undergoing coronary artery surgery

	No. of patients	Operative deaths
Single vein graft	32	0
Double vein graft	16	3
Triple vein graft	1	0
Total	49	3 (6%)

follow-up. Most of these were sudden deaths due to arrhythmia, or progressive congestive heart failure–both related to myocardial disease. There are two important aspects of Figure 22.7, one is that the incidence of emboli is extremely low, the chance for a patient having an embolic episode

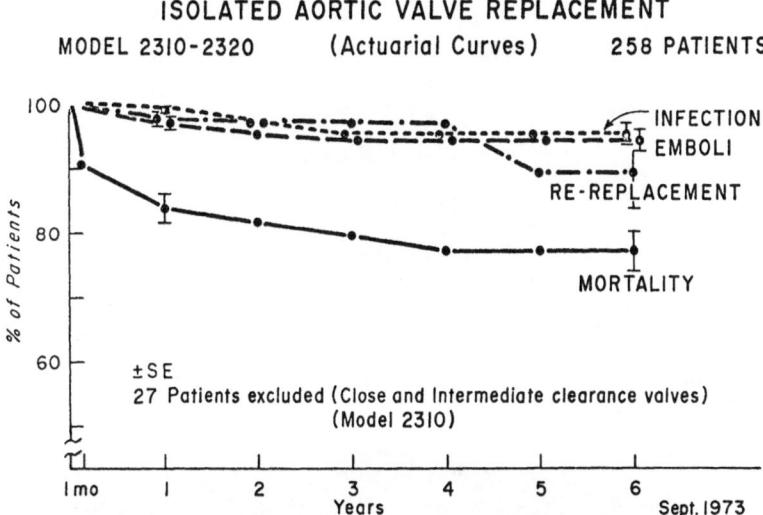

Figure 22.9 The results of aortic valve replacement (in an actuarial display) using composite seat prostheses

by the end of six years being about 4 or 5%. Notice however there is a significant re-replacement rate suddenly becoming noticeable at the 4th year after operation. Figure 22.10 explains the reason for the reoperations in the group of aortic cloth-covered prostheses. It shows an example of very extreme cloth tear of the Model 2310 valve which was covered by two layers of Teflon. Actually, with the 2320 valve covered by polypropylene, cloth tear would occur without the cloth leaving the strut. It would appear to be a denuded strut on its inner portion, but this much displacement of the cloth would not occur.

This kind of problem led to the reoperation of nine patients out of the first 350 patients operated upon with these cloth-covered composite seat aortic prostheses. Of these nine patients, seven were found at operation to have cloth tear. Gradual stenosis of the prosthesis has never been observed in either the aortic or the mitral position. One patient was operated on primarily for a gradient across the prosthesis due to thrombus material and three patients were reoperated for peribasilar leak. These actually were relatively small leaks, but they can result in haemolytic anaemia with cloth-covered prostheses. This reoperation rate then, in actual terms, was 2.6% of the cases that have been operated on, but in the actuarial display which gives a much more accurate indication of what the true risk is for a patient entering the series, the reoperation rate was about 8–10%. This, again, shows the display to guide the development of medical and surgical

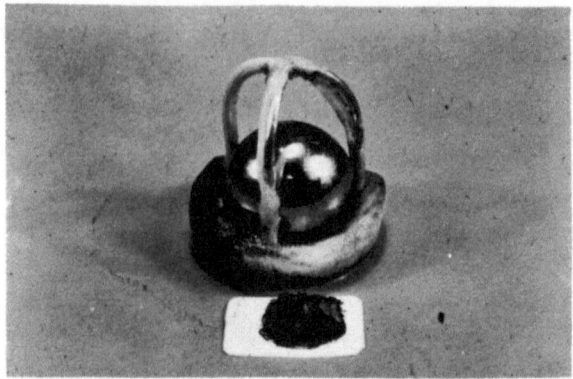

Figure 22.10 An example of very extreme cloth tear of the Model 2310 valve which was covered by two layers of Teflon

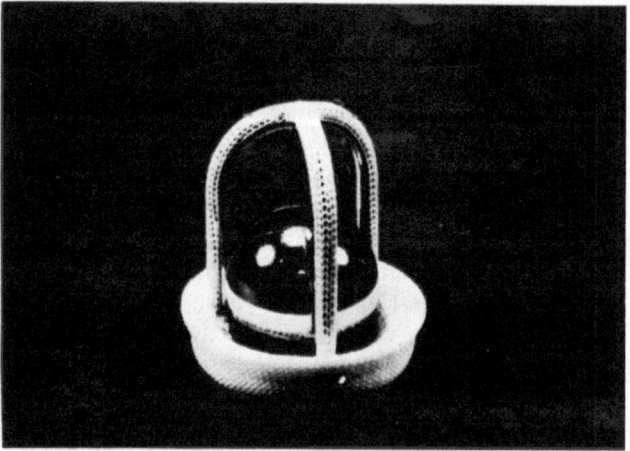

Figure 22.11 The composite seat-track valve—Model 2400

thinking rather than simple percentage expressions (Figure 22.9). It seemed logical then to make modifications of the aortic prosthesis to effect those particular problems that were observed over a significant period of time without introducing any new and unexpected problems. This was done with what is called the track valve (Figure 22.11). This valve has an inner track on the inside of each strut which makes it possible to change the configuration of the cloth on the strut from a double layer to a single layer of finer material because cloth injury is no longer feared. As a result, this valve has a much smaller diameter strut then the previous cloth-covered valves. One of the disadvantages of the cloth-covered valve compared to the non-cloth-covered valve is the thickness of this strut. The changes in the seat had been minimal in changing from the non-composite seat to the composite seat configuration.

Table 22.4 The mortality rate of patients undergoing aortic valve replacement with cloth-covered composite seat prostheses. University of Oregon medical school August 1968–January 1974

Valve Model	No. of Patients	Operative Deaths	Late Deaths
2310	121 (35%)	10 (8%)	19 (16%)
2320	172 (49%)	16 (9%)	18 (10%)
2400	57 (16%)	2 (3·5%)	3 (5%)
Total	350	28 (8%)	40 (11%)

Table 22.4 shows the mortality rate in percentages of these patients. Fifty-seven patients with the Model 2400 valve had been operated upon. Notice the very low operative mortality; this shows the effect of selecting cases on the operative mortality of aortic valve replacement since most of these patients who have the composite seat-track valves were in the younger age groups because it was in this group that the problem of cloth tear and haemolytic anaemia was feared most.

The extent of haemolysis in patients selected at random from the follow-up of all the patients was studied and thus 123 patients of these 350 patients were called in. They were randomly selected without any knowledge of the presence or absence of any complications and had haematocrit determinations (Table 22.5). The haematocrits were only

Table 22.5 Randomly selected patients for haemolysis study

	2310	2320	2400
Hct.	43 ±0.8	41 ±0.7	42 ±0.8
Retic. count	1.6 ± 0.2	1.7±0.2	1.4±0.2
LDH	745* ±70	844* ±62	485* ±40
No. pts. $\frac{123}{350}$ Total	$\frac{45}{121}$ (37%)	$\frac{55}{172}$ (32%)	$\frac{23}{57}$ (40%)

*$p<0.01$
All data ± ISE

slightly decreased from normal and the reticulocyte count slightly increased. The LDH levels which indicate intravascular haemolysis were greatly elevated in all three groups of patients. The maximum in the author's laboratory is 200. So there were fourfold increases in serum LDH associated with the 2310 and the 2320 prostheses. However, with the track

Table 22.6 The difference in the incidence of embolism, measured in episodes per 1000 months of follow-up

Anticoagulant Status	Valve model	Emboli 1000 months	Total 1000 months
Yes	2310 2320 2400	0 0 0	0
No	2310 2320 2400	2.1 5.6 0	4.5
Discont.	2310 2320 2400	14.8 54.1 0	18.7

valve, the LDH level was elevated only twice above normal. It could be said then that all these patients have a haemolytic state which is almost always compensated. It could also be said that the amount of haemolysis seems to be significantly less with the Model 2400 valve. In further analysing this data, the reason for this must be that there are many patients in this asymptomatic group with elevated LDHs who have cloth injury as a cause for their elevated serum LDH. When a difference in the thromboembolic potential of these various composite seat aortic prostheses, the 2310, 2320 and 2400 is looked for, no statistical difference is found unless the patients are arranged according to the anticoagulant programme that they have been receiving. Thus, the patients can be divided into three groups; those that have been receiving Warfarin or Coumarin, those receiving no Coumarin and those in whom Coumarin was discontinued. The difference in the incidence of embolism is measured in episodes per 1000 months of follow-up and is striking and statistically significant in these three groups of patients. Thus, 0.0 episodes in patients who are receiving anticoagulants, 4.5 episodes in those that have never received anticoagulants and an extremely high incidence of embolism in those patients in whom anticoagulants were discontinued (Table 22.6). The model 2400 valve has had no embolic episodes thus far, which again shows how difficult it is to evaluate the thromboembolic potential of a prosthesis, whose follow-up is relatively short—in this case almost 23 or 24 months. The timing of these embolic episodes is of some interest (Figure 22.12). Of these 18 episodes in 350 patients, the distribution between the first, second and third postoperative years can be seen. During the first year after operation no patient had an embolic episode who was receiving anticoagulants. During the second year, there were three episodes and one patient was receiving

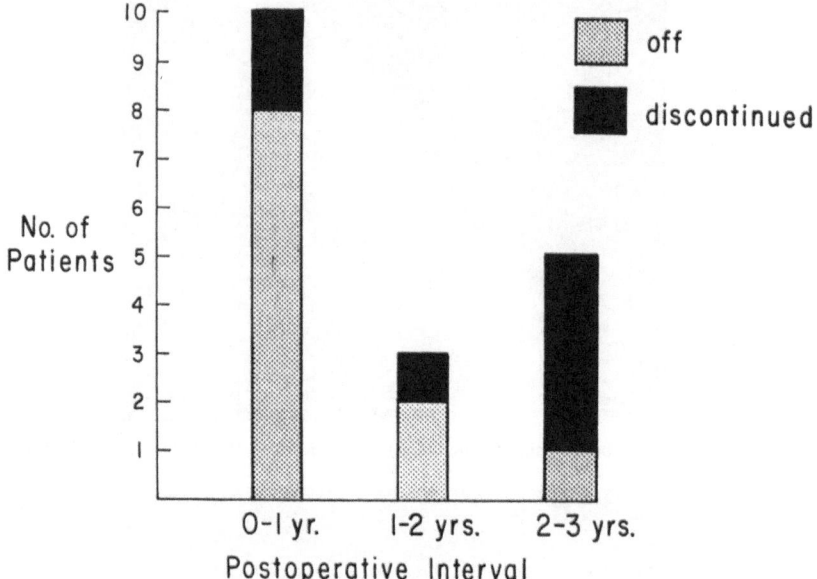

Figure 22.12 The timing of postoperative emboli

antiplatelets. The other two were in different categories; one had had anticoagulants discontinued and the other had never been placed on anticoagulants. Notice that by the third year most of the embolic episodes are in patients in whom anticoagulants were discontinued. The embolic threat tapers off with increased follow-up and then these patients emerge as the dominant factor producing the thromboembolic complications.

Cloth-covered prostheses provide a method of allowing autogenous material to cling to the surface producing a relatively non-thrombogenic surface. It is possible that in the future this may be achieved with materials other than cloth. For example; metallic beads can be plastered onto the surface of a prosthesis. Figure 22.13 shows a very high magnification of such beads. There has been a very extensive animal implantation programme of such valves. This has shown how a metallic surface can become completely covered by autogenous and non-thrombogenic material. As a result one can then design ball-valve-type prostheses containing these metallic spheres to reproduce the cloth surface, at the same time as retaining a track and a metallic seat for seating a silicone rubber poppet. In this kind of configuration this would be a safe poppet to use since this valve is identical to the Model 1200 valve, the prosthesis in which fatty infiltration of the silicone rubber poppet has never been seen.

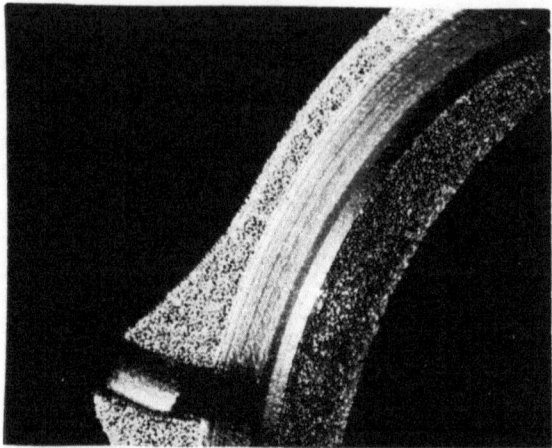

Figure 22.13 Metallic beads (highly magnified) plastered onto the surface of a prosthesis

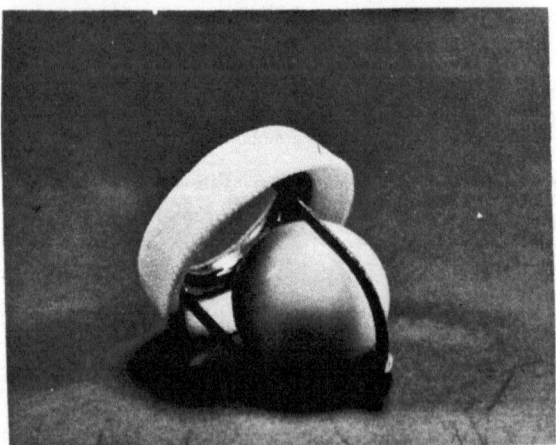

Figure 22.14 Model 1200, showing a metallic surface around most of the strut leaving a smooth inner track for the surface of the ball to impinge upon

Figure 22.14 shows another view of that prosthesis, showing the metallic surface around most of the strut leaving an inner track smooth for the surface of the ball to impinge upon. This type of valve can be made into a disc valve as well. With this kind of orifice, metallic beaded, the beads can be carried down part way, or they can be carried all the way across the struts. These prostheses have provided long-term survival in animals beyond one year and are very promising for some clinical investigation during the next year or two.

Therefore, in summary, there is a rapidly changing field in valve replacement. Yet, at the same time, there is considerable information upon which to base clinical judgement with regard to the selection of patients for valve replacement. In the author's group, the mitral problem has been relatively well-solved. A prosthesis is available that is used almost uniformly. This provides a very low incidence of thromboembolic complications in anticoagulated patients and a very respectable late death rate, with 80% of the patients alive six years after operation. This figure is in fact 88%, but actuarially projected is 80%. With aortic valve replacement, the problem is greater because the problem of haemolysis and cloth tear is encountered, yet the overall results of aortic valve replacement with these cloth-covered prostheses are very attractive. With the development of the track on the inside of each strut, it is very likely that the major problem with those prostheses, namely haemolysis due to cloth injury on the strut, has been solved. This is not just projection, because this prosthesis has actually been used in the author's unit for almost two years and other centres are beginning to use it in increasing numbers.

These prostheses are still relatively bulky, and the use of cloth in the future may not be the most sophisticated and the most ideal method of obtaining a healed surface. For this reason further explorations in animal laboratories are necessary. For the present, however, in ordinary clinical practice, the cloth-covered prostheses are used with the knowledge that they are still in an evolutionary phase, and the non-cloth-covered valves are used to a very wide extent in many clinics because much is known about them and they have their attractions.

23

Five years experience with the Björk–Shiley disc valve in aortic, mitral and tricuspid valvular disease

V. Björk

The Björk–Shiley tilting disc valve has a freely rotating pyrolytic carbon disc in a Stellite ring with a Teflon sewing ring. The disc which tilts to open to 60 degrees permits a central and nearly laminar flow. The disc is thus washed on both sides. The disc will also rotate which results in an even distribution of the wear. One of the most important features of this construction is that the disc is not overlapping but fits within the ring of the prosthesis. This design feature, eliminating the overlap, means that a round 2 mm valve orifice diameter is gained for a given tissue diameter. There is no other valve available today which has such a big blood path for the same outside diameter. This is most important, especially in narrow aortic roots. The other advantage of the fact that the disc is not overlapping is the low haemolysis rate. As the disc does not hit the ring on closure there is less crushing of red blood corpuscles and there is only about half the amount of haemolysis as compared with a valve with an overlapping disc (e.g. Lillehei-Kaster valve). Radio-opaque markers have been mounted into a Delrin disc to prove and demonstrate the rotation of the disc. From January 16th 1969 to the present date, over a period of more than five years, 757 Björk–Shiley tilting disc valves have been inserted at the Thoracic Surgical Clinic of Karolinska Hospital. Of these 470 were introduced into the aortic area, 245 in the mitral area and 42 in the tricuspid area. There are five important criteria regarding an artificial heart valve which must be studied carefully:

1. Durability
2. Haemolysis
3. The gradient during forward flow
4. Regurgitation
5. Thromboresistance

All these five factors will be evaluated in terms of the Björk–Shiley tilting disc valve.

DURABILITY

The valve has been tested in an accelerated life tester at a speed of 1000 cycles/min with an average diastolic pressure of 90 ± 10 mmHg. After 1020 million cycles which is equivalent to 27 years of cycling at 72 beats/min, there is still no visible wear of the pyrolytic carbon disc. The contacting surface of the disc was merely polished in some areas and the surface wear on the pyrolite disc is so slight and evenly distributed that the depth is inmeasurable without a profilometer and was found to be less than 0·025 mm.

The wear on the orifice ring is comprised of slight polished flats on the disc contacting areas of the lower leg and hook. The maximum depth of this wear of the lower leg is 0·025 mm. The projected wear life is calculated to be 794 years assuming a constant wear rate. An excellent disc rotation and uniform wear were indicated by lack of static wear patterns. Edge chipping to a depth of 0·1 mm was caused by excessive pressure due to tester failure, but this chipped area did not increase during a continued observation period which was equivalent to another six years cycling at 72 beats/min.

During a period of more than five years of clinical experience with the Björk–Shiley tilting disc valve, not one single case of mechanical failure has been encountered.

HAEMOLYSIS

In order to obtain the least amount of mechanical trauma of the blood corpuscles, the Björk-Shiley tilting disc valve is so constructed that the disc is not overlapping and does not hit the valve ring during the cycling. The resulting haemolysis is low in the test chamber with a physiological valve function in a minimal volume of human blood, 70 ml. This non-overlapping principle was compared to the overlapping disc of the Lillehei–Kaster valve and only found to have about half the rate of haemolysis. In other words, 0·24% of the red cells were destroyed per hour compared to 0·50% in the Lillehei–Kaster valve with an overlapping disc. This erythrocyte destruction can be converted to *in vivo* conditions. In a postoperative patient with a blood volume of 4800 ml, 0·08% of the red cell volume will be destroyed in 24 h by the non-overlapping disc of the Björk–Shiley valve and 0·18% by the overlapping closing mechanism of the Lillehei–Kaster valve. In a single valve replacement, the normal erythrocyte production rate of the bone marrow will have to increase by 10% and 22% each day, respectively, in order to prevent the development of anaemia. In multiple valve replacements the stress on the bone marrow will increase further and more markedly as a result of the mechanical crushing produced by an overlapping occluder.

Paraprosthetic leaks have long been recognised as a cause of haemolytic anaemia and the author has studied intravascular haemolysis due to a paravalvular leakage in 102 patients. These patients were examined by means of postoperative thoracic aortography and arranged in four groups according to the degree of regurgitation from the aorta to the left ventricle. Quantitive estimates of the red cell destruction were made by studying the serum lactic dehydrogenase activity and the serum hapto-

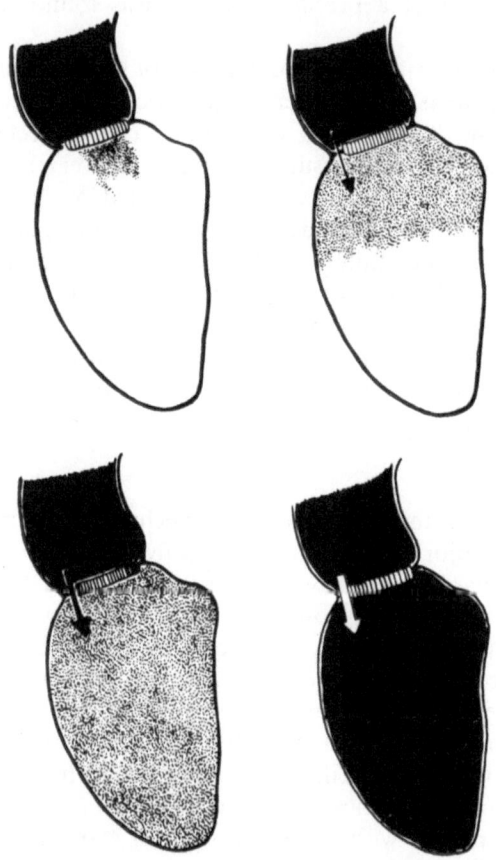

Figure 23.1 The results of aortography showing four grades of perivascular leakage

globin concentration. Serum lactic dehydrogenase was nearly normal (275 ± 42 units/l) in the patient group with grade I regurgitation i.e. an excellent local result after valve replacement. The upper normal range of LDH was 270 units/l which indicated that almost 50'₀ of these patients had normal enzyme activities. The LDH increased when paraprosthetic leakage was present. Figure 23.1 illustrates the anatomical result of aortography in the four groups: in group I there was subvalvular leakage, in group II half the ventricle was visualised by contrast, in group III the whole ventricle was visualised by contrast but the density was less than in the aorta and in group IV there was the same density of contrast in the aorta and the left ventricle. Figure 23.2 shows how the LDH activity and the haptoglobin were related to the grade of aortic regurgitation after

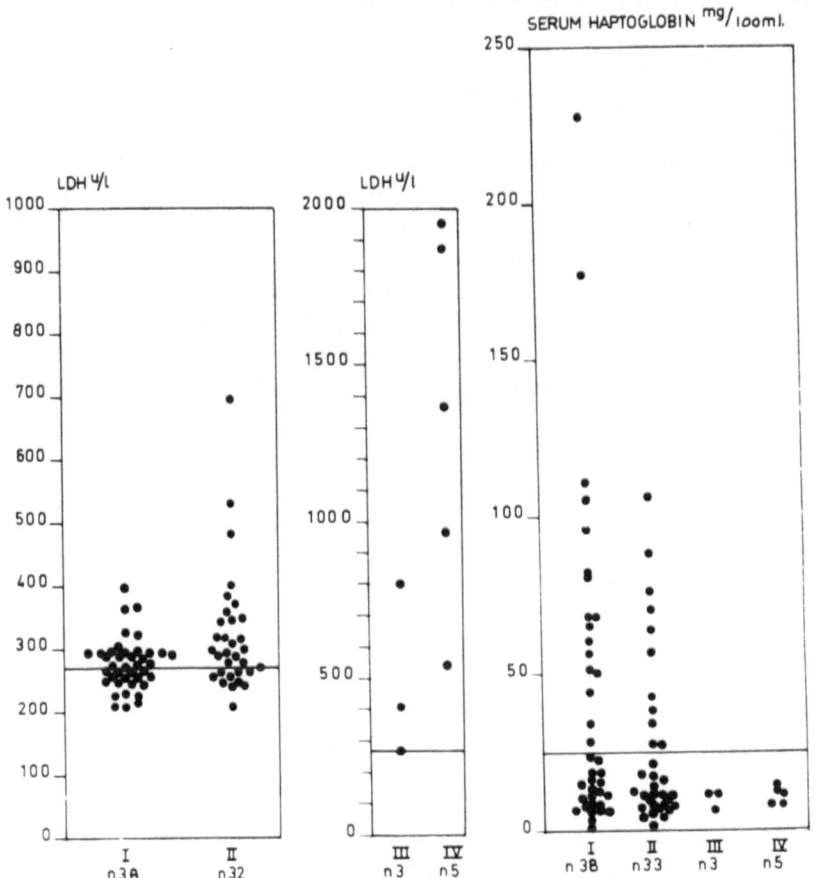

Figure 23.2 Left-hand two columns compare the LDH activity in groups I & II, and III & IV. Note that the vertical scale is compressed in groups III & IV. In the right-hand column, the serum haptoglobin concentration is compared in the four groups

surgery. Group I exhibit normal LDH activity and in group II LDH activity is high in a few valves. In group III and group IV all valves exhibit very high LDH activity. On the other hand the serum haptoglobin is more within normal limits in group I and II, but significantly below the value for normal valves in group III and IV. This very small amount of red blood cell trauma is in all probability related to the non-overlapping closing mechanism of the Björk–Shiley tilting disc valve, which minimises mechanical crushing of the cells.

THE GRADIENT ACROSS THE VALVE

Enlarging the angle of the tilting disc from 50–60 degrees in the mitral valve results in only a marginal decrease in the pressure difference across the valve in a 25 mm prosthesis in flows up to 16 l/min. Increasing the angle above 60 degrees will not diminish the gradient of the prosthesis; it will only delay the closure of the disc with increasing insufficiency during closing. As the pressure fall or gradient varies directly with the square of the flow and inversely with the fourth power of the radius of the valve orifice, it is important that the prosthesis has the greatest possible orifice:tissue diameter ratio to provide optimal conditions of the low resistance to forward flow. The *in vivo* rheology of the Björk–Shiley aortic prosthesis has been determined by heart catheterisation including trans-

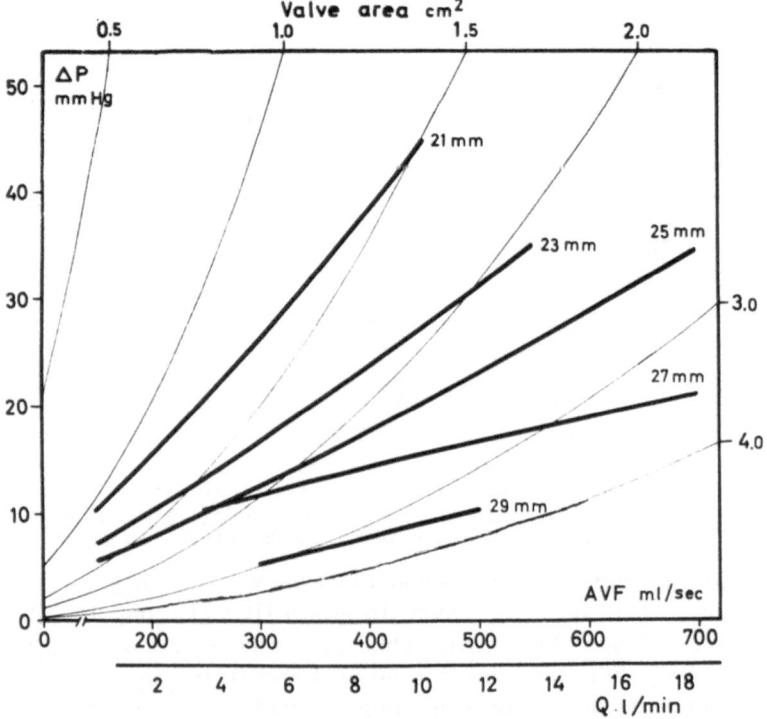

Figure 23.3 Shows the flow/pressure relationships of Björk-Shiley valves between 21 and 29 mm in diameter

septal approach of the left heart at rest and during exercise in 100 patients. The mean prosthetic pressure differences were obtained by planimetry on the pressure tracings and related to aortic valve flow and cardiac output up to 16 l/min for the different valve sizes. The *in vivo* flow driving pressure fall relationship for the Björk–Shiley aortic prosthesis was almost linear with a pressure difference at rest of less than 10 mmHg for the 25, 27 and 29 mm valves and about 12 mmHg for the 23 mm valve, and a gradient of 20 mmHg for the 21 mm valve (Figure 23.3). With increasing flow during exercise, the pressure fall increased almost linearly

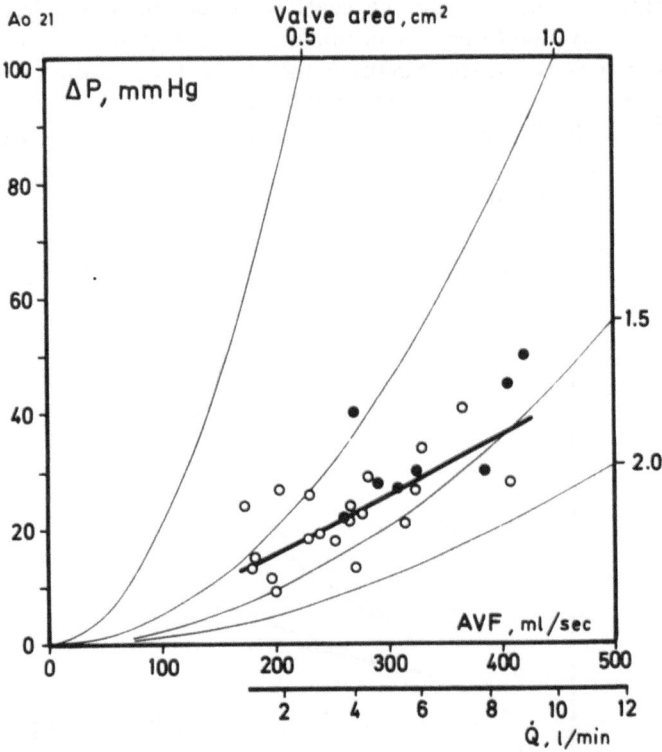

Figure 23.4 The relationship between the mean pressure difference across a 21 mm valve and the mean aortic valve flow

and the slope of the line became steepest for the 21 mm valve. Figure 23.4 shows the relationship between the mean pressure difference across a 21 mm Björk–Shiley aortic prosthesis and a mean aortic valve flow in ml s^{-1} of the cardiac output. This value for the 21 mm Björk–Shiley can be compared with a No. 8 A Starr valve, which gives about double the gradient from 40–70 mmHg in narrow aortic roots.

REGURGITATION

All cardiac prosthesis valves have some regurgitation at the moment of valve closure. The mass and shape of the occluder and the design of the closing mechanism as well as the driving pressure at the beginning of diastole, are major determinants of this regurgitation. The Björk–Shiley valve is still slightly regurgitant after valve closure due to its non-overlapping tilting disc. There have been some discussions about the magnitude of this regurgitation and some doctors have measured the regurgitation on a fibrillating heart with suction in the left ventricle, where falsely high values can be obtained. The magnitude of regurgitation through the circular space between the seated disc and the valve ring was evaluated in an experiment which utilised human whole blood, prostheses of 21, 23, 25, 27, and 29 mm in diameter and a pyrolytic carbon disc.

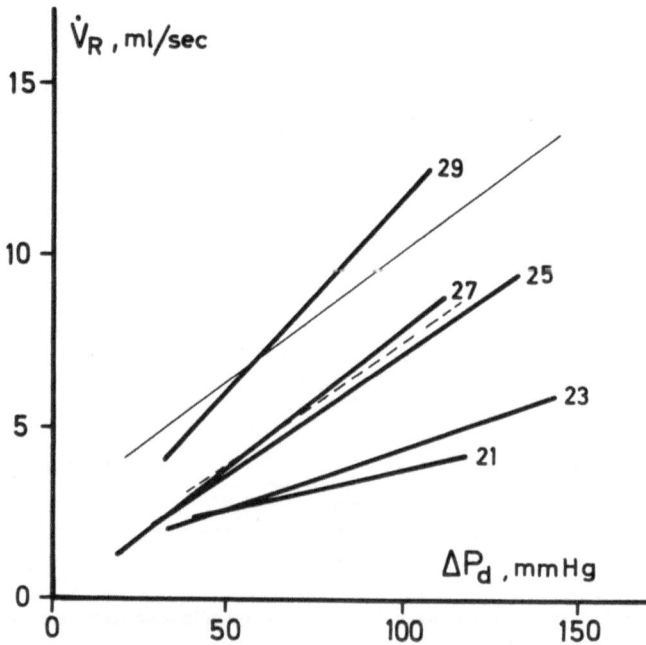

Figure 23.5 The relationship between regurgitation and diastolic pressure difference, showing the correlation with valve diameter

It was found that the regurgitation after valve closure increased linearly with the diastolic pressure difference (Figure 23.5). The slope of this line became steeper with increasing valve size. The relative magnitude of this regurgitation can be calculated by applying the average stroke volume of 80 ml and a heart rate of 78 beats/min and a mean diastolic pressure of 67 mmHg at rest, observed in the postoperative patient after prosthetic valve replacements. For patients with 21 and 23 mm valves it would be 2% of the forward stroke volume, for patients with 25 and 27 mm valves the corresponding percentages would be 3% and for the 29 mm valve 5% of the stroke volume. Regurgitation would diminish with the haemodynamic changes during exercise. This physiological regurgitation is minimal and appears at thoracic aortography as a sub-valvular reflux of contrast medium, which is defined as a grade I aortic regurgitation.

THROMBOEMBOLISM

Although adequate anticoagulant treatment in the form of Dicumarol has been very effective in preventing thromboembolism, it has been in itself a source of significant mortality. The author has encountered six deaths following massive intracerebral haemorrhage in the whole series of patients treated with Dicumarol. This is equivalent to a mortality of nearly 3%. Therefore, in the first of 117 patients with a Delrin disc on Dicumarol and a mean follow-up of 24 months, there was not one single thrombo-embolic episode, but when in 32 cases Dicumarol was withdrawn, there were five thromboembolic episodes during a 12 month follow-up. A pyrolytic carbon disc was then used in 27 patients without anticoagulant treatment on half a year follow-up and here there were two cases of thromboembolic episodes, including one case of encapsulation. Following this, in a series of 30 cases with the pyrolytic carbon disc and a 12 month follow-up with Dicumarol treatment, there was only one case of thrombo-embolic episode. In this case anticoagulants proved to be ineffective with a thrombotest of 38% (therapeutic range 6–15%). At the present time the author has a series of 30 cases with pyrolytic carbon disc having 100 mg of Persantin/day and 1 g of aspirin, after initial heparin treatment, for a week. *

The greatest number of thromboembolic episodes was found in the group where Dicumarol was withdrawn. Furthermore, the best result was obtained with an adequate Dicumarol treatment, which, however, carried a certain mortality as high as 3%. Thromboembolism has accounted for a total mortality of 1–2% of 160 patients. A successful emergency thrombectomy has been performed in a patient with encapsulation of the valve who did not have anticoagulant treatment. This patient died 20 months later because of recurrent valve thrombosis despite Dicumarol medication, which however, was found to be ineffective.

*This treatment was ineffective and abandoned in favour of Wafarin treatment

Another case of fatal thrombotic encapsulation was encountered in a patient receiving Persantin–aspirin. This patient had suffered from infection, probably endocarditis, one month prior to death.

OPERATION

The valve is sutured in place with 30 isolated sutures of Thycron on the beating heart at 30 °C utilising both right and left coronary artery perfusion during the procedure.

Results of the operation

Single aortic valve replacement was performed in 161 cases which were then followed-up for 2–5 years. The hospital mortality in this group was 5% and total accumulated mortality up to five years was 14%. The group consisted of 65 cases of aortic stenosis, 48 cases of combined aortic stenosis with insufficiency and 48 cases of pure insufficiency. The mean follow-up was 30 months. The causes of late death were: thromboembolism in one case, cerebral haemorrhage in four cases, myocardial in five cases, malignancy in three cases, and infection in two cases. The clinical improvement included elimination of syncope, relief of angina pectoris and reduction of dyspnoea. The absence of such improvement was due either to significant coronary artery disease seen in two patients or to paraprosthetic leakage seen in five patients. The operative closure of these paraprosthetic leakages involved no mortality. The postoperative relief of disability correlated with the highly significant increase in working capacity and reduction in cariomegaly, as well as the haemodynamic improvement.

The haemodynamic investigation was carried out in four different groups of patients. There were 22 cases of the pure aortic insufficiency, 37 of pure aortic stenosis and 19 cases had narrow aortic roots, where only a 21 mm prosthesis could be placed. In 12 cases the age was more than 60 years.

In the group with aortic incompetence there was a high incidence of heart decompensation before operation. This was indicated by large blood volumes and markedly elevated left atrial and right heart pressures. The main response to aortic valve replacement was an increase in effective stroke volume and a shift to a more normokinetic circulation, both at rest and during exercise. The large preoperative blood volumes as well as the pressure elevations in the left atrium and right heart were on an average normalised, indicating that the cardial decompensation was eliminated. Markedly elevated left ventricular end-diastolic pressures returned to almost normal levels after surgery. The patients with acute aortic insufficiency due to septic endocarditis and with a rupture of a valve, in whom myocardial impairment had not advanced to an irreversible state, demonstrated the most pronounced haemodynamic improvement.

The volume load of the left ventricle was thus eliminated by aortic valve replacement in patients with aortic incompetence. In the group with aortic stenosis the pressure load of the left ventricle was eliminated following valve replacement. The left ventricular systolic pressure and stroke work as well as the left ventricular end-diastolic pressure and diastolic work of filling was markedly decreased. Stroke volume and kinetics of central circulation remained unchanged. Heart incompensation was uncommon in this group before operation. In patients with narrow aortic roots the haemodynamic response was similar to that of the group with aortic stenosis.

A comparison of patients over and under the age of 60 years, all with aortic stenosis, showed that the left ventricular end-diastolic and systolic pressure as well as the systolic stroke work diminished to the same extent at rest and during exercise in both groups as a response to aortic valve replacement. Stroke volume or stroke index were significantly lower in the older age group as was the change in stroke volume per change in left ventricular end-diastolic pressure on transition from rest to exercise. There was an almost fourfold increase after surgery in the younger group, but it remained mainly unchanged in the patients over 60 years. The myocardium in the over 60-year-old group lost some of its resiliency and ability to recover from prolonged overwork but aortic replacement brought about an unloading of the left ventricle and a haemodynamic improvement, which is comparable to that in younger age groups. The pulmonary hypertension was mainly normalised after operation. In all four groups this resulted from simultaneous decreases in pulmonary vascular resistance and left ventricular end-diastolic pressure.

At present 65 consecutive long-term surviving patients have been re-examined twice after periods of eight and 25 months after surgery. The initial decrease in heart volume and improvement in physical working capacity were maintained, while haemolysis showed a slight but probably significant decrease with the passage of time. There was an adequate prosthetic function in all patients. Fourteen of these patients have now been followed up for the third time after five years after the valve replacement. The clinical improvement has been maintained and no thromboembolic episode has occurred in this group, receiving continuous Dicumarol treatment.

A careful analysis has shown the response to aortic valve replacement in the different groups with pure aortic insufficiency, pure aortic stenosis, narrow aortic roots and patients above and below the age of 60 (Figure

23.6). A group of normal young individuals has been compared with a group of normal old people between the age of 60–80 years in respect to the relation between left ventricular end-diastolic pressure or pulmonary capillary pressure and the stroke volume at rest and during exercise. The more horizontal is the line beetween the resting and exercise values, the more insufficient is the myocardium. Figure 23.6 also shows the response in cases with pure aortic insufficiency, pure aortic stenosis and very narrow aortic roots. In these cases the line becomes more like the one obtained from old normal individuals. In cases with aortic insufficiency the stroke volume is increased both at rest and during exercise as a result of aortic valve replacement, which is not the case in patients with pure aortic stenosis. The end-diastolic pressure diminishes both at rest

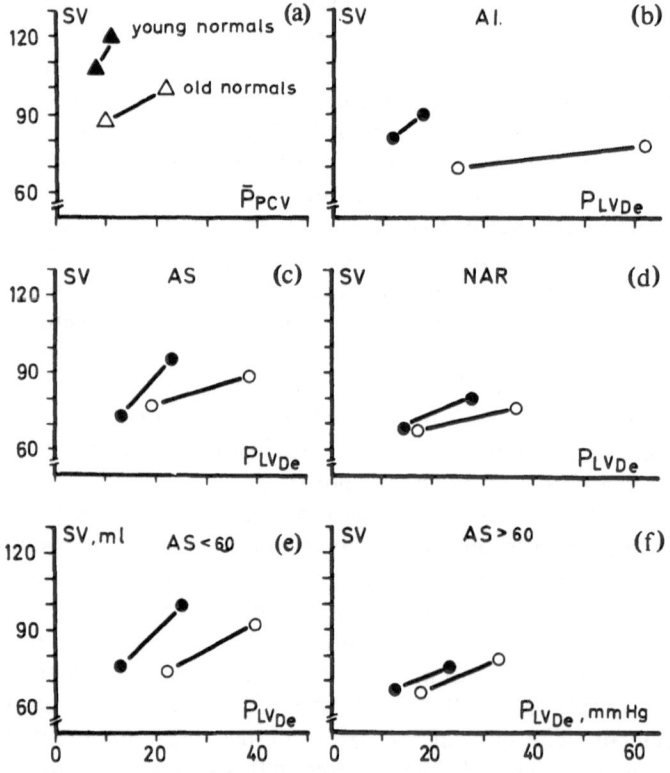

Figure 23.6 The relationship between the left ventricular end-diastolic pressure or pulmonary capillary pressure with the stroke volume at rest and during exercise in (a) old and young normals, (b) aortic insufficiency, (c) aortic stenosis, (d) narrow aortic rest, (e) and (f) aortic stenosis with a gradiant less than and more than 60 years of age respectively.

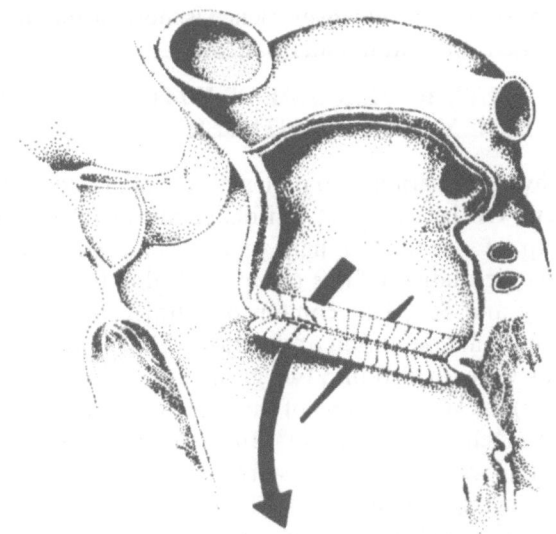

23.7

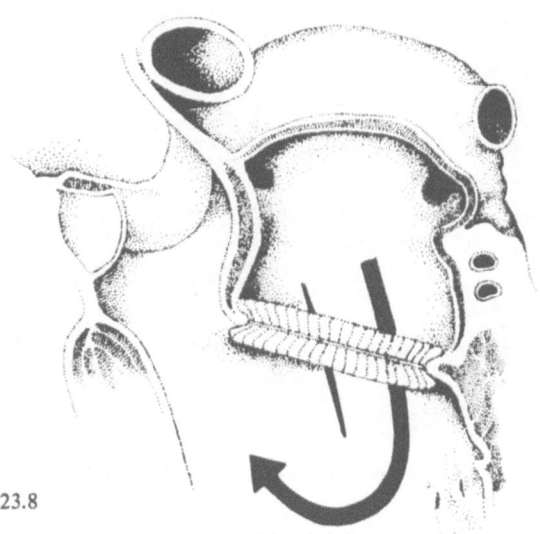

23.8

Figures 23.7 and **23.8** Show the position of the valve in 44 cases and 31 cases respectively

and during exercise in all groups of patients. It is also seen that myocardial hypertrophy or myocardial insufficiency is more pronounced in cases with narrow aortic roots and in older patients.

MITRAL VALVE REPLACEMENT WITH THE BJÖRK–SHILEY TILTING DISC VALVE PROSTHESIS

During a five year period, 250 patients were operated on for mitral valve replacement. Of these the first 75 isolated mitral valve replacements with a follow-up of one and a half years were chosen for postoperative haemodynamic studies. Of this group 7% had mitral stenosis, 35% mitral insufficiency and 58% had combined mitral valve lesions. In order to study the optimal orientation of the Björk–Shiley mitral valve prosthesis, the patients were divided into two groups. In the first group of 44 cases, (Figure 23.7) the large opening of the valve was orientated anteriorly and the disc of Delrin opened 50°. In the second group of 31 cases the larger opening was orientated posteriorly and the disc of pyrolytic carbon opened 60 degrees (Figure 23.8). The two groups of patients were comparable when judged from the preoperative clinical data regarding age, presence of fibrillation, heart size and maximum working capacity before operation. The haemodynamic examination before operation also showed that the two groups were comparable. The arterial venous oxygen

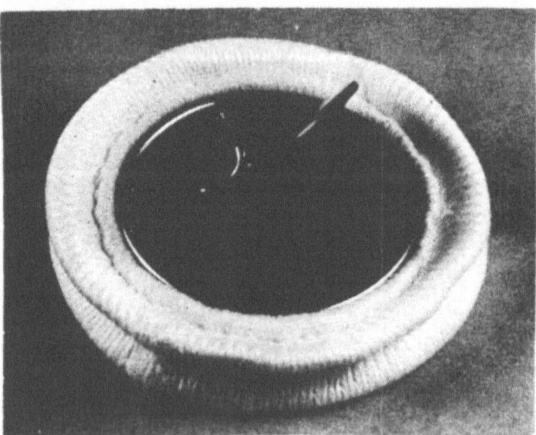

Figure 23.9 The valve in the open position showing the pyrolysed carbon disc and supporting structure

difference both at rest and during exercise was the same in the two groups, as was the cardiac output, stroke volume and pulmonary vascular resistance. Also the left ventricular end-diastolic pressure, the V wave and the mean left atrial and mean pulmonary artery pressure were similar both at rest and during exercise in the two groups. The differences found postoperatively were therefore due to the difference in technique used. Figure 23.9 shows that the mitral valve prosthesis is identical with the aortic valve prosthesis with a freely rotating pyrolytic carbon disc. The only difference is that the Teflon sewing ring has two flanges to allow a variation in suturing technique i.e. supra, infra or intraannular fixation (Figure 23.10). Buffering the sutures over both flanges is of advantage in friable or calcific valve bases to prevent cutting through or embolisation of calcific particles from the bases of the mitral leaflets.

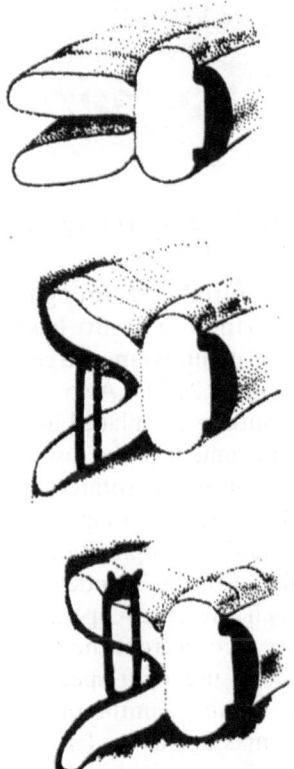

Figure 23.10 Compares infra—and supra—annular fixation of the Teflon sewing ring for mitral valves.

Mitral valve replacement is performed through a median sternotomy with the heart beating and with venting of the left ventricle. The aorta is crossclamped for only a few minutes when the atrium is opened and the valve evaluated and excised. On a flaccid heart in anoxic arrest it is tempting to choose a valve which is too large. Therefore, after the excision of the mitral valve the aortic clamp is released and the obturator used for measuring should now pass easily down into the left ventricle of the beating heart. This avoids using a prosthesis which is too big. For fixation, the author prefers a subannular fixation of the prosthesis with 20 isolated mattress sutures. The valve is positioned in the valve holder and rotated about 10 times to ascertain free rotation within the sewing ring. The

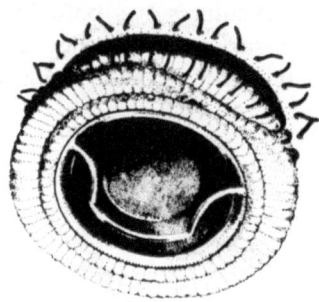

Figure 23.11 Shows the method of introducing mattress sutures through the lower portion of the sewing ring into the mitral valve ring

mattress sutures are then introduced through the lower portion of the sewing ring, passed through the mitral valve base from the ventricular side, starting in the antero-lateral commissure and continuing along the anterior rim of the mitral valve (Figure 23.11). Also starting in the antero-lateral commissure all posterior sutures are placed in a similar fusion. When the valve is in position, free movement of the disc is checked and if necessary the valve holder is reintroduced to rotate the valve within the sewing ring to a more favourable position. Air embolism remains a problem and great care is taken to avoid this complication.

The patient is then placed in the Trendelenburg position and a Foley catheter is passed through the small opening of the valve to keep it incompetent. Continuous suction from the ascending aorta to the heart–lung machine is applied by use of a special needle connected to the coronary sucker. There is also continuous suction through the left ventricular vent. Manual massage of the left ventricle and the left atrium with its appendix which is invaginated is performed. The lungs are inflated with free bleeding from the remaining portion of the left atrial incision before removal of the Foley catheter. These steps are routine and are taken to avoid air embolism before going off bypass.

RESULTS

There was no difference in the early mortality in the two groups but late mortality was higher in the first group than in the second. Thromboembolism was also higher in spite of the fact that adequate anticoagulation was higher in the first group than in the second group. In the second group there was an incidence of 7% thromboembolism, corresponding to two patients with transient signs of embolism who both recovered without sequelae. All instances of thromboembolism occurred within the first year following operation and those patients with thromboembolic episodes and a known thrombotest index at the time of the episode, were all above the therapeutic level. The subjective improvement was the same in both groups.

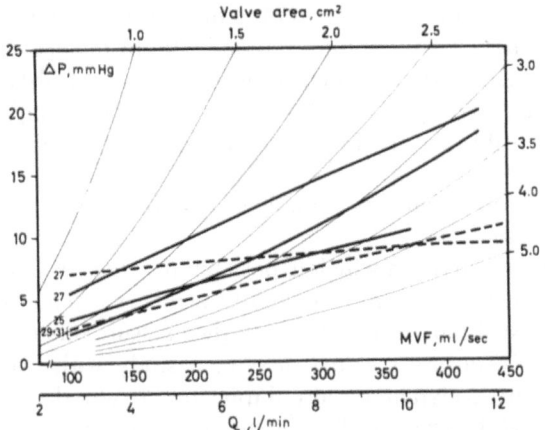

Figure 23.12 Compares the driving pressure across the mitral valve *in vivo* in ml/sec

COMPLICATIONS

Haemolytic anaemia did not occur in any patient and lactic dehydrogenase and serum concentrations were within normal limits. In the two groups there was no paravalvular leakage although two of the whole group of 250 mitral valve replacements had a leakage. One was reoperated on and the other died before reoperation. Four cases had serum hepatitis within 3–6 months after operation and one had a septicaemia but recovered without sequelae after treatment with antibiotics. Prior to operation, the two groups were similar and comparable, both in clinical and in haemodynamic respects. The differences encountered in clinical and haemodynamic results after surgery may be ascribed to the technical difference in the surgical procedure in the two groups. The improvement in central haemodynamics was of the same order for both groups at rest. However there was a much more marked improvement in the second group during exercise, both regarding arterio-venous oxygen difference, cardiac output, stroke volume, pulmonary and systemic vascular resistance, left atrial and pulmonary artery pressures. In spite of the general improvement in central haemodynamics a prominent V wave was observed in the left atrial pressure curve in both groups and this V wave was not due to paravalvular leakage but was related to an increased mean left atrial pressure. The pressure difference across the mitral valve prosthesis, as well as the difference calculated according to the Gorlin formula, were similar for both groups at rest but more favourable for the second group during exercise. Figure 23.12 shows the driving pressure across the mitral valve prosthesis *in vivo* in relation to the mitral valve flow in ml s $^{-1}$ and cardiac output in l/min after mitral valve replacement at rest and during exercise. There is a much more favourable gradient with the big opening orientated posteriorly in group II. The relationship between mitral valve flow and cardiac output and the gradient showed a linear relationship. Four factors may be responsible for the improved results in group II with posterior orientation.

1. The disc angle which is possibly only partially responsible.
2. The disc material.
3. The disc orientation which is possibly the most important factor.
4. The influence of the movement of the left ventricular septum.

The influence of the opening angle on the pressure difference across the prosthesis has been investigated, first in a study with continuous flow and also in a hydrodynamic pulse duplicator. It was demonstrated that only a marginal decrease of the pressure difference across the valve was obtained when the angle was increased from 50–60 degrees in a 25 mm prosthesis in flows up to 16 l/min. The cardiac output in these groups never exceed 8 l/min and 79% of the cases had a prosthesis of 27 mm or larger. It is, therefore, concluded that the effect of the change of the opening angle could only to a minor degree be responsible for the improved pressure flow relationship observed in the second group of patients.

A change from Delrin to pyrolytic carbon did not influence the pressure flow relationship of the prosthesis in a haemodynamic pulse duplicator. Pyrolytic carbon with its excellent thromboresistant properties may have contributed to the reduction in thromboembolic complications, although we believe that thrombus formation does not start on the disc but rather in the groove between the metal and the Teflon of the sewing ring.

The orientation of the prothesis in the second group directs the main blood stream towards the parietal wall of the left ventricle instead of directing it towards the septum and, therefore, less turbulence, less vortex formation and less loss of energy with the smaller gradient during exercise was obtained in group II. The observed movement of the ventricular septum during the cardiac cycle with a bulging of the upper portion of the septum into the left ventricular cavity during the ventricular filling period

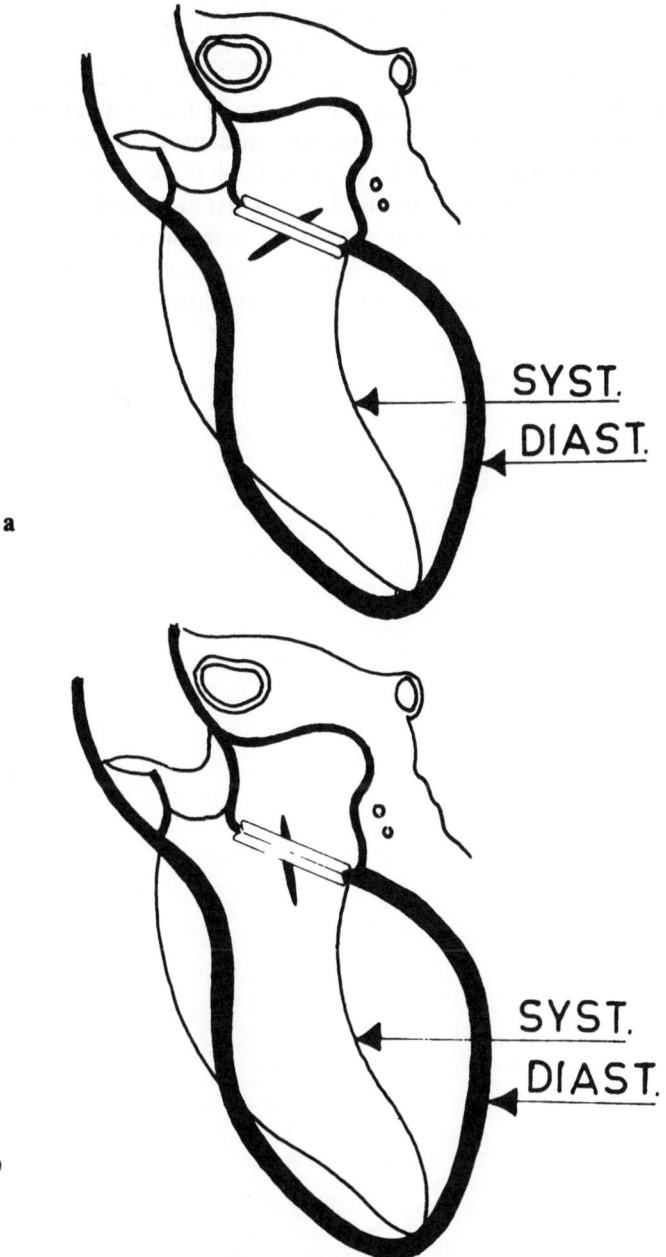

Figures 23.13a and **b** Compare the freedom of flow through the mitral valve with the disc directing the flow to the septum or the parietal wall of the heart

may also influence the pressure–flow relationship in the prothesis by slightly narrowing the inflow tract (Figure 23.13). The rotation of the prosthesis directing the blood stream towards the parietal wall (Figure 23.13b) instead of towards the septum (Figure 23.13a) would tend to reduce the obstructive effect of such a bulging and probably also result in a smoother flow pattern in the left ventricle. Both these effects would reduce the energy loss in the prosthesis. In conclusion, therefore, the Björk–Shiley mitral valve prosthesis should be orientated with the opening posteriorly (Figure 23.13b) in the mitral orifice and in the tricuspid orifice with the big orifice towards the diaphragmatic surface of the right ventricle.

24
The Australian experience with prosthetic valves
H. D. Sutherland

It is a difficult task to cover a topic as general as this, however, the matter will be approached from several aspects in the hope that justice will be done to the subject. Table 24.1 shows the total experience in Australia with valve replacement from 1963 to the end of 1972 taken

Table 24.1 The total experience with valve replacement in Australia from 1963 to the end of 1972 (3814 operations)

COLLECTIVE AUSTRALIAN FIGURES: 3814 OPERATIONS *1963-1972*			
	Aortic	*Mitral*	*Multiple*
Prosthetic	1242 (12%)	1314 (10%)	579 (23%)
Tissue	358 (17%)	121 (28%)	?
42 p.a.			
1972			
	Aortic	*Mitral*	*Multiple*
Prosthetic	244 (10%)	255 (5%)	77 (14%)
64 p.a.			

from the National Heart Foundation of Australia annual reports on cardiac surgery. The present case-load position is indicated by the figures for 1972 alone. As expected these 1972 figures show an increase of valve replacements per Unit with a very significant decrease in mortality. This introduces the essential theme of this presentation, namely that the valves are better, the surgery is better and that continued use of prosthetic valves is justified.

Both in Australia and New Zealand there has been considerable experience with tissue valves of all types hence it is necessary to make some reference to this. It can be seen that the total numbers in Australia (New Zealand figures are not included) for tissue valves are very much smaller than for prosthetic valves and the mortality has been greater. The cause for the higher mortality is not evident but it seems unlikely that this difference is in any way due to valve selection.

The main topic will be developed in three steps, firstly, a detailed review of the whole Australian experience which was done for a meeting in Melbourne in 1971. Secondly, this analysis was advanced for a meeting in New Zealand in 1972. Thirdly, a more detailed analysis has been made of the total experience of our own Unit in South Australia which carries through until the end of 1973.

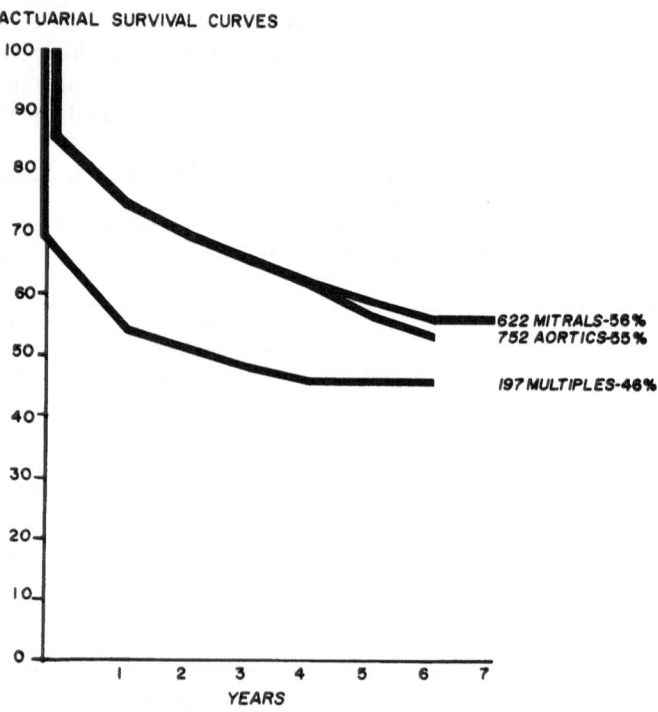

Figure 24.1 Actuarial profiles for survival compiled from Units predominantly or wholly using Starr valves

Figures 24.1–24.4 give the actuarial profiles of survival compiled from Units with sufficient numbers of cases and predominantly or wholly using Starr valves up to that time (1971). In all there were 1581 operations performed in all the Units included and these totals were used in Figure 24.1, but in Figures 24.2, 24.3 and 24.4 the returns from some Units with only small numbers of cases were omitted from the graph. In spite of the stability of the actuarial curves it can be seen in Table 24.2 that the range of mortality in the different Units was very wide of the mean and in general the mortality was highest in the Units with the smallest numbers and thus the least experience.

It can also be seen from these curves that if the variation in operative mortality is excluded and the variations in the one year survival are also excluded that the survival rate as indicated by the slope is remarkably constant. The variation in operative mortality probably gives an indication of variation in team skill and case selection of cases and to some extent the first year survival is also related to these two factors. Having survived

Table 24.2

	Cases	Hospital & Operative mortality	%	
Multiple	197	68		18-55
Aortic	752	118	1	10-32
Mitral	622	96	16	6-25

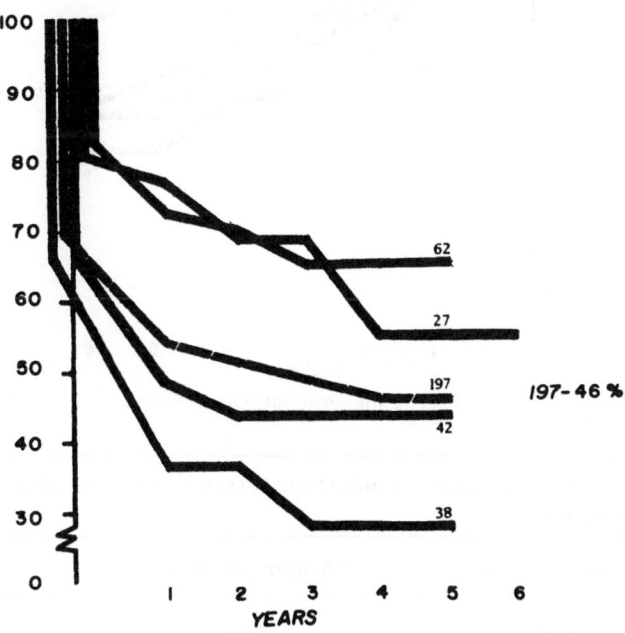

MULTIPLE VALVE REPLACEMENTS

Figure 24.2 Actuarial survival curves for multiple valve replacements

these two hazards the remainder of the curve is an indication of expected survival with the Starr prosthesis.

The incidence in the whole series of infection which was severe enough to cause death or valve dehiscence is shown in Table 24.3. For the most part these occurred within six months of operation suggesting that the infection probably occurred at the time of operation. It is now clear that better surgical technique and better application of antibiotic therapy have reduced this incidence but there are no figures available to support this contention.

Table 24.4 shows the incidence of perivalvular 'leak' from the 1971 analysis. 'Leak' is defined as dehiscence sufficient to require reoperation.

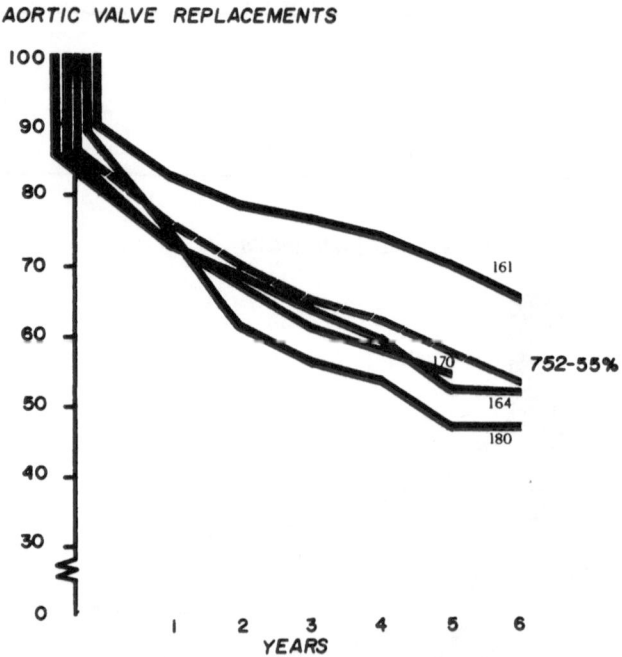

Figure 24.3 Actuarial survival curves for aortic valve replacements

Table 24.3 The incidence of infection severe enough to cause death or valve dehiscence

Operative survivors	Blood stream infections	%
1286	48	3·7

Again there is considerable variation demonstrated between Units. Two Units with the most experience had an incidence of less than 1% of all cases, whilst a second group of four Units with less total experience had an incidence of greater than 6%. It has to be accepted that this difference is due to variations in surgical skill.

By 1972 the South Australian Unit was using the cloth-covered Starr valves as they became available. As this was the only major change in technique up to that time it was thought that the new valve might have

MITRAL VALVE REPLACEMENTS

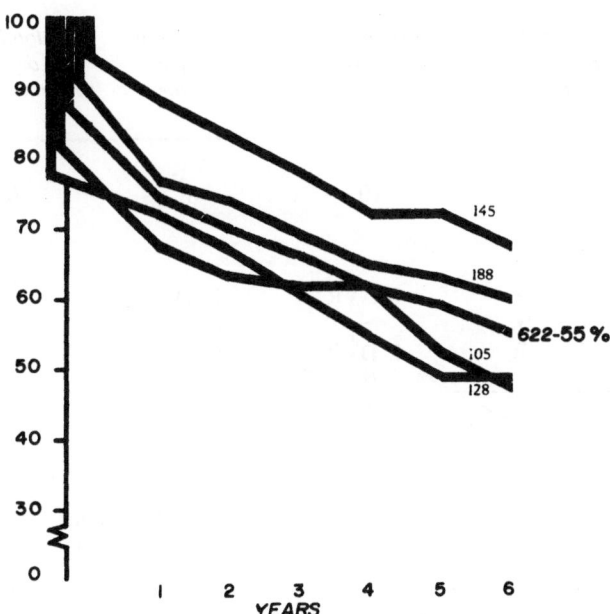

Figure 24.4 Actuarial survival curves for mitral valve replacements

Table 24.4 The incidence of perivalvular 'leak' (1971)

	Valves	*'Dehiscence' or 'Perivalvular leak'*	%
2 Units	663	5	< 1
4 Units	908	55	> 6
Totals	1411	60	4.3

been the cause of haemolysis which was appearing to be more prevalent in management.

In order to get further data on this, an analysis was made of a group of 364 valve replacements and from these the patients who, six months after valve replacement, had haemoglobin levels persistently below 12 g% were studied in detail. A summary of the findings are shown in Table 24.5.

Table 24.5· The results of an analysis of a group of patients who six months after valve replacement had haemoglobin levels persistently below 12 g% (July 1963–June 1971)

Total	*Anaemia* *Hb<11.0 gm%* *after*	*Haemolysis* *major* *factor*	*Haemolysis* *minor* *factor*	*Blood loss* *Fe deficiency* *systemic infection*
	24	10	8	6
364				
	15 AVR	8 AVR	4 AVR	
	6 MVR	—	3 MVR	
	3 DVR	2 DVR	1 DVR	
	3 Repeated transfusion	6 Controlled Fe, folate, B12	1 Correcting himself	

There were 10 cases where significant cell damage was thought to be due to valve function or dysfunction. As known by the experience of others the aortic valve was the chief culprit, but in our experience only one case of the ten finally required reoperation and all but one of the other nine cases have fully recovered with the passage of time. The valve (Starr model 2300 Size 8A) of the case reoperated had a fracture of the cloth on the struts and a minor leak at the valve ring. The cloth was removed and a single suture closed the perivalvular leak. This was thought to be adequate as the patient was by then over 70 years of age. The haemolysis ceased with the reoperation. It was noted that there was virtually no evidence of fibrin formation or pseudo-endothelialisation on the cloth of the valve. It is postulated that the absence of this reaction leaves the cloth unprotected and more liable to fracture and is also a possible explanation of the gradual remission of haemolysis in the others as the fibrin deposition becomes effective, albeit a much slower rate than for the majority.

By 1972 it was possible to carry the analysis of 1971 a year further along. The numbers operated on were increasing. It was not possible to review the work in detail of all the Units incorporated in the 1971 study

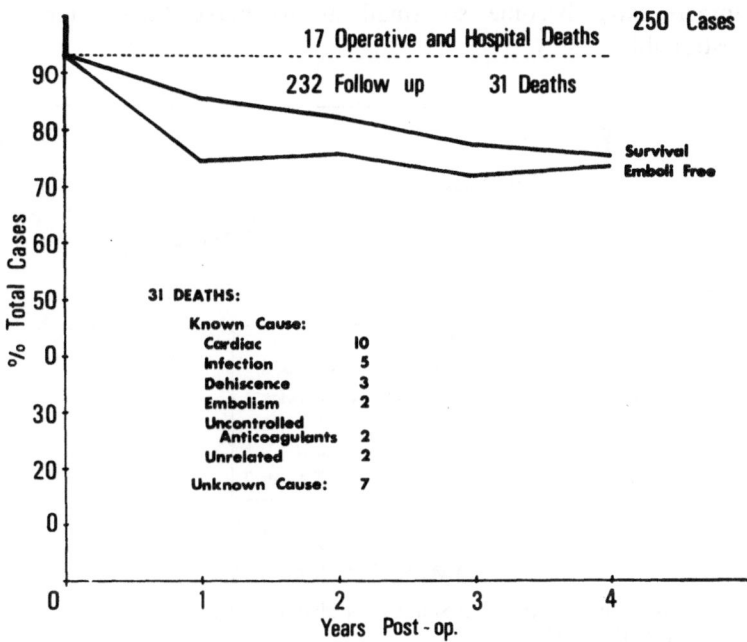

Figure 24.5 The combined figures for aortic valve replacement from the Royal Adelaide Hospital and St. Vincent's Hospital, Sydney. January 1967–December 1971

but one further analysis was possible as shown in Figure 24.5. In this the figures for aortic valve replacement from the Royal Adelaide Hospital and St. Vincent's Hospital, Sydney were combined for the valves used after the Starr Model 1000 was superseded. The actuarial survival curve for the 250 cases demonstrated a reduced operative mortality and a reduction in the slope of the curve compared with the 1971 figures. It is believed that these two facts were indicative of improved selection and management plus an improvement in valve function.

At the height of tissue valve promotion in 1970 the South Australian Unit had a brief but unpleasant experience with tissue valves. The details are shown in Table 24.6. The small numbers do not warrant analysis but needless to say tissue valves are no longer considered.

From mid-1963 to the end of 1973 a further series of analyses (using the actuarial method) of the total South Australian experience was carried out. This made use of several subgroupings of the cases seen during this time and represents a total of 641 Starr valves inserted into 579 operative cases. Figure 24.6 summarises this total experience, shows the operative mortality for the three main groups and again demonstrates the stability of the survival curves. The dotted lines in years 8 to 10 indicate that the numbers have become so small as to make their interpretation questionable.

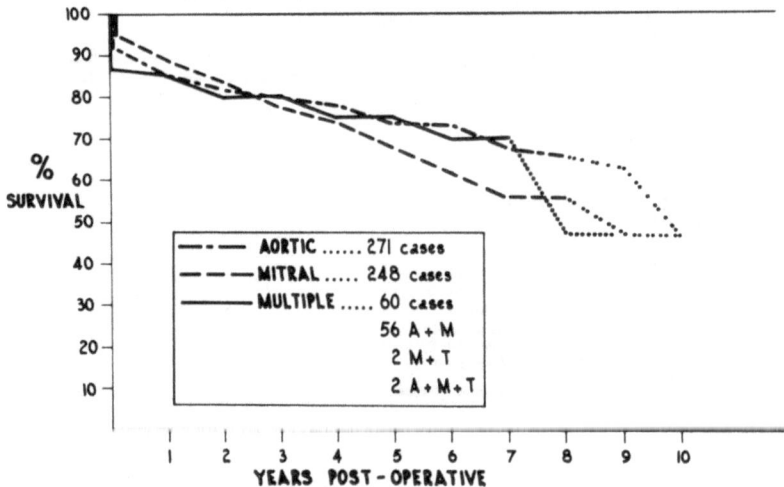

Figure 24.6 Analysis of the total South Australian experience with Starr–Edwards valve replacements, 1963–1973

Table 24.6 Experience with tissue valves at the Royal Adelaide Hospital in 1970

	Type	Number	Replaced	"Good"	"Poor"	Died
Aortic	Pig	6	5	–	1	–
	F.L.	1	–	1	–	–
Mitral	Homo-graft	1	1	–	–	–
	F.L.	8	3 (+1)	3	1	1
Totals		16	10	4	2	1

Figure 24.7 demonstrates the actuarial survival profile of the whole series of aortic valve replacements up to the end of 1973 and compares this with the survival curve for cases using the cloth-covered models 2300 to 2320. At the same time the curve for valve replacements up to the time the 2320 valve was used is also displayed. The curve for the cloth-covered series extends over the last five years. In this group

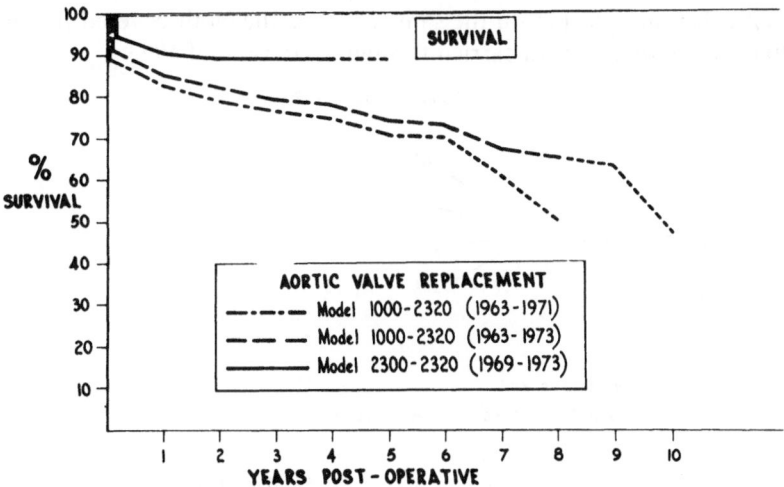

Figure 24.7 The actuarial survival profile of the whole series of aortic valve replacements in South Australia, 1963–1973

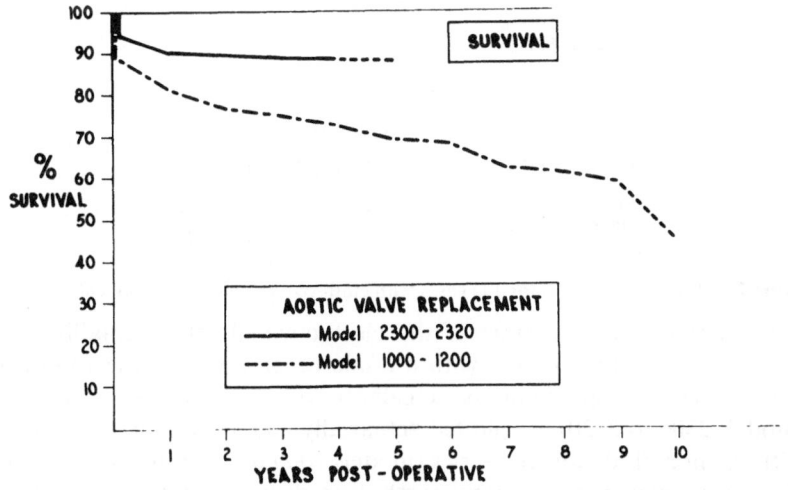

Figure 24.8 Actuarial survival curves for aortic valve replacement using non-cloth-covered and cloth-covered valves in South Australia, 1963–1973

the operative mortality has been lowered and there is a significant flattening of the slope of the survival curve. It must be remembered that each of the subgroups is a series of sequential cases which form a part of the whole. The improvement in mortality and survival are two of the reasons why the use of the Starr valve will be continued. This situation is perhaps more clearly demonstrated in Figure 24.8 on which the survival curves of the non-cloth-covered (model 1000 and 1200) valves are plotted on the same chart as the cloth-covered (models 2300 and 2320) and both carried through to the end of 1973.

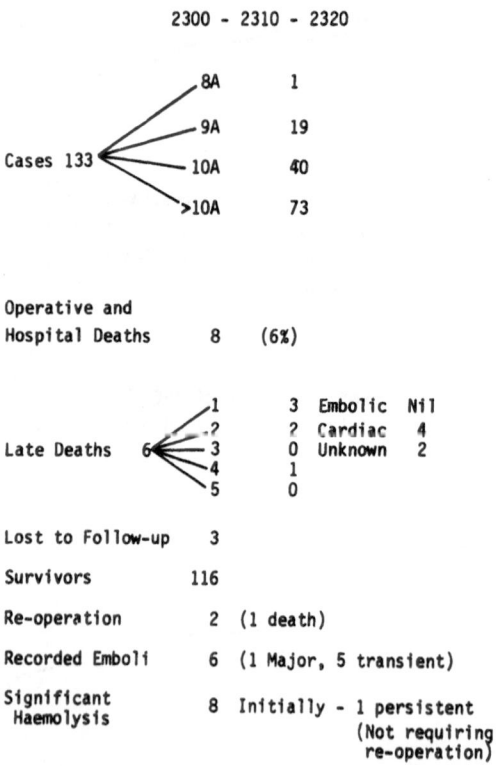

Figure 24.9 Follow-up figures for 133 cases with cloth-covered valve replacements

A more detailed analysis of the cloth-covered series, totalling 133 cases is seen in Figure 24.9 with a crude break-down of the follow-up figures. The thromboembolic incidence of the cloth-covered series (models 2300 to 2320) are plotted actuarially and are seen in comparison with the non-cloth-covered series (models 1000 to 1200) in Figure 24.10. The lower incidence of thromboembolism demonstrated is, we believe, significant and in keeping with the experience of others.

The comparison of the survival curves in our mitral valve replacements divided up into similar subgroups is seen in Figure 24.11, the survival of both cloth- and non-cloth-covered valves being almost identical. However, there is a dramatic difference in the incidence of thromboembolism as seen in Figure 24.12. A more detailed analysis of the follow-up of the cases with cloth-covered valves is seen in

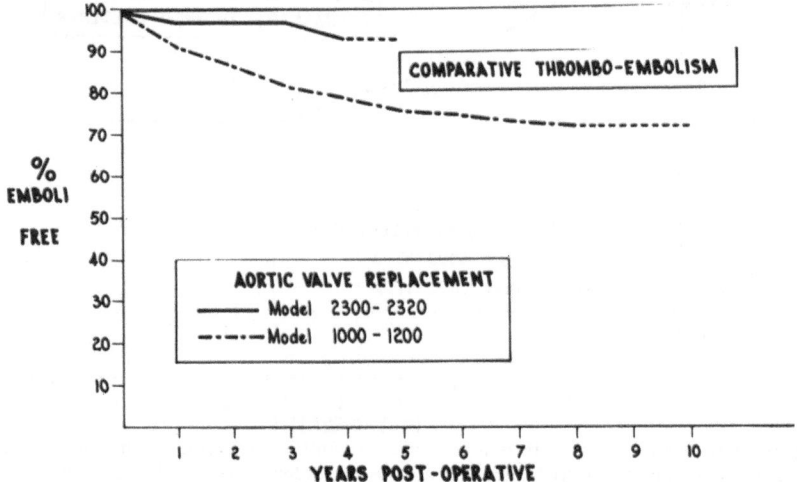

Figure 24.10 The incidence of thromboembolism in aortic valve replacement when cloth-covered and non-cloth-covered valves are used. Royal Adelaide Hospital, 1963–1973

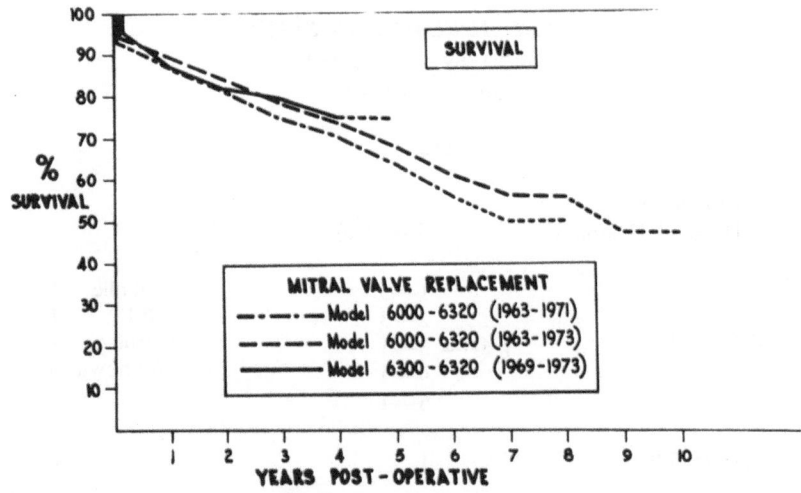

Figure 24.11 Actuarial survival curves for mitral valve replacement when cloth-covered and non-cloth-covered valves are used. Royal Adelaide Hospital, 1963–1973

Table 24.7. The sizes of the valves used are not shown because this factor was not thought to have any direct bearing on the outcome but it should be said that no size MI Starr valves were used and rarely size M4.

Some reference should be made to other Units in Australia and some general remarks on these Units may be of interest.

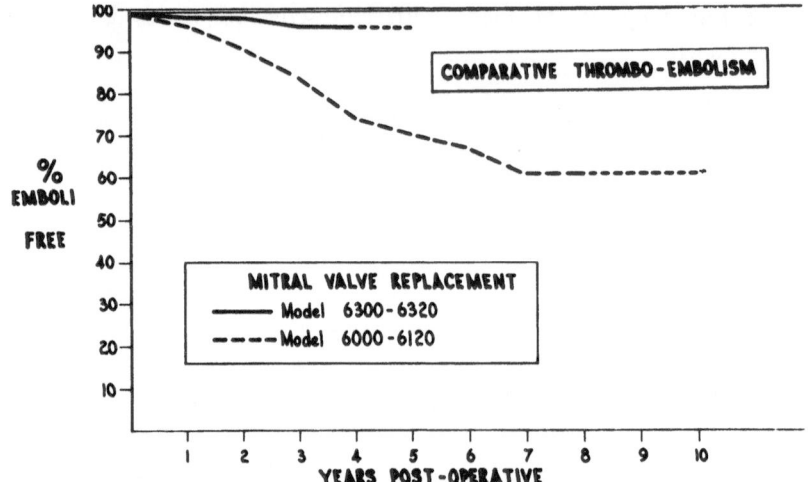

Figure 24.12 The incidence of thromboembolism in mitral valve replacement when cloth-covered and non-cloth-covered valves are used. Royal Adelaide Hospital, 1963–1973

Table 24.7 Follow-up figures for 114 cases with cloth-covered valve replacements

ROYAL ADELAIDE HOSPITAL
6.2.1969 to 31.12.1973
6300 — 6310 — 6320

Cases	114	
Operative and Hospital Deaths	5 (4·4%)	
Late deaths	8 ⟨ 1—3, 2—3, 3—1, 4—1, 5—1	Embolic 1, S.B.E. 1, Cardiac 1, Unknown 5
Lost to follow-up	1	
Recorded embolic incidents	2	

The Alfred Hospital in Melbourne has in the past had more experience with fascia lata valves than the South Australian Unit. Mr Eric Cooper has kindly given permission for their experience to be quoted. This can be summarised as 27 aortic valve replacements, 14 mitral valve replacements and 5 double valves. Of the 46 patients, 17 died at or near operation. Of the 29 survivors, 14 were classed as 'alive and well'. Of the other 15 cases, 5 had died late deaths and 10 had the fascia lata valves replaced with Starr valves at the time of review. This dismal picture explains why they no longer use fascia lata valves in any position. However, in common with the experience of others, some of those with surviving fascia lata valves are among their best cases in all respects. As long as they survive and remain well, tissue valves continue as a challenge.

St. Vincent's Hospital in Melbourne have given up tissue valve replacements almost entirely but still select certain patients for stent-mounted aortic valve homografts in the mitral position. There are two surgical groups at the hospital, one using Starr valves and the other Bjork–Shiley valves. The surgeons involved believe there is little detectable difference between the two series of cases.

St. Vincent's Hospital in Sydney who have had a lot of experience of valve replacement first used Starr valves in all cases. About two years ago they began using Björk–Shiley valves for small aortic roots. They have now gradually swung over to using the latter for virtually all cases and say that they can detect no obvious differences in the management for follow-up of the cases.

Mr Mark O'Brien, who has had a lot of experimental and clinical experience with tissue valves, told the author recently that he was restricting his use of tissue valves. He believes that the mechanical prostheses have improved steadily, hence making the preference for tissue valves harder to sustain. He believes that any form of denatured protein in valves is fallible and should not be used, that non-valve tissue such as fascia lata will not function as valve tissue for prolonged periods and so should be abandoned and that stent-mounted tissue carries too high an infection rate and should not be used. This leaves him with the choice between mechanical prostheses and tissue viable unmounted homografts in the aortic position; hence they are only applicable to small aortic roots – a small percentage of the total requirement in this whole field of work.

In summary, the South Australian Unit believes that the mechanical valves are functioning better and better. It is prepared to continue to use the Starr valves available and it may be encouraged to use the Starr track valve when it has had a longer clinical trial.

25
The use of Starr-Edwards composite seat valves (models 2320 and 6320) in the aortic and mitral positions

W. P. Cleland

The author started using these valves on a regular basis and as a matter of preference in 1970, when experience with frame-mounted homografts had shown that, in the long term, these were proving unsatisfactory even though, in the short term, they had given excellent results.

Prior to 1970 the author had used composite seat valves irregularly and they had given satisfactory service. They had the advantage of a metallic poppet which had eliminated risks of ball variance, even though personal experience with the latter had been limited to a trifling number of cases. Cloth covering of all exposed metal also seemed a desirable goal in the prevention of thromboembolism. Limited experience up to 1970 with the composite seat valve had been satisfactory so it seemed logical to continue with this prosthesis.

The continued use of the prosthesis would depend upon the results obtained and any decision to change would only be on the demonstration of superiority by an alternative prosthesis over both the short and the long term. From January 1971 to December 1973 the composite seat valve has been used as a first choice with only relatively few exceptions.

Table 25.1 Aortic valve replacement – model 2320. 1971–1973

	Group I	Group II	Group III
Total	131	79	44
Early deaths	15	9	6
Late deaths	6	2	4
Embolism	2	0	2
Haemolysis	4	2	2
Leak	9	3	6

Table 25.1 indicates experiences with single aortic valve replacements. Group I includes total experience on the author's service whilst Group II refers to his personal series and Group III to operations carried out on

his behalf. There are minor differences in the three groups regarding early mortality and the incidence of early diastolic murmur probably related to technical problems but the figures indicate that there are no special problems related to the technical aspects of insertion.

Of 116 patients available for follow-up two have had embolic problems – both cerebral – and both have recovered. Four patients have developed anaemia but none has required more than iron to maintain an adequate haemoglobin. Nine patients have an audible EDM but in no case has reoperation been required because of a significant leak.

Table 25.2 shows experience with single mitral valve replacements with a similar division into personal and non-personal patients. Of nearly 100 patients available for follow-up there have been two embolic episodes, both cerebral and both minor with full recovery. Six patients have an apical systolic murmur suggesting a paraprosthetic leak but in no instance has there been a haemodynamically significant regurgitation. Haemolysis of moderate degree is occurring in two of these patients with a paraprosthetic leak.

Table 25.2 Mitral valve replacement – model 6320. 1971–1973

	Group I	Group II	Group III
Total	115	65	50
Early deaths	18	7	11
Late deaths	7	5	2
Embolism	2	0	2
Leak	6	3	3
Haemolysis	2	2	0
Infection	5	3	2
Rhythm disorders	4	3	1
A/C problems	1	1	0

There have been five instances of blood stream infection three of which proved fatal. There have not been any fungal infections in this series. Rhythm disturbances serious enough to be responsible for an early death were encountered in four patients. This complication occurred only with the mitral valves and is possibly related to irritation of the left ventricle endocardium by the cage of the prosthesis. However, in none of the patients was the left ventricular cavity small and in all four the dominant lesion was regurgitation with considerable dilatation of the ventricle and it is possible that the rhythm disorders were related to ventricular disturbances rather than the prostheses.

Control of coagulation often proved difficult and actually led to complications but in only one instance was it thought to be responsible for death. This was in a patient who had a massive cerebral haemorrhage three months after mitral valve replacement at a time when she was moderately overcoagulated.

Table 25.3 indicates the effect of previous surgery on the early and late mortality of mitral valve replacements. The figures are, of course, small but may be significant. Better results have been obtained with second operation in the latter part of the experience.

Table 25.3 Mitral valve replacement – model 6320. 1971–1973

	No previous surgery	*Previous closed valvotomy*	*Previous valve replacement*
Total	74	25	16
Early deaths	9	5	4
Late deaths	4	2	1

I should mention that the figures given are not completely up to date. This is an 'on-going' investigation and inevitably there is some delay in obtaining up to date details. The incidence of complication thus represents the minimum and only that known at the time of writing.

Experiences with composite seat valves during the period 1971 to 1973 have been satisfactory with an acceptable level of complications related to the type of valve. The author cannot see any need to change at present until convinced that an alternative prosthesis is better. A disadvantage of the composite seat valve for some patients is the noise made by the prosthesis. This annoyance is usually only of a temporary nature and most patients readily accept the clicking noise. So far, in patients under review there has been no evidence of strut cloth wear. There has not been any occasion as yet to remove one of these prostheses and so there is no evidence about the strength of the cloth on the struts.

However, the author does have certain reservations about the caged ball type of prosthesis in the following circumstances:

1. In a small aortic root. The composite seat valves are seriously obstructive and better haemodynamic results are probably obtainable from the Björk–Shiley type of valve.
2. Similarly in patients with a small left ventricle, the larger size of the composite seat valve which should be used may be too large for the ventricle and cause damage to the endocardium and possibly be responsible for rhythm disorders.

3. Finally, in the tricuspid position the shape of the right ventricle is such that a caged ball valve will not fit comfortably under any circumstances.

26
Mitral valve replacement
S. C. Lennox

In the absence of the perfect prosthesis one is left to select the valve whose qualities one regards as being the most important.

Having used, until 1970 at the Brompton Hospital, mounted homograft valves for mitral valve replacement, I decided that durability was the most desirable quality to obtain, the reason being that although the homograft valves were functionally good and the patients were free of embolic or anticoagulant problems, they had a high late failure rate. As a result I decided to return to the valve of which at that time we had the most knowledge. That was the Model 6120 Starr valve.

From January 1971 to December 1973 I performed 169 open mitral valve operations and in 23% of these at least one other valve procedure was undertaken. 48 of these patients had had previous operations. Ten patients have died, giving a combined early and late mortality rate of under 6%.

In this series there were 94 patients with a Model 6120 Starr valve inserted for lone mitral valve disease. The majority of these patients had a No. 3 valve inserted, although more recently I have tended to use a No. 4 prosthesis. Smaller valves had to be inserted in children and in one four year old girl a No. 1 valve was used.

Undoubtedly this valve works well and in the majority of cases the patients have gained considerable benefit. There have, however, been some problems. Three patients died from the low output syndrom. Two of these had mitral regurgitation from so-called "papillary muscle dysfunction" and in one a left ventricular aneurysm had been resected previously. In these patients the mitral valve looked macroscopically normal, but in view of the known mitral regurgitation, was replaced.

Echocardiography shows that the Starr valve produces a paradoxically moving ventricular septum. This appears to be of little importance in those patients who have good left ventricular function. However, in those patients with dysfunction of their free wall, the added burden of a paradoxically moving septum is probably too great; therefore it seems that the Starr valve, and any other valve which produces abnormal septal movement, should not be used.

Like others we have had difficulties with patients who have had beta blockers prior to operation. The dangers of these drugs were clearly seen in one young boy who required large doses of Practolol to control his heart rate before operation. Following valve replacement we had considerable difficulty in weaning him off cardiopulmonary bypass. His condition, however, improved and he was well until 48 hours after operation when he again developed a persistent tachycardia. Further doses of Oxyprenalol were given and this resulted in circulatory failure from which he could not be resuscitated. Another interesting problem arose in a patient who, apparently having had a routine valve replacement, started to bleed from behind the heart following discontinuation of cardiopulmonary bypass. The exact site was difficult to locate as it could only be seen by lifting the heart forward. Despite numerous attempts to suture the bleeding area haemostasis could not be achieved. This bleeding was found to occur from the back of the left ventricle and not through the anulus. A number of similar cases have now been reported, but the exact cause of the bleeding is still not clear.

Bacterial endocariditis has not been a problem, but it resulted in death in the only case in this series six months after valve replacement. A further late death occurred in a patient who had a valve replacement for cardiomyopathy and who died from her disease eighteen months later, and two patients later died from their pre-existing lung disease.

During this period only two patients have had recognised embolic episodes and this is about 1.1 per thousand months. One has, however, to be careful in assessing the instance of embolic episodes because it is too easy to describe any minor neurological episode as being due to an embolus when the patient has a mechanical valve. Similar episodes in a normal person would be dismissed without thought. Only one patient in the whole series had a prosthetic leak and this was through the centre of the valve, presumably due to obstruction of the poppet. This patient has been much improved since inserting a larger valve.

In conclusion, although the Model 6120 Starr valve is far from perfect, it appears to function haemodynamically adequately for most patients and if their anticoagulants are well controlled the risk of embolic episodes appears to be low. Its main virtue, however, appears to be that it is extremely durable and is associated with a very low late failure rate.

27
The use of Starr-Edwards valves (model 1260)
M. F. Sturridge

At the London Chest Hospital and the Middlesex Hospital the model 1260 is the valve which has been used for patients who are acutely ill and for patients in whom one cannot fit a homograft in the early stages. This valve has been found very satisfactory when used in these circumstances.

From 1966 to the present only 100 patients aged between 23 and 75 years have been operated on. The majority of these patients were in the older age group because initially the tendency was to use the homograft valve in younger patients. Nine patients were congenital cases, usually under the age of 40 with a valve that showed very little normal architecture, 23 were rheumatic, 46 had bicuspid valves which were predominantly stenotic, 15 had already had homograft operations and 19 of the patients in this series had already had a total of 23 bypasses. In most of these the larger size valves had been used because again the elective operation in the first few years was to put in a homograft and if the homograft was not large enough, a Starr valve was used.

There were eight hospital deaths in the 100. Four of these deaths were in the first 20 and four in the last 80. Of the late deaths, there were four from bacterial endocarditis at 5, 8, 12 and 22 months postoperatively. Nearly all these were patients from the East end of London where perhaps general health is not as good. Three of the aortic patients died from dissection or rupture at 14 months, 15 months and 33 months after the operation; these deaths were not associated with infection. Two patients died from haemorrhage; one a cerebral haemorrhage and one a massive retroperitoneum haemorrhage. Apparently both of these haemorrhages were spontaneous but the patients were all on anticoagulants. One patient died from congestive cardiac failure, one died suddenly after four years and one from carcinoma. This patient had the condition before operation, but was quite well at the time and therefore it was considered worth operating.

Of the 80 survivors, four have diastolic murmurs; two of these are audible but apparently not significant and two are definitely significant and will without a doubt have to be replaced. One of these developed on operation and the other one developed some months after the operation.

There were three cases of thromboembolism in a total of two per 500 patient months. One patient developed a transient blindness and another developed a VSD one year after valve replacement and had a hemiplegia a few months after that was repaired. One patient haemorrhaged, which makes a total of three haemorrhages; these plus the cases of embolism must be considered as anticoagulant problems. There are four patients in heart block, in three of these this occurred before operation, and in one it occurred a year after operation. Three patients have had myocardial infarction since operation, three have angina, two still have some congestive cardiac failure and one patient developed endocarditis and had his valve successfully replaced.

Therefore basically this valve has performed satisfactorily, but when considering embolism and perhaps more especially the haemorrhage rate on anticoagulants, it might be preferable to think in terms of other valves.

28
The use of Braunwald Cutter valves: Part I
J. E. C. Wright

The specification for a perfect valve prosthesis has changed little since Harken outlined his list of desirable features many years ago. So far no valve fulfills all his criteria.

The author used the bare cage, silastic ball Starr valve for some time but turned away from it because of the undoubted incidence of thromboembolic complications. He then inserted a series of 50 composite seat Starr valves into the mitral position using long-term anticoagulation. There were only two minor transient episodes of thromboembolism and so far no evidence of cloth wear such as reported by others. There were however several incidences of complications due to the anticoagulants including one major haemothorax. In addition, there is a worrying noise problem with the composite seat Starr valve such that on occasion the patient's relatives have refused to stay in the same room as the patient. Biological valves do of course remove both the problems of thromboembolism and noise although they are perhaps a little suspect in their long-term fate, particularly in the mitral position. Tissue failure and calcification is a definite worry.

The concept of tissue encapsulation offers a prospect of freedom from thromboembolism, or relative freedom from thromboembolism and may remove the need for anticoagulation. The Braunwald Cutter valve appealed rather than the Starr valve because it retained the silastic poppet and a low noise level. The cage is covered with Dacron and the seat, a fine polypropylene mesh, has been shown experimentally to produce a thin layer of neo-endothelium, which should avoid the tissue ingrowth problem encountered with some earlier types of cloth-covered valves.

The series to be considered is a selective series in that there is no bias one way or another, the most appropriate valve being used in each case, e.g. the biological valve, a homograft, is still used for a small aortic root and when faced with a small left ventricle. In other patients, the Braunwald Cutter valve is used. There is no significant gradient problem in the size of valves used.

A total of 71 valves have been inserted. Forty-two Braunwald Cutter valves have been inserted in the aortic position, using conventional normothermic bypass, coronary perfusion and interrupted stitches. Twenty-nine were placed in the mitral position using a continuous suture technique and the left atrial appendage was removed. Five double replacements were performed. There was no hospital mortality (30 days). No anticoagulants were used for patients with aortic prosthesis and anticoagulants were discounted after three months in patients with mitral valves. There were two late deaths, one occurring in the only case of endocarditis in this series and one from left ventricular failure due to widespread ischaemic heart disease. One patient has clinically important haemolytic anaemia, controlled by iron. There were two minor and transient embolic episodes. The mean survival time is seven months the total patient months being 512. This gives a 3·9/1000 patient month incidence of thromboembolism. The author therefore considers the value to be quite satisfactory.

Table 28.1 The London Chest Hospital. Braunwald Cutter valve

Anticoagulant policy –
  Aortic: None
  Mitral: 3 months on warfarin

No. of embolic episodes	2
Total patient months	512
Episodes/1000 patient months	3·9

Table 28.2 The London Chest Hospital. Braunwald Cutter valve (Sept 1972 to present)

	Total	Hospital mortality	Late mortality
Aortic	37	0	2
Mitral	24	0	0
Double	5	0	0
Total	66	0	2

1 endocarditis
1 left ventricular failure

29
Experience with the Björk-Shiley prosthesis: Part I

J. G. Bennett

Over the past 18 months 188 patients have been subjected to operation using Björk-Shiley prosthesis, their ages ranging from 12 to 78 years. For a mitral valve replacement, the aorta was clamped and ischaemic arrest after a short period of cooling was used. The valve was sutured with two layers of continuous prolene sutures and when in position, root perfusion through a coronary cannula was used. The atrium was closed with a beating heart and the left atrium was vented. In the aortic position, coronary perfusion and interrupted ethiflex sutures were used for implantation of the valve. These sutures were placed in the lower half of the valve ring. No anticoagulants were used postoperatively in either aortic or mitral valve replacement and 27% of the 188 patients had had previous operations.

Fifty tricuspid plications were performed. Five of these patients died from organic lesions of the tricuspid valve. One hundred and thirty-seven patients underwent mitral valve replacement. During the follow-up period of only 18 months, the figure for overall mortality was 17%, with an embolism rate of 4·4% with two deaths. These deaths were caused by thromboses on the ventricular surface of the valve which completely interfered with valve action. Another patient died as a result of infection. This patient had two valve replacements for infection and at postmortem it was found that the vegetations were completely covering the valve. There were three cases of mechanical defect; two patients were subjected to reoperation because it was considered that in one case the aortic and in the other case the mitral valve replacement, was regurgitating. They did not survive their operation. In the third patient the valve appeared to be regurgitant at the time of operation and was replaced satisfactorily with a similar valve. There were three cases of perivalvular leak: the first was subjected to reoperation, the second was not and the third died from what amounted to a dehiscence of the valve. There were no cases of haemolysis requiring particular treatment. These complications related to the valve only involve those operations where mitral valves were implanted together with other valves. They do not apply to aortic valve replacement and therefore only concern 137 patients.

Therefore the Björk–Shiley prosthesis can be used as a low-profile valve. The haemodynamics are extremely good owing to the nearly central flow, the large orifice diameter in relation to the tissue diameter, the opening to 60 degrees and the low mass of the disc. There is also little blood damage, rather low thrombogenecity, and as tested it is durable.

30
Experience with the Björk-Shiley prosthesis: Part II

G. H. Smith

The Northern General and United Sheffield Hospitals began to use the Björk–Shiley valve in 1971 and have to date inserted 198 mitral prostheses and 65 aortic prostheses. They were attracted to the prosthesis for several reasons; first the effective area for forward flow seemed to be large in comparison with the external diameter of the valve, and Professor Björk himself has published detailed comparisons with other valves in respect of this feature showing that Björk valve compares very well. This seemed to be important in terms of cardiac output, especially during exercise, and also in the possible prevention of haemolysis. Secondly, the central flow characteristics of the valve were a good feature and finally, it was hoped that thrombus formation might be inhibited by the 3–5% of built-in regurgitation. Anticoagulants have been used on all patients after surgery.

Of 198 mitral valve replacements, hospital mortality has been 14, or 7%. Mostly, this hospital mortality was due to the consequences of low-output syndrome but two cases were due to posterior heart disruption, occurring after the excision of a heavily-calcified mitral valve and no surgical cure has been found for this disaster as yet. These patients have been followed-up for periods from six months to two years and eight months with an average follow-up of 10 months. Seven patients have developed paravalvular leaks, again usually after the excision of calcified valves and all of these have had a second replacement. Of these, two have again developed leaks. There have been two early definite episodes of thromboembolism, and one definite incident after leaving hospital. This gives a total thromboembolic rate of nearly 2000 patient months. No cases of mechanical failure have been found and no valves have thrombosed.

The functional results have been encouraging. However, the length of follow-up has been very short and therefore many of the patients are probably still improving from this point of view as their pulmonary vascular changes regress. Experience with aortic valve replacement has been largely similar. The total number of patients having the prosthesis was 65 and there was a large hospital mortality of 12. This was largely due to myocardial infarction and to a lesser extent to technical hazard. The late mortality has been only one from congestive cardiac failure and there have been no episodes of late valve failure or thromboembolism. However, early in the aortic valve experience there were some valve-related problems during the operation. These difficulties arose with both the Delrin and the Pyrolite discs and the circumstances under which three patients were damaged were all broadly similar. Briefly, under certain conditions of non-pulsatile perfusion during operation and cardio-pulmonary bypass, some Björk–Shiley valves in the aortic position would permit an excessive amount of regurgitation. This was subsequently demonstrated in the laboratory to make quite sure the valves were being properly inserted and this regurgitation appeared to be related to excessive clearance between the disc and the valve ring. Representatives from Shiley laboratories confirm that the tolerances of manufacture had possibly been rather lax in the early days. Apparently the firm is now applying much tighter tolerances and also testing all the valves in the way described. It therefore appears unlikely that this problem will cause any future trouble.

31
The use of the Braunwald Cutter valve: Part II

J. K. Ross

The Southampton Unit started using the Braunwald Cutter valve in January 1973. Seventy-one valves have been put in to date; 24 in the aortic position, 42 in the mitral position and five in the tricuspid position. Forty were lone aortic or mitral valve replacements and 31 multiple in various permutations and combinations, including 3 triple valve replacements. At the present time, the mortality for isolated aortic valve replacement is running at just under 4%, for isolated mitral valve replacement is just under 7% and for multiple valve replacements between 10 and 12%. The relatively small number of aortic Braunwald Cutter valves reflects the policy still adhered to, i.e. to use homograft valves in the aortic position whenever possible. None of the aortic Braunwald Cutter valves have been anticoagulated and the mitral valves have been routinely anticoagulated. There have been no valve-related hospital deaths and there is no known major systemic embolism to date. There has been one known perivalvular leak in the mitral position in a woman who had had a previous valvotomy. This is a group which is particularly prone to this type of complication particularly if the previous valvotomy had extended out into the perivalvular tissues and ruptured them. There was also one other suspected perivalvular leak. Possibly because the cage is not quite so big as in the composite seat Starr valve, these valves in the tricuspid position seem to be giving a very good performance although the Unit still believes the frame-mounted homograft to be the best tricuspid substitute.

Part 4

Tissue Valve Replacement and Repair

32
Viability of homografts
and problems of long-term storage
N. Al-Janabi

Clinical experience at the National Heart Hospital during the last decade indicates that homograft aortic valves are an excellent valve substitute. At the same time it has become clear that their long-term function relates to the methods of sterilisation and storage.

The choice of method of sterilisation and storage depends on whether or not it is necessary to have viable cells in the graft. If it can be shown that non-viable grafts perform and function as well and as long as viable grafts, most of the sterilisation and storage problems will be solved.

Although it is difficult to compare the long-term function of viable v. non-viable homograft valves, some factors are known. Studies by Hudson[1] of ethylene-oxide sterilised valves and by Smith[2] of betapropiolactone-treated valves show that ingrowth of host tissue has not effectively replaced or covered the non-viable cusps. The cusps remain acellular and become focally thinned, fenestrated, torn or ruptured. In 1969 D. N. Ross concluded that the best chance of permanent cusp survival without late degeneration is if the tissue is not only completely fresh but is also viable at the time of insertion, i.e. that the cellular components (fibroblasts) of the valve cusp not only continue to survive *in vitro* but, after transplantation, are revived and will themselves undergo cell division. For this reason antibiotic solutions have been advocated for sterilisation and preservation of fresh homografts and cell viability has been postulated as the prerequisite for the maintenance of implanted homograft heart valves.

Human aortic valves are collected from routine autopsy material under unsterile condition within 48 h after death (Figure 32.1). The size of the valve is measured and the valve is sterilised and preserved. Therefore it is important:

1. To assess the viability of such grafts
2. To find an antibiotic mixture for rapid and complete sterilisation of heavily contaminated valves without impairing their viability
3. To select a storage method that will preserve the valves in a viable state for a realistic period of time.

By using a radioactive technique and utilising tritiated thymidine, it has been shown quantitatively that fresh valves sterilised in antibiotics remain viable for varying periods, i.e. they have living fibroblasts capable of synthesising deoxyribonucleic acid[3] and also these fibroblasts are capable of synthesising protein[4]. Preservation of these two metabolic systems provides a means of self-repair of the valve structure and offers the prospect that the valve could become a permanent replacement.

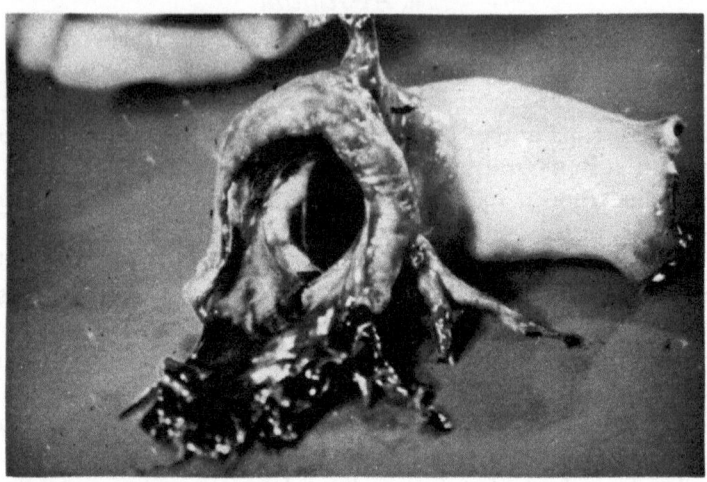

Figure 32.1 Aortic valve allograft collected from routine autopsy material under unsterile conditions within 48 h after donor death

Currently, at the National Heart Hospital the use of antibiotic-treated fresh aortic valves to replace diseased heart valves is now a routine practice. The erratic supply of these valves does not meet the demand. Over the past three and half years, two methods of preservation have been used. Both methods involve the use of National Heart Hospital formula of antibiotic[5] with either (1) or (2) below:

1. Hank's solution for method (1). Valves preserved by this method were used from June 1970 to January 1972.
2. Nutrient medium (medium 199 + 10% calf serum). Valves preserved by this method have been used from January 1972 to the present time.

RESULTS

The viability of valve tissues exposed to the antibiotic in Hank's (Figure 32.2) showed that 73% of fibroblasts studied actually took up thymidine during the first 24 hours of preservation. The valves showed a steady decline in thymidine uptake after four days of storage, which became more pronounced after 18 days.[3]

Compairing the viability between valve tissues exposed to antibiotic in Hank's solution with those exposed to antibiotic–nutrient (Figure 32.3) solution shows that active metabolism in valves placed in the nutrient medium persisted for a longer storage time. The percentage of viability in

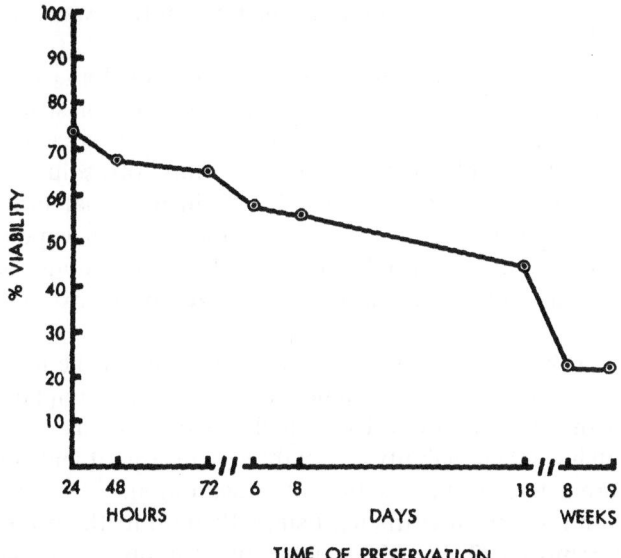

Figure 32.2 Thymidine uptake representing duration of survival of fibroblasts in valves stored in Hank's antibiotic solution at +4 °C

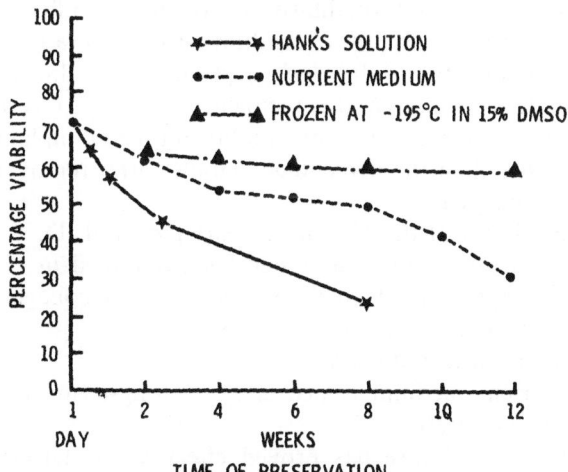

Figure 32.3 Comparison of thymidine uptake as an index for viability. Period of viability is greatly extended when the valves are stored in nutrient medium (at +4 °C) or frozen at −195 °C in 15% DMSO

211

homograft valves preserved in nutrient medium at eight weeks is comparable to the percentage viability of valves preserved in Hank's solution at eight days. These indicate that valves stored in a nutrient medium have a definite advantage over those stored in Hank's solution. As a result of these findings, a nutrient medium storage was introduced for clinical use in January 1972.

As a projection of this it seemed desirable to look for a method of storage offering maintained viability and preservation of structure for longer or even an indefinite period of time. That is achieved by adding 15% dimethylsulphoxide to the nutrient–antibiotic solution and by freezing the valves by 1 °C/min to −70 °C in a special programme cabinet and storing them at −195 °C in liquid nitrogen vapour.[6] The survival curves (Figure 32.3) indicate that a large percentage of metabolically active fibroblasts persist in valves frozen up to five months at −195 °C.

Pieces of aortic homograft wall and anterior leaflet of the mitral cusp have been received for viability studies from each valve implanted and it is also planned that any valves which have to be removed subsequently will have their viability and pathology measured and compared with the figure determined at the time of implantation.

From around 400 fresh grafts used since 1970 up to the present time eleven were removed (Table 32.1) at the time of surgical replacement at intervals of 23 to 1001 days after implantation. The viability and histological changes found in these fresh allografts in the present study are quantitatively and qualitatively somewhat different from those chemically sterilised. In these antibiotic-treated grafts the number of viable donor fibroblasts did decline progressively during the time the valve was functioning in the recipient but not to zero extent. The difference between percentage of viability at time of implantation is about 20–30% higher than the percentage viability after removal except in the longest surviving case.

The pathologist at the National Heart Hospital, Dr E. Olsen, found that the most severe alterations had been obtained in Hank's solution in the mitral position, which showed particularly collagen degeneration and calcification in one patient.

In summary, it would seem that:

1. A nutrient medium is necessary, if long-term storage of viable valves is desirable.
2. Antibiotic mixture has proved effective in sterilising the valves without impairing their viability.
3. Storage of valves at −195 °C allowed keeping the valves viable for a longer period of time.

Table 32.1 Details of eleven fresh antibiotic-treated allografts removed three weeks to three years after implantation

Details of antibiotic-treated aortic valve allografts

	Donor		Recipient		Ster. & Pres. time days in Antibiotic		Pos. of Homogft.	% Viability		Days in patient	Cause of removal
Case No.	Age	Sex	Age	Sex	Hank's	Nutr.	Valve	Before insertion	After remov.		
1	–	–	38	M	–	12	Ao.	–	35%	23	Dehis. of valve and became loose along the whole of the right coronary sinus.
2	–	–	41	F	–	10	Ao.	–	–	151	Notes not available.
3	29	M	14	M	–	37	Ao.	55	40	27	Perf. of 1·5 cm in diameter at the base of right coronary sinus.
4	41	M	62	M	–	32	Ao.	60	45	81	Dehis. of right and non-coronary cusp areas and around the left and non-coronary cusp areas.
5	73	F	13	M	35	–	Mit.	60	35	553	Valve prolapse and calcium with three cusps thickened.
6	15	M	13	M	40	–	Mit.	60	40	93	Gross Mitral Regurgitant and dehis. below the pericardial patch of the mitral ring.
7	66	F	27	M	20	–	Ao.	53	46	195	Perfor. at two sites in the upper suture line of the left coronary sinus & leakage at coronary cusp level.
8	–	–	62	F	20	–	Mit.	42	20	272	Mitral regurgitation.
9	–	–	62	M	–	–	Ao.	35	20	606	Some prolapse of the non-coronary cusp allowing regurg. which was not severe.
10	52	M	52	F	10	–	Mit.	45	35	685	Dehis. of vlave—peripheral lesion.
11	–	–	41	M	–	–	Mit.	cusp is acellular		1001	Chronic rheumatic heart disease—homograft was reported competent.

These three factors have allowed the establishment of an adequate bank of fresh and living homograft valves for clinical use in the National Heart Hospital.

References

1. Hudson, R. E. B. (1966). Pathology of the human aortic valve homograft. *Brit. Heart J.* **28,** 291
2. Smith, J. C. (1967). The pathology of human aortic valve homografts. *Thorax,* **22,** 114
3. Al-Janabi, N., Gonzalez-Lavin, L., Neirotti, R. and Ross, D. N. (1972). Viability of fresh aortic homograft: A quantitative assessment. *Thorax,* **27,** 83–85'
4. Al-Janabi, N., Gibson, K., Rose, J. and Ross, D. N. (1973). Protein synthesis in fresh aortic and pulmonary allografts. *Cardiovasc. Res.,* **7 (2),** 247–250
5. Lockey, E., Al-Janabi, N., Gonzalez-Lavin, L. and Ross, D. N. (1972). A method of sterilisation and preservation of fresh aortic homografts. *Thorax,* **27,** 398–400
6. Al-Janabi, N. and Ross, D. N. (1974). Long-term preservation of fresh viable aortic valve homografts by freezing. *Brit. J. Surg.,* **61,** 229–232

33
Problems of sterilisation
in homograft preparation

Eunice Lockey

The well-prepared and properly inserted homograft has many advantages and like the people who make prosthetic valves, those in the homograft field are constantly trying to improve their product. The author will deal here only with the antibiotic method of sterilisation and to a large extent her presentation is self-critical.

Sir Brian Barnett-Boyes pioneered the technique but it was found that the antibiotic formula which he recommended in 1969 failed to sterilise almost 50% of the valves used. This was probably because these valves were obtained from public mortuaries under totally non-sterile conditions and were very heavily contaminated. Therefore, with the help of Professor B. W. Lacey, a formula of cidal antibiotics designed to kill very heavy inocula of the widest possible range of micro-organisms was evolved. This formula contained:

Methicillin 10 000 μg ml^{-1}
Erythromycin Lactobionate 6000 μg ml^{-1}
Gentamicin 4000 μg ml^{-1}
Nystatin 2500 units ml^{-1}

The method of testing for sterility was to place pieces of donor aorta, about 2 mm by 10 mm in size, in with the valve being sterilised. These were removed after 24 h at 4 °C and a piece of each was placed in serum broth – Brewer's medium and Sabaraud's medium. After 24 h and 72 h incubation at 37 °C subcultures were taken from these liquid media and the plates were incubated for up to five days. At least 500 valves were tested in this way and all were found to be sterile. Over 300 of them were inserted and with only one possible exception they were all apparently trouble free from the infection point of view.

Two major factors, however, made it necessary to re-think the antibiotic combination and method of testing. One was a patient from whose valve a gentamicin resistant pseudomonad was isolated when it was excised three months after implantation; the other was the increasing complexity of the procedures to which the valves were being subjected before use, with at the same time, increasing pressure from the surgeons to reduce the concentration of antibiotics used, in the belief that this would render the valve even more 'viable'.

The work the author now presents is the result of a study done by Miss Waterworth and Dr Berry at University College Hospital and Miss Pearce and the author at the National Heart Hospital and is shortly to be published in detail in *Thorax*.

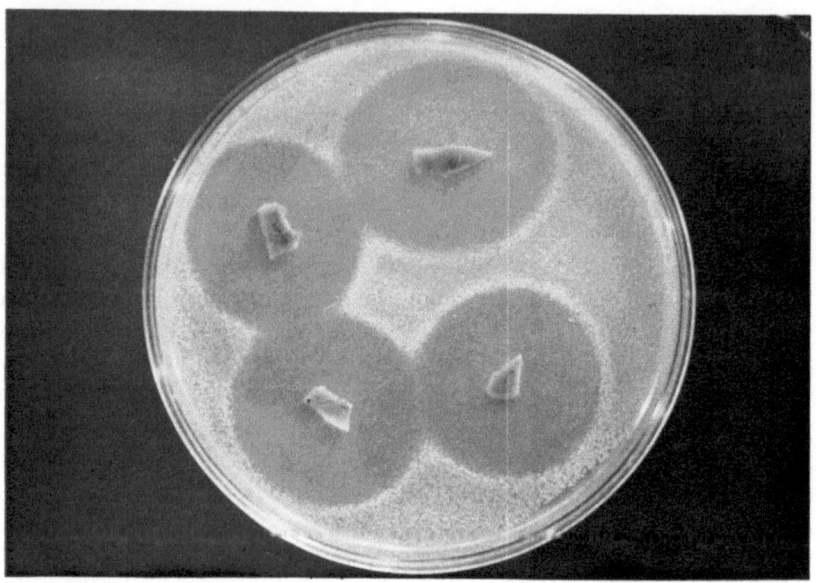

Figure 33.1 Pieces of tissue on blood agar plates seeded with either staphylococci or pseudomonads

First the sterility testing method that had been used was assessed by subjecting the pieces of aorta which had been in the antibiotic mixture with the valve for 24 h, to 30 min agitation in eight successive 100 ml portions of physiological saline. These pieces of tissue were then placed on blood agar plates seeded with either staphylococci or pseudomonads and as Figure 33.1 illustrates sufficient antibiotic was still adherent to the tissue to inhibit growth over a wide area. Manifestly this test for sterility had been invalid. Any joy derived from the thought that so much antibiotic had been implanted with the homo-graft was tempered by the thought of patients allergic to any of the antibiotics.

The next step was to attempt to find a proper method of testing and as this was not one which could be easily and quickly done in a busy routine laboratory the chief aim was to search for a combination of antibiotics which would be unfailingly bactericidal so that sterility testing could be dispensed with. In these experiments organisms isolated from homografts before sterilisation and also 'stock' organisms of known antibiotic resistance patterns were used to inoculate the antibiotic solutions. After incubating for 24 h at room temperature 2 ml of the solution were syringed through a Swinnex-25 filter, followed by 25 ml of sterile water. The filter was then removed and incubated in nutrient broth at 37 °C for 3 days. If growth occurred then the antibiotic combination under examination was not effective. If no growth occurred the efficacy of the antibiotics was confirmed by reinoculating the broth with the same organism. If growth was still inhibited then sufficient carry-over of antibiotic had occurred to render the test of antibiotic efficacy invalid.

Many combinations of antibiotics were tried but the best antibacterial results were obtained with the following mixture:

Penicillin 1000 μg ml^{-1}
Gentamicin 1000 μg ml^{-1}
Polymixin B Sulphate 10 μg ml^{-1} (100 units ml^{-1})
(Nystatin 2500 units ml^{-1})*

This combination had no effect on human embryonic fibroblasts exposed to it for 17 days.

* The nystatin was not added during the testing because it does not go into solution and clogs the pores of the Swinnex filter

Table 33.1

Organism	Number of strains	Number sterilised
Staph. aureus	7	6
Strep. faecalis	7	1
E. coli	6	5
Klebsiella spp.	4	4
Proteus spp.	6	3
Providencia	9	0
Serratia marsescens	4	4
Ps. aeruginosa	7	7
Achromobacter	1	1
Acinetobacter	1	1
Alkaligenes	3	3
	—	—
	55	35

N.B. 20 *Not* sterilised

However even with this antibiotic formula a considerable number of organisms were not killed (Table 33.1). Of course the tests being applied are extremely stringent but as there is virtually no organism which can be regarded as non-pathogenic and most have been incriminated as the cause of bacterial endocarditis, small comfort can be derived by microbiologists from this fact.

The bactericidal action of penicillin is greater at higher temperatures and certainly incubation at 37 °C greatly improved performance against *Strep. faecalis*. Therefore, the author would recommend that the valves should be incubated for 24 h at 37 °C in their antibiotic solutions, before being refrigerated.

Counts of surviving organisms after exposure to the antibiotic formula, were also made and in most cases a 99·9% kill was achieved, but those organisms such as certain members of the Providencia which are resistant to gentamicin and polymixin showed a much higher survival rate.

In summary, perfection in this area is probably impossible but the author does not think antibiotics can be relied on unfailingly to sterilise homograft tissues.

34
Tissue valve preparation
A. Carpentier, J. Relland and Ch. Dubost

At the first workshop on tissue valves[1] held in 1969 in Silverado, California, the general impression, as summarized by D.C. McGoon was that the fascia lata valves appeared to have the most promising future followed by fresh homografts, preserved homografts and last of all xenografts valves. The facts did not confirm this prediction. Fascia lata valves were rapidly abandoned and both preserved and fresh homografts valves progressively led to disenchantment.[2,9] The initial results with xenograft valves were discouraging.[3,4] However there was a renewed interest in this field when, in 1968, we introduced glutaraldehyde in the preparation of these valves, and found that this product significantly improved their durability.[6]

A – FACTORS AFFECTING GRAFT VALVE DURABILITY

Three factors affect the long term durability of a tissue valve. These are: valve selection, valve mounting and valve preparation.

I – Valve selection
From an immunological point of view, it would appear to be preferable to place greater confidence in descending order in autograft valves, followed by homograft valves and least of all xenograft valves.

However, the use of an autologous tissue such as fascia lata or pericardium, the structure of which is not adapted to valve function, led to the deterioration and shrinkage of the leaflets. The use of the patient's pulmonary valve as suggested by D. Ross is a valuable biological alternative but far from the ideal solution because of the additional time required to carry out the procedure and also because a homograft valve must still be placed in the pulmonary position.

In fact, the choice is limited to three types of tissue valves: fresh homograft, preserved homograft and preserved xenograft. All three grafts possess important advantages: decreased risk of thrombo-embolism, avoidance of anticoagulation, and the progressive nature of the occasional valve failure permitting elective reoperation under optimal conditions.

Advantages incumbent to xenograft valves are: easy availability, wide range of sizes and the possibility of commercial production assuring perfect standardization of the valves and accurate quality control in the laboratory of both valve structure and valve function.[5]

Whatever the type of graft used, quality control of valve structure is a critical point. A large percentage of valves must be discarded due to abnormal cusp configuration, cusp fenestration, areas of weakness, infection or calcification. There is no doubt that some cases of valve failure in both homograft and xenograft valves have been due to improper valve selection in the early series. For example, at the present time at Edwards and Hancok laboratories, initial selection leads to the elimination of 70% of the valves harvested at the slaughter house.

II – Valve mounting

One of the most important advances in the use of tissue valves was the introduction of frame mounted valves. This was done in order to eliminate the potential errors in valve implantation. In addition, valve function can be tested in the laboratory ensuring excellent mechanical performance. The disadvantages inherent in this technique are: the reduction of the ratio of the internal and external diameters and the rigidity of the stent. The use of flexible struts (Reis–Hancok) and the recently introduced incorporated flexible stent by Edwards laboratories are important advances in the solution of this problem.

III – Valve preparation

From our early experience with xenograft valve implantation (1965–1968), we learned that the most important factor affecting valve durability was that of the method of preparation.[6] This is true not only for xenograft valves but also for homograft valves. While homograft valves induced a less important graft–host reaction than the heterograft valves, both types of grafts were confronted with the problems of collagen degeneration. The reason being that collagen turnover, which is responsible for the continuous regeneration of normal valves, either ceased completely in preserved homografts or xenografts[5] or at best became severely altered in fresh homografts.[2] On the other hand, the theoretical possibility of valve regeneration by host fibroblast infiltration failed to materialise in both homografts and xenografts.[5]

(1) – Homograft valve preparation
There are two ways of using a homograft valve:

    (a) the living grafts are preserved in such a way that the cells are alive at the time of implantation. The valve is kept in a tissue culture medium at 4 °C for periods of less than three weeks. The durability of a living homograft valve is based in theory on the possibility of cells retaining full metabolic function assuring a normal turnover of the collagen.[2] In practice, this has been shown not to be the case.

(b) Preserved homografts are valves preserved in a high concentration of antibiotics in saline for periods of more than three weeks. They may be frozen but this is responsible for modification of the collagen structure. The durability of a non-living homograft valve is based on the theoretical possibility of valve regeneration by host cell ingrowth but this in fact does not occur.

(2) – Xenograft valve preparation
Important advances have been made in the past 5 years in the knowledge of the factors involved in the graft–host reaction and in collagen degeneration leading to appropriate changes in valve preparation.

(a) Cellular factors: As already stated, the theoretical regeneration of a graft by the infiltration of host fibroblasts failed to materialise. Moreover, that cellular ingrowth which did occur proved to be more harmful than beneficial as the cells invading the graft tissue were most often inflammatory in nature. This led to the concept of "Greffe Protégée"[6] in which the aortic sheath was enveloped in a fabric covering in order to protect it from cellular ingrowth.

(b) Chemical factors: At the histological level, a valve is made up of collagen fibres, elastin fibres, ground substance and cells. At the molecular level, the components are: the collagen, with a triple helix configuration, the elastin, the mucopolysaccharides, the glycoproteins and the soluble proteins. All of these components have different antigenic powers: collagen and elastin for example appear to be much less antigenic than are mucopolysaccharides, glycoproteins, and soluble proteins.[6,5] Thus it seemed logical to try and eliminate most of the antigenic determinants.[6] Soluble proteins and some mucopolysaccharides were eliminated by washing the valve in Hank's solution for 4 hours.[6] Collagen degeneration which is the result of a slow hydrolytic reaction or enzyme digestion could be delayed by the introduction of cross linkages between the collagen molecules. Various cross linking factors such as dialdehyde starch, mercurial salts, formaldehyde were tried for heterograft valve preservation with disappointing results because of the reversible nature of the cross linkages.[4,5] The introduction, in 1968, of glutaraldehyde was an important advance in valve preparation.[6] The true chemical action of this product is somewhat complex and can be summarised as follows: As a tanning agent, glutaraldehyde gives the tissue increased stability by forming irreversible cross linkages between collagen molecules.

These cross linkages are probably of the Schiff base type which is the binding between one aldehyde group of the glutaraldehyde and one free amino group of the collagen molecule:

$$COH + NH_3 \rightarrow CH = N \text{ or}$$
$$COH + NH_3 \rightarrow CH_2—NH \text{ (hydrated form)}.$$

The fact that the glutaraldehyde molecule possesses 2 free aldehyde groups allows the same molecule to bind two amino groups of two adjacent collagen molecules. In fact, the nature of intermolecular binding may be more complex with the formation of an intermediate compound linked to the collagen molecules by covalent bonds and hydrogen bonds. On the other, hand, by the blocking of the reactive free prosthetic groups extending from the body of both collagen and glycoprotein molecules glutaraldehyde significantly reduces the antigenicity of the tissue.

This chemical treatment leads to drastic changes in the tissue so that the valve must be considered more a prosthesis made from biological material than a graft *stricto sensu*. The term "bioprosthesis" which we proposed in 1969[5,6] is better adapted to this type of frame mounted chemically treated graft valve. It permits a clear distinction between the non-treated grafts, the durability of which is supposed to be due to tissue regeneration and the bioprosthesis such as the glutaraldehyde preserved heterograft, the durability of which is based on the stability of the biological material.

B – GRAFT EVOLUTION

Graft evolution is a result of the competition between constructive reactions and destructive reactions. Constructive reactions are the result of cellular metabolism in living grafts, or of the activity of host fibroblasts in non living grafts. Destructive reactions are the result of inflammatory cell penetration or of collagen degeneration.

I – Evolution of living homograft valves
Since we have had no personnal experience in living homograft valves, we will summarise Dr Angell's work on this subject.[2] The valve cusps invariably become thickened and the donor cells progressively disappear. The thickening of the cusps is both due to the presence of a fibrinous platelet sheath covering the surface of the valve and to areas of active fibroplasia which may indicate malfunction of the cellular metabolism. Areas of hyalinization and sometimes necrosis may appear later and are usually the cause of valve failure.

II – Evolution of preserved homografts

Preserved homograft valves usually show degenerative changes in the tissue structure i.e.: hyalinization, elastin fibre fragmentation and necrosis. Most fibroblasts may be encountered in localised areas but never have these fibroblastic ingrowths been able to assure regeneration of the valves.[9]

III – Evolution of xenograft valves

(1) Preserved xenograft valves showed two types of graft disease occurring 6 months to 2 years after implantation: inflammatory reaction and collagen degeneration. Inflammatory reaction seemed to be the host's response to foreign tissue and could take the form of non specific inflammatory reactions with polymorphonuclear leucocytes, hysticocytes, and macrophages, or the form of a typical immunological reaction with mononuclear pyroninophilic cells of the lymphocyte and plasma cell series. Both reactions may disappear after several months or become extensive leading to cusp perforations. Collagen degeneration may take different aspects such as necrosis, hyalinization, or calcification leading to valve failure.

(2) Glutaraldehyde preserved xenografts showed a completely different evolution. Inflammatory reactions never occurred or were limited to transistory foci of 10 to 2 cells localized on the surface of the cusps. Collagen degeneration was delayed and limited both in its extent and its importance 6 years after implantation in the mitral area, valve had a perfectly preserved structure with only limited areas of hyalinization and collagen fragmentation since these lésions were predominantly located at the central part of the cusps which is also the hinged portion, it seems logical to conclude that they were due to the repetitive flexion of the leaflets.[7] Thus, because of excellent biological tolerance, glutaraldehyde preserved valves are going to be confronted with long-term fatigue-induced lesions which did not exist with previous types of xenografts because of their relative short durability. At the present time, the incidence of valve failure at five years is 10% in our experience which has been extensively reported elsewhere.[7]

This failure rate may depend upon the nature and physical characteristics of the "encapsulation" of the graft. A process we have observed in two specimens recovered after 5 years. This is a process of complete covering of the graft by a sheath of fibrin and collagen extending from the host over the exposed surface of the valve. The thickness of this sheath is about 50 to 100 microns on both sides of the leaflets. The structure of the sheath is that of collagen and elastin fibres oriented to the axis of the valve and a remarkably small number of active fibroblasts. Because of this well adapted structure and reduced thickness, the valves remained perfectly pliable. The sheath was perfectly adherent to the cusp surfaces and there was no penetration of the tissue composing the sheath into the cusp tissue itself. Thus, this process of "encapsulation" appears to be essentially different from that of host cell ingrowth and valve regeneration. This may well turn out to be an extremely important factor in improved valve durability as the valve structure is itself reinforced.

CONCLUSION

More than 6 years follow up in the different types of tissue valves allow certain conclusions:

1. Autograft valves made from fascia lata or pericardium must be abandoned because of inadequate adaptation of the tissue to valve function.
2. Homografts are still in use but the practical difficulties of obtaining them and a somewhat high incidence of valve failure at 5 years limits their use.
3. Glutaraldehyde-preserved frame-mounted xenografts appear to have the greatest durability to date. This is in large part due to the importance of the method of preservation.
4. The failure rate with glutaraldehyde-preserved xenografts at 5 years is 10% due mainly to fatigue induced lesions.
5. The process of "encapsulation" which we have observed after 5 years may be the critical factor in achieving long term durability for these valves.

References

1. Proceedings of the First International Workshop on Tissues Valves (F. Gerbode, Editor), *Ann. Surg.*, Suppl. to Vol. 172 No. 1
2. Angell, W. W., Shumway, N. E. and Kosek, J. C. (1972). A Five Year Study of Viable Aortic Valve Homografts. *J. Thorac. Cardiovasc. Surg.*, **64**, 329
3. Binet, J. P., Carpentier, A. and Langlois, J. (1975). Implantation de valves hétérologues dans le traitment des valvulopathies aortiques. *CR. Acad. Chir. Paris*, **261**, 5733
4. Carpentier, A. (1966). Les greffes valvulaires hétéroplastiques. *Foulon Paris*, Ch. 13.
5. Carpentier, A. (1972). Principles of Tissue Valve Transplantation in Chapter 22 and I: From Xenograft to Bioprosthesis (Evolution of Concepts and Techniques in Valvular Heterograft Valves) in Biological Tissue in Heart Valve Replacement. Butterworths, London 1972.
6. Carpentier, A. (1969). Biological Factors Affecting Long Term Results of Heterograft Valves. *J. Thorac. and Cardiovasc. Surg.* **18**, 467
7. Carpentier, A., Deloche, A., Relland, J., Fabiani, J. N., Forman, J., Camillieri, J. P., Soyer, R. and Dubost Ch.,: Six Year Follow up of Glutaraldehyde Preserved Heterografts (1974), *J. Thorac. Cardiovas. Surgery* **68**, 771

8. Reis, R. L., Hancock, W. D., Yarbrough, J. W., Glancy, D. L. and Morrow, A. G, The flexible Stent (1971). A new concept in the Fabrication of Tissue Heart Valve Prosthesis. *J. Thorac Cardiovasc. Surg.* **62,** 683

9. Wallace, R. B., Londe, S. P. and Titus J. L. (1974). Aortic Valve Replacement With Preserved Aortic Valve Homografts. *J. Thorac. Cardiovasc. Surgery*, **67,** No.

10. Zuhdi, N. M.: discussion of Dr Walace's paper (See Ref. 8) and Dr Carpentier's paper (see Ref. 7).

35
Mechanical characteristics of vena cava and a technique for its use, unsupported, for mitral valve replacement

B. T. Williams

The currently available mechanical heart valves have reached a position of relative reliability, but all have the disadvantage of poor haemodynamic characteristics. This will only be improved when a material is developed which allows a completely new valve design.

MECHANICAL CHARACTERISTICS OF VENA CAVA

These closely resemble those of normal valve cusps in several important respects; when stressed, elongation of the tissue occurs easily at first and later 'locking' of the tissue ensues, a situation in which large increments of force produce little increase in length. The percentage elongation when 'locking' supervenes varies with the alignment of the tissue for both vena cava and valve cusp.

Figure 35.1 is a graph of stress *v.* percentage elongation for a normal aortic valve cusp. When stress is applied in its transvere axis, locking occurs at 10% elongation compared with 25% when the force is applied in the longitudinal axis of the cusp: with fresh vena cava similar shapes of curve are obtained (Figure 35.2). However, the absolute values for percentage elongation when the tissue locks are higher overall for vena cava than for valve cusps. This greater extensibility is a critical factor when using the tissue as a material for valve cusp replacement.

THE USE OF SUPERIOR VENA CAVA (SVC) FOR VALVE REPLACEMENT

Complete resection of the SVC in patients has been made possible by the development of a new vascular prosthesis of woven silicone rubber (Ashton). This provides the possibility of using the patient's own superior vena cava for valve replacement with the theoretical advantages of having not only the correct mechanical characteristics, but being fresh, living, endothelialised and immunologically inactive. The experimental technique for this operation is in two stages:

1. Resection of the SVC. The vessel is first dissected free of attachments

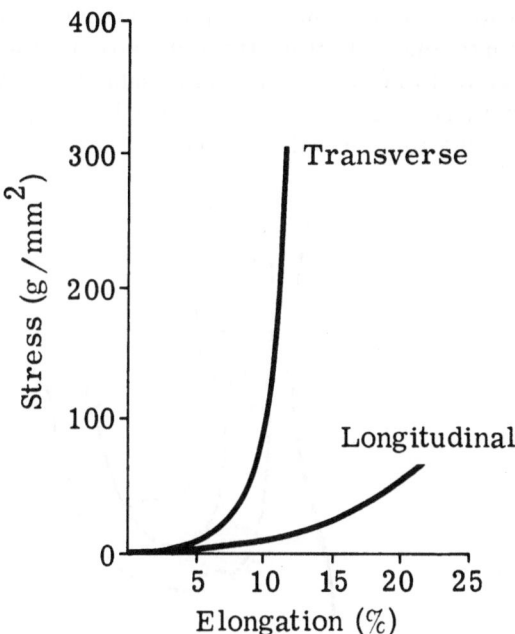

Figure 35.1 Stress–strain curves for normal aortic valve cusp

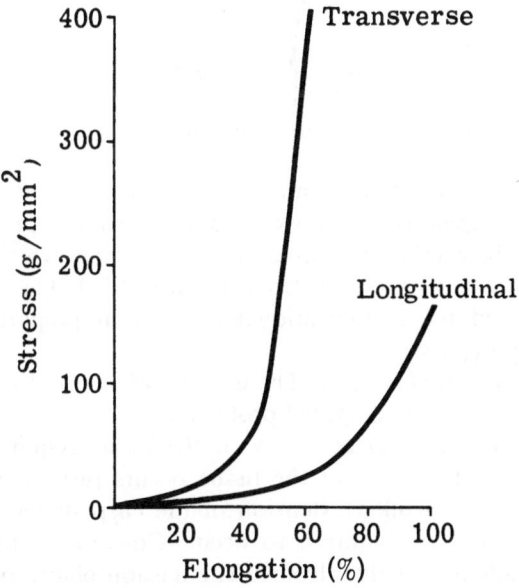

Figure 35.2 Stress–strain curves for vena cava

throughout its length. A jointed cannula bearing a side outlet hole is introduced into the SVC from the right atrium (Figure 35.3a). This allows SVC blood to be conducted to the right atrium, whilst the SVC is resected between closed tapes (Figure 35.3b), leaving a cuff of vein above and below to anastomose to the prosthesis.

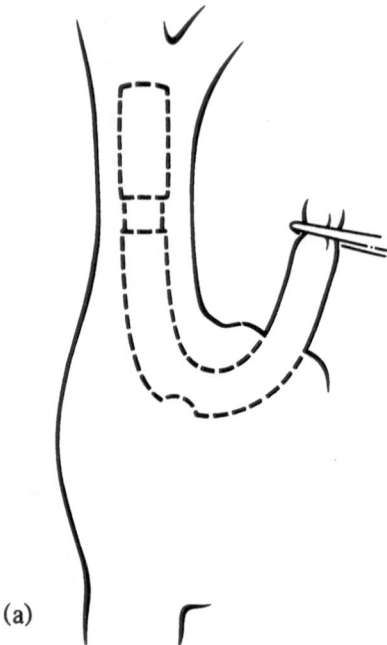

(a)

Figure 35.3 (a) Technique of resection of the superior vena cava

The connection in the cannula allows the segment of SVC to be removed and replaced by the woven silicone rubber prosthesis with only transient obstruction to blood flow, following which the upper and lower anastomosis are completed (Figure 35.3c). The jointed cannula is then replaced by a conventional cannula in preparation for cardiopulmonary bypass.

2. Mitral valve replacement. The use of SVC tissue for the construction of a valve presents two special problems.

Firstly, the great extensibility of the tissue requires that it is preloaded, so that locking of the tissue occurs just as the cusps oppose. Excessive, uncontrolled extension of the cusp under load allows prolapse and free regurgitation to occur. Conversely, premature locking precludes adequate valve closure. The tension placed on the valve cusps during insertion is therefore critical.

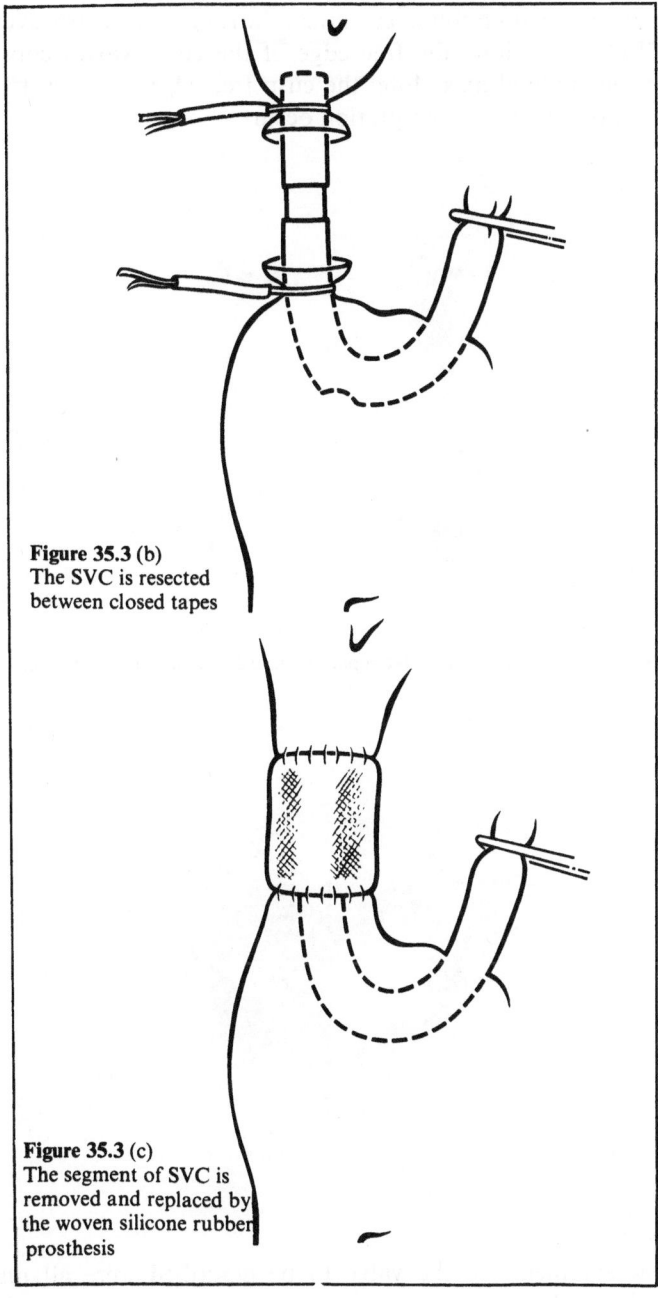

Figure 35.3 (b)
The SVC is resected
between closed tapes

Figure 35.3 (c)
The segment of SVC is
removed and replaced by
the woven silicone rubber
prosthesis

Secondly, it has been found essential to arrange for the transverse axis of the SVC to tie along the free edge of the cusp; valves constructed with the longitudinal axis along the cusp free edge continue to extend until cusp prolapse and regurgitation occurs.

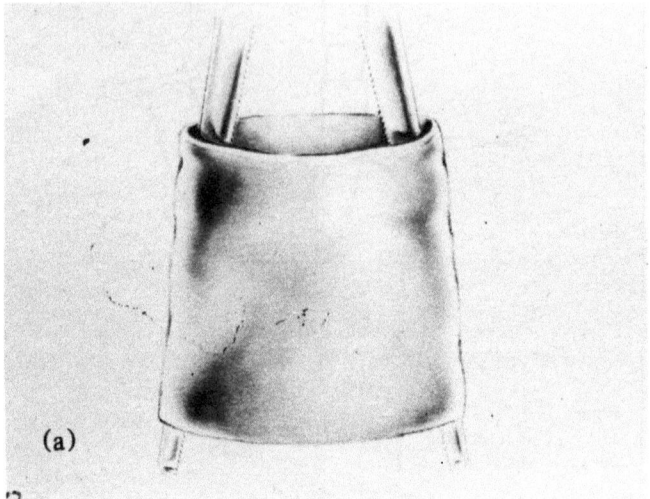

(a)

Figure 35.4a Technique of mitral valve replacement using a cuff of superior vena cava

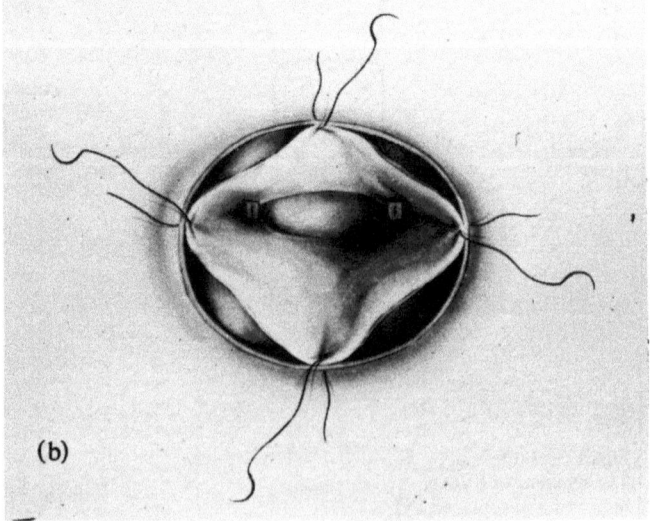

(b)

Figure 35.4b

The measurements in the valve to be described were all made on tissue under load.

Figure 35.4a shows the simple technique of placing the cuff of SVC under load using a large pair of forceps; the width is measured, the diameter calculated and this figure used to match the cuff to the mitral cannulas. Longitudinal traction allows the cuff to be trimmed to the correct length; the ratio of length : diameter has been found experimentally to be 1·5 : 1.

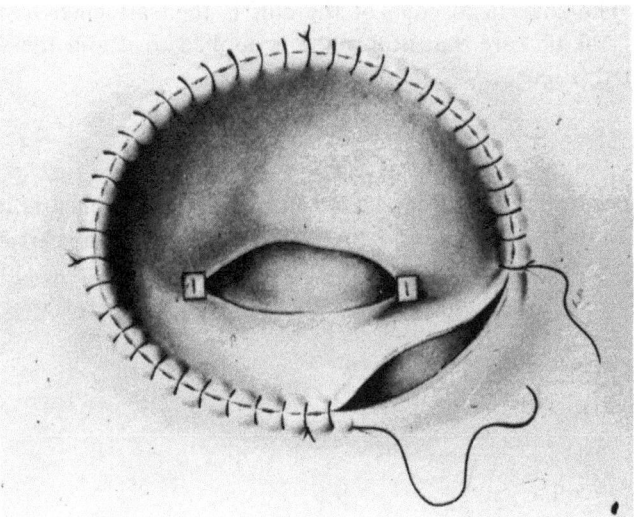

Figure 35.4 c

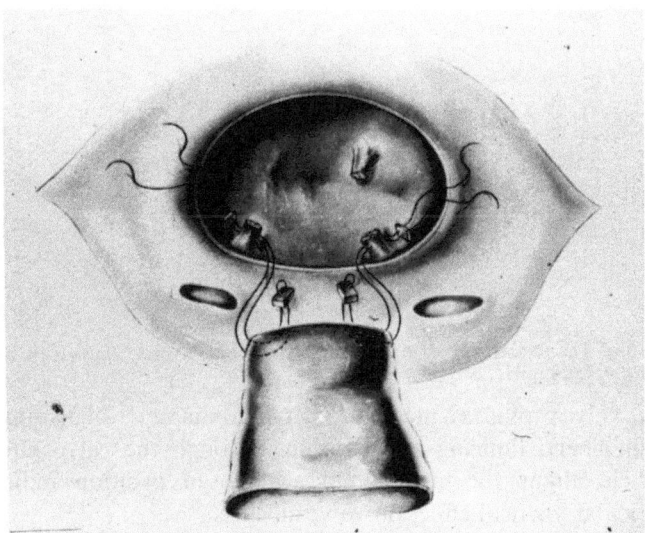

Figure 35.4 d

After excision of the mitral valve, the left ventricular cavity is carefully inspected and two groups of papillary muscles on the ventricular wall selected so that their distance apart approximates to the diameter of the SVC cuff. The lower end of the cuff is attached to these papillary muscles, reinforcing the attachment with Teflon felt pledgets (Figure 35.4b). The superficial edge of the cuff is then attached to the mitral annulus, taking care that no torsion is applied to it and the suture line completed (Figures 35.4c and 35.4d).

RESULTS

This procedure was first conducted in twenty cadaver hearts in order to establish its feasibility and has subsequently been carried out in experimental animals.

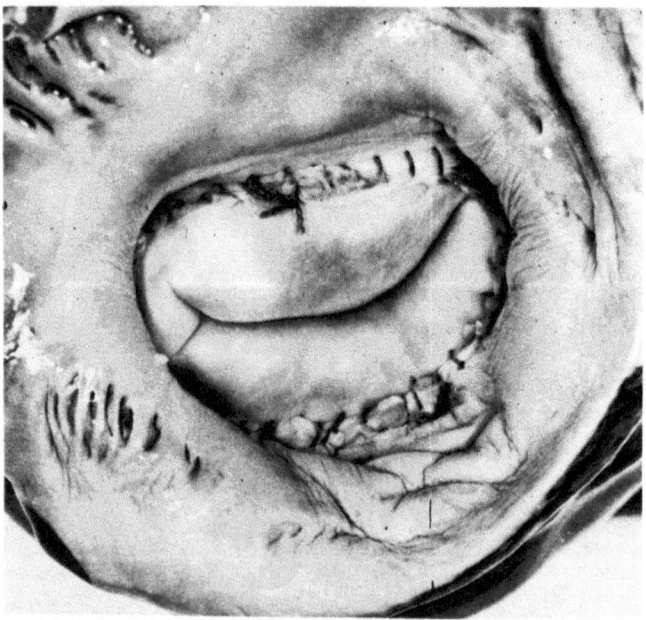

Figure 35.5 The closed valve from the left atrial aspect (human); the ventricular pressure = 150 mmHg

The valve provides a mean unobstructed diameter of 34 mm in the adult human heart. Pouring a fluid bolus through the valve into an empty ventricle aligns the cusps in a semiclosed position indicating good ventricular vortical effect on valve closure.

Valve competence has been tested by pressurising the left ventricle with water up to 200 mmHg. Figure 35.5 shows a valve subjected to a left ventricular pressure of 150 mmHg. Its competence and a configuration closely mimicking a normal mitral valve can be clearly seen.

The attachment of the lower end of the SVC cuff to the lateral wall of the ventricle was designed to obviate outflow tract obstruction. This has been confirmed by palpation of a valve under pressure through the aortic root.

36
Homograft and autograft replacement of the aortic valve

D. N. Ross

In assessing the long-term results of an operation, it is conventional to present statistics in terms of operative mortality and late mortality. From the patient's point of view he is likely to want to know his prospects after the operation and in particular he will want to know the quality of life he is going to lead. Surgeons have to become more sophisticated in the presentation of their results and make a greater effort to find ways of presenting results so that they are comparable. There is a need for agreed and established criteria for assessing the results of various surgical procedures if surgeons are going to benefit from their cumulative experience in cardiac surgery. It goes without saying of course that they should not delude themselves in presenting their results, nor should they mislead one another since it is the patient who matters and not the surgeon's statistics.

The first point the author would like to consider is the much abused term 'long-term results'. After six to 18 months, results have been presented as long-term results and three year results are considered by some to be very long-term. As in the cancer statisticians' books, long-term results could be presented in multiples of five years, i.e. five year long-term results or 10 year long-term results, ,or communications could simply be headed as an 18 month experience or a three year experience. Dr McGoon of the Mayo Clinic has introduced the use of actuarial survival curves as a medium for presenting results. Nevertheless, there are still great difficulties in arriving at agreed criteria on how to compile actuarial curves and it may be safer to talk rather of survival curves. It could be preferable not to include the operative mortality in presenting survival curves but rather to give the operative mortality separately. The survival curve would then start from 100% and exclude the operative mortality which lowers the take off point of the graph. This is because the chief interest is in knowing what happens to the patient once he leaves hospital and a curve may look worse than it really is because it started from a lower point which may not reflect the current operative mortality and may be misleading in relation to other results.

Dr Kirklin has presented survival curves showing homograft together with Starr valve results. There is a higher mortality in his Starr valve replacements which makes the survival census look worse, but the author believes that if the operative mortality was excluded and they all started from 100%, the curves would indicate more usefully what happened to the valves. There is a degradation in the curve for the

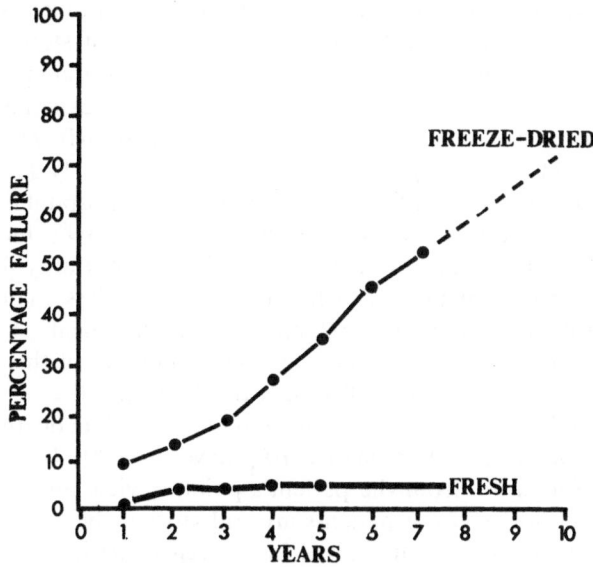

Figure 36.1 Survival curves excluding operative mortality. The first five years using freeze-dried valves are compared with the results from 1967 to date.

Starr valve which is not apparent in Dr Kirklin's homograft results. He has also tried to iron out some of the difficulties of comparison by trying to select a group of Starr valves with a mean age comparable with the mean age of the patients with homografts. There still appears to be a greater fall off in the Starr valves when compared with the homografts. In the light of these curves why is Dr Kirklin not using homografts since he seems to have proved that they are better valves? Perhaps the curve has been misinterpreted and this emphasises the need for agreed criteria. Furthermore, it is important to have a uniform sample of valves, on a curve, because modification and improvements are made and if they are added to the sample they tend to make the results appear better. Similarly, if earlier valves and earlier experience are added to recent results, whether they be homograft or mechanical, the results tend to look poorer.

With this general background in mind the author has tried to review his homograft replacements over a period of 10 years, and, to keep the sample as uniform as possible, he has included only isolated aortic valve homografts inserted by a single surgeon and in one hospital. All the valves have been in for at least a year and there are 311 patients in this series. The design of valve of course has not changed over the years since it was introduced, nor has there been any significant change in the technique of insertion, all being free-sewn valves without a supporting frame. The only alteration has been the technique of sterilisation and storage. Freeze drying was certainly a denaturing and damaging process and was therefore stopped in 1967 after the first five years experience (Figure 36.1). In the subsequent five years all the valves have been frozen, or kept at 4 °C. Of the 311 patients operated upon, there were 42 early deaths, within the first 30 days of surgery. That represents an overall hospital mortality of 13·5% which has fallen over the past five years to a 3·9% mortality, so that on this basis it is fair to say that the operative mortality for isolated aortic valve replacement with a homograft is now less than 4%. This compares satisfactorily with prosthetic valve replacements. Late deaths may or may not be related to the valve, but a number of them certainly are. There have been a total of 44 late deaths from all causes over the 10 year period under review and that represents 14% late deaths or about 1·4% year. Of the 14% late deaths, 10% have probably been related to the valve. Therefore, from the patient's point of view one can say that 72% of the entire group of patients are still alive at the end of 10 years, but of course not all of the valves have been in patients for 10 years although all have been in for at least 1 year. The obvious is stated in order to emphasise some of the problems in presentation. Since giving up the freeze-drying process of the valve the long-term results look more favourable with an incidence of only 2·9% of late deaths over the past six years, or $\frac{1}{2}$% year. Figure 36.2 shows a survival curve to indicate the difference between earlier survival probabilities and more recent survival probabilities using fresh homografts. Again the curves are influenced adversely by the increased operative mortality of the past, compared with the operative mortality of the present. This is ironed out because the two curves are started at the same point.

Failure of the valve, or the homograft, should be distinguished from other forms of postoperative complication. The term 'valve failure' also requires definition. Valve failure is defined as a major deterioration of the valve requiring its replacement or causing death of the patient. It is relevant to add at this point that valve failure in a homograft certainly does occur, but it is a slow process. There is generally a slow clinical deterioration over a period of about two to three years, which gives plenty of time and warning for the need for valve replacement. This contrasts, in the author's experience, with valve failure in mechanical valves, which are usually sudden and often fatal. This is a point worth emphasising. There have been a total of 52 failed valves in the series of 311 patients, which is 16% of the total group of valves inserted. Put in another way, 62% of the patients survive with their original valves in

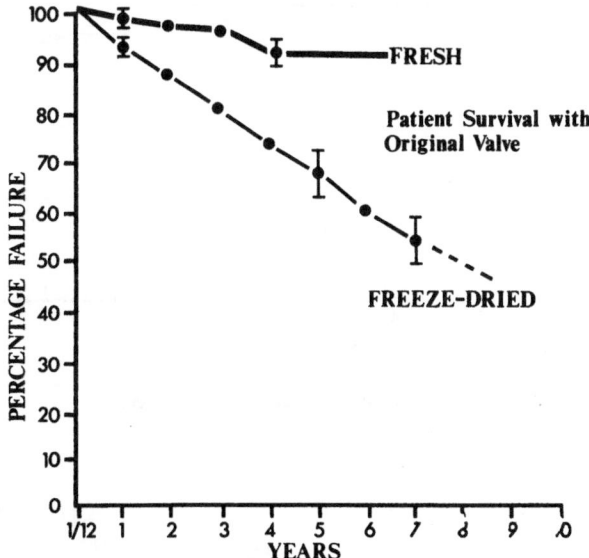

Figure 36.2 Actuarial curves relating the incidence of failure with the method of storing the valve.

place. This is over a 10 year period and it is not known how well the valve survival curve would compare with a series of 10 years of mechanical valve replacement. Results can be presented in many ways and it was thought that perhaps the best way to present them was in years (Figure 36.3a). For instance, if the survival per year is examined one can at least be sure that all the patients in that year have had their valve in for that length of time. On this basis one can see what has happened to the valves inserted each year. The curve for 1968 represents a half-way situation with all the valves in that group in for five or more years. In 1968 the preparation technique was changed and the freeze-drying process was abandoned. It looks as though there was an improvement from that time, but all subsequent valves have been in a shorter period of time. Since 1968 there has apparently been a zero failure rate.

With regard to the initial question posed – what is the quality of life the patient can expect to lead after the operation? – this is important and

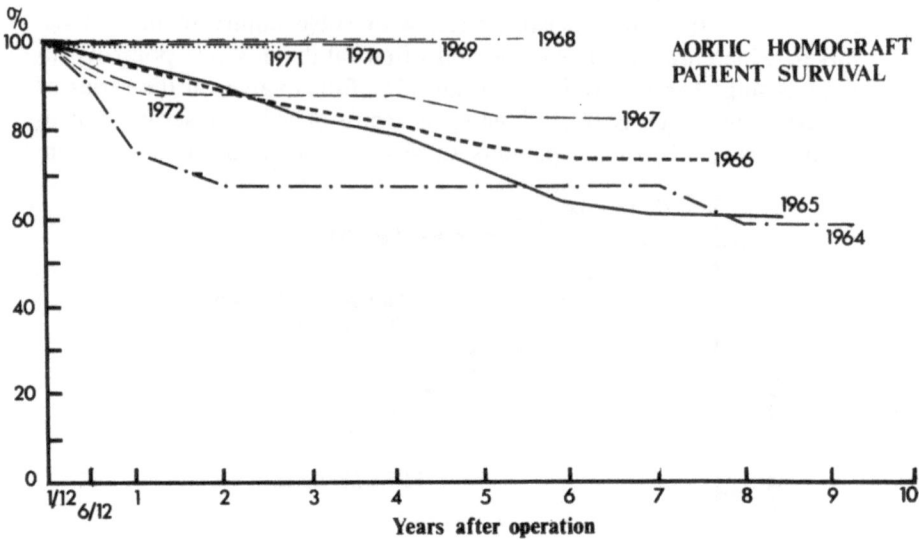

Figure 36.3a Patient survival curves related to year of valve insertion.

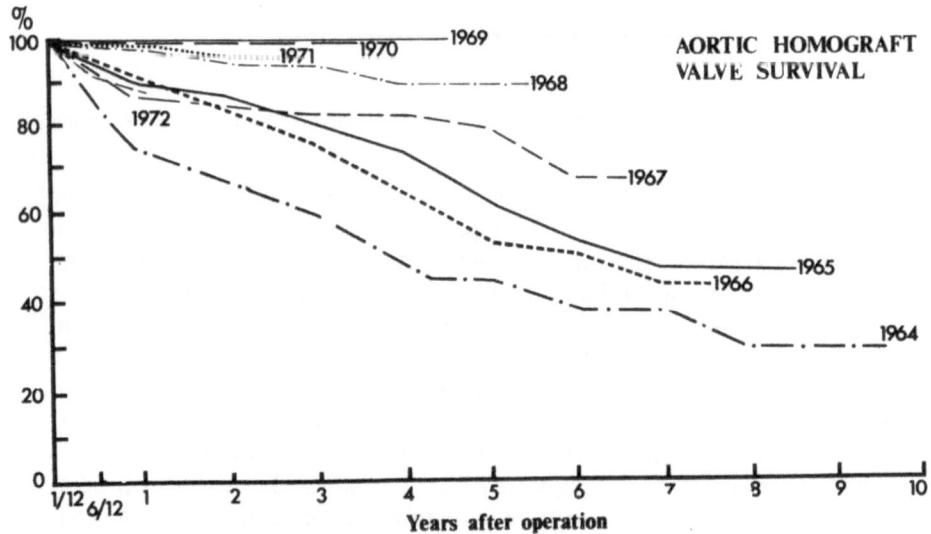

Figure 36.3b Survival curve for the original homograft valve.

the question can be answered immediately. The quality of life after a successful homograft operation is excellent. The incidence of embolism is zero. The need for and therefore the dangers and inconvenience of anticoagulants and the complications attendant upon their use, is also zero. Haemolysis does not normally worry patients but anaemia can and this of course is entirely absent with homografts. Surviving patients have been graded by conventional clinical criteria on the New York Heart Association grading. About 75% of the original group are now in class 1 and 2, whereas an equal number were in class 3 and 4 preoperatively. There is a relatively high proportion ungraded here because they represent people who are not in the country, but presumably a comfortable proportion would be in each group.

Of the observed complications, diastolic murmurs are still the most common feature in homograft work. Although there is a significant number of diastolic murmurs in the author's series – only 2·5% – they are judged to be haemodynamically important from a point of view of widening of the pulse pressure, or requiring a further operation. The current early incidence of audible diastolic murmurs is 25% and these seem to be stable with no tendency to progress to clinical regurgitation. The late onset of a murmur usually means valve failure. Infection has not been a problem and rupture and calcification has not been apparent over the past five years. In fact, the early and late deaths, failures and complications have all fallen dramatically since changing from the chemically preserved type of homograft to antibiotic sterilised fresh homografts. Fresh and frozen homografts have now been in use for six years with few problems.

THE AUTOGRAFT OR PULMONARY SWITCH OPERATION FOR ISOLATED AORTIC VALVE DISEASE

This operation (Figures 36.4 & 36.5) is generally reserved for patients under 40 years of age. The rationale is to insert a permanent and non-deteriorating replacement of the aortic valve for patients in this young age group. They represent a selected group and are not entirely comparable with the homograft or prosthetic series. To date 117 cases have been operated upon at the National Heart Hospital between 1967 and 1973 and they represent a seven year long-term follow-up, again with all valves in place for at least one year. The hospital mortality has been 14, or 12%, which again reflects the problems of introducing a new technique. Valve-related late deaths have been 3, or 2·8%, which is low. If these figures are compared with homografts inserted over the six year period it can be seen that currently there is a higher operative mortality but a reduced late valve failure incidence. The problem however is that over the past five years since using fresh valves the failure rate is more comparable so that the dilemma is to know whether to put in a homograft or an autograft. The known low incidence of valve failure in the autograft encourages perseverance with it as a method of valve replacement and now that the mortality of the homograft and autograft is the same it will form an interesting basis for comparison. Probably, living autografts will eventually prove to be the

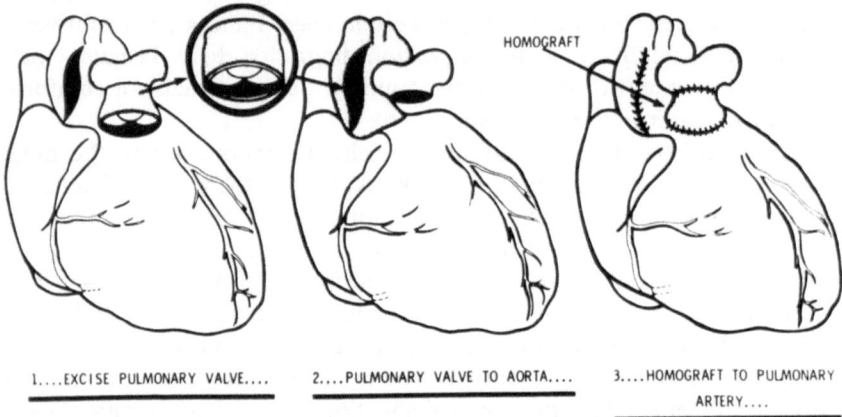

1....EXCISE PULMONARY VALVE....   2....PULMONARY VALVE TO AORTA....   3....HOMOGRAFT TO PULMONARY ARTERY....

Figure 36.4 Diagram of the main stages of the pulmonary autograft operation.

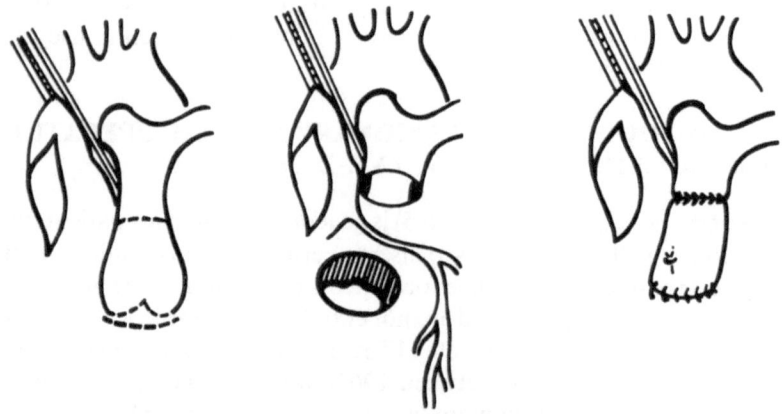

PULMONARY VALVE EXCISED
RIGHT VENTRICULAR OUTFLOW
RECONSTITUTED WITH HOMOGRAFT

Figure 36.5 Pulmonary autograft operation showing excision of the pulmonary valve and reconstitution with homograft.

best. Incidentally, the switch operation involves a homograft replacement of the pulmonary valve, and in contradistinction to the results that have been reported in children it does not appear to calcify in this site. Why there is this age difference is not understood and the homograft valve in this position is not an important source of mortality or morbidity. There has been only one pulmonary valve requiring replacement.

In summary, the homograft valve is fully competitive with current prosthetic devices, both from the point of view of mortality and patient survival. The problem of late valve failure seems currently to be under control. Also, most important from the patient's point of view, it offers a superior quality of life. Autografts may well offer additional advantages in the long term.

Table 36.1 Isolated aortic homografts—311 patients, 10 year follow-up period

Incidence of valve failure	16% (52 patients—20 died)
Surviving patients with original valve	62% (193 patients)

Table 36.2A Clinical grading of patients surviving with aortic homografts

Class I	60%
Class II	14.3%
Class III	3.1%
Class IV	0%
Uncertain	23.6%

Table 36.3 Late deaths in 311 isolated aortic homografts

Related to homograft	28	(9%)
Uncertain	8	(2.6%)
Unrelated	8	(2.6%)
Total	44	(14.2%)

Table 36.4 Isoaortic homografts—311 patients, 10 year follow-up

Hospital mortality	13.5%	(42 patients)
Late deaths (all causes)	14%	(44 patients)
Surviving patients	72.5%	(225 patients)

Table 36.5 Isolated aortic homografts—311 patients, 10 year follow-up

Incidence of late death from all causes	1.4% per year
Incidence of late death related to the valve	0.9% per year
Incidence of valve failure	1.6% per year

Table 36.6 Incidence of complications in isolated aortic homografts

	10 year follow-up	*5 year follow-up*
Diastolic murmur	33.1%	24%
Infection	3.2%	2%
Perforation of rupture	.9%	0%
Calcification	.9%	0%

Table 36.7 Isolated aortic homgrafts—10 year follow-up hospital mortality

	Total	Deaths	
1963	1	–	
1964	18	4	
1965	50	9	*Freeze-dried*
1966	70	13	
1967	45	11	
1968	27	3	
1969	4	0	
1970	4	0	
1971	28	0	*Fresh and frozen*
1972	32	1	
1973	32	1	
Total	311	42	

Overall mortality 13.5%
Over last 5 years 3.9%

Table 36.8 Aortic autografts—117 patients, 1967–1973 (7 year follow-up)

Early mortality	14 patients (12%)
Late mortaility	7 patients (6%)

Table 36.9 Aortic autografts—117 patients, 1967–1973 (7 year follow-up)

Surviving with Original Autograft	93 patients
Surviving with Another Valve in Aortic position	2 patients
Surviving with another valve in pulmonary position	1 patient
Total survivors	96

Table 36.10 Aortic homografts—311 patients, 10 year follow-up (1963–Oct. 1973—

Early mortaility	14%	44 patients
Late mortaility	13.5%	42 patients*

*Composed of 24 without re-operation and 18 after re-operation

Table 36.11 Biological valves (comparison with mechanical prostheses)

1. Central flow unobstructed orifice
2. No thromboembolism
3. No anticoagulants
4. No haemolysis
5. Low cost
6. No noise audible to patient
7. Comparable mortaility
8. Low incidence late deaths

Table 36.12 Biological valves—homografts and autografts 1967-1973

	Homografts		*Autografts*	
Total	172		106	
Hospital deaths	16	(9.3%)	13	(12.2%)
Late deaths	5	(2.9%)	3	(2.8%)
Valve failure	15	(8.7%)	3	(2.8%)

37
Experience with heterografts
C. G. Duran

As yet a haemodynamically correct heart valve substitute has not been found. No prosthetic valve, so far, fulfils all the ideal requirements, and therefore tissue valve grafts with their haemodynamic advantages and non-thrombogenic properties deserve study as an alternative procedure.

Although originally the author worked with homoglogous valves,[1, 2] the practical difficulties of obtaining them necessitated studying the possibility of using animal valves or xenografts. A simple relationship between the size of the human aortic valve and the domestic animal aortic valves has universally centred the choice on the porcine valve.

Initially it was assumed that the fresh pig aortic valve would elicit an intense rejection and that the best possible antigenic attenuation would be obtained at the expense of the tissue viability. Therefore, the behaviour of freeze-dried valves transplanted into the dog was studied.[3] The immunological difference between the valve cusps which maintained perfect anatomic conditions and the aortic wall which ruptured a few months after its transplantation was immediately obvious. This problem was solved by inserting the xenograft with a minimum of aortic wall within a prosthetic tube.[4] This principle has also been successfully applied in the reconstruction of the right ventricular outflow tract, in Rastelli's technique and also in total cardiac prosthesis. When examined microscopically the acellular cusps were always observed with integrity of collagen structure.

Encouraged by these results in 1965, a small clinical series was started with the help of Dr Binet.[5] Although the initial results were similar to those obtained with homografts, it was soon observed that the transplanted cusps became progressively thinner and some of them ruptured. The similar results observed by other authors with different methods of preparation and storage of the valves, as for instance with the use of formaldehyde, discredited the use of xenografts in clinical practice.

Later, Carpentier introduced the use of glutaraldehyde as a more stable method of producing cross-linking between the collagen fibres.[6] These valves were mounted on an eccentric prosthetic ring which supports the right coronary cusp which in the pig is myocardial (Figures 37.1 and

37.2). The fact that these valves are produced by a commercial laboratory permits standardisation in their preparation and comparable results between the different authors and centres, which could not be done when each centre prepared its own valves. 46 Carpentier-Edwards xenografts have been used in a limited series of 43 patients. 31 were

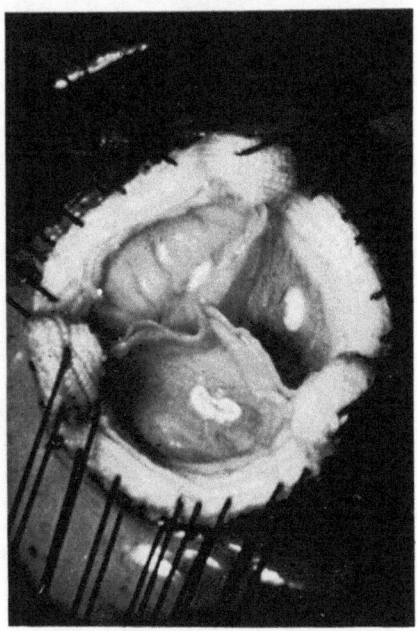

Figure 37.1 Carpentier–Edwards aortic xenograft. The right coronary sinus myocardial base is supported by the stent. The aortic wall edge is covered by Dacron.

single valve replacements and 12 were multiple valve replacements. There were eight hospital deaths. The sizes of valves used were mainly 27 and 29mm in diameter in the aortic area and 32mm in the mitral area. Only 44 months have elapsed since the first xenograft was placed in July 1970 into a 12-year-old gipsy boy. The late mortality was of six cases: two of **SBE**; one of bronchopneumonia; one of a possible arhythmia; one of a massive haemorrhage eight months after graft placement and one of valve failure.

There has been no incidence of thromboembolic phenomena and anticoagulants were only used in the mitral or tricuspid patients for about two months postoperatively. Six patients presented insufficiency murmurs very soon after surgery; two mitrals and three aortics had a short murmur which has not changed since. One aortic patient with a grade III/IV diastolic murmur was recatheterised and reoperated on for a perivalvular leak eight months after graft implantation. The valve was resutured without difficulty but 10 days after surgery the patient died due to a massive haemorrhage from the level of the aortic cannulation site. At postmortem no evidence of infection was found, although this was thought to be the cause of death as the valve was in perfect condition,

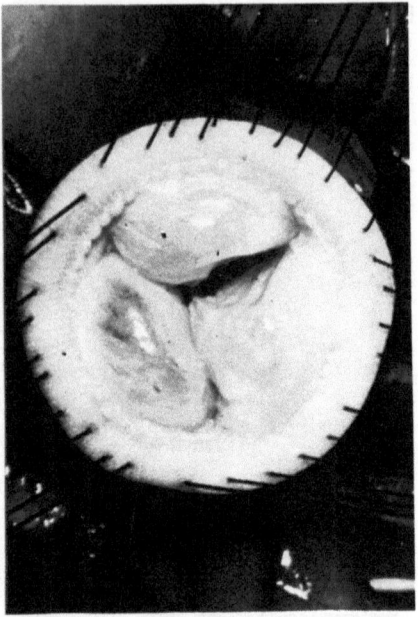

Figure 37.2 Carpentier–Edwards mitral xenograft.

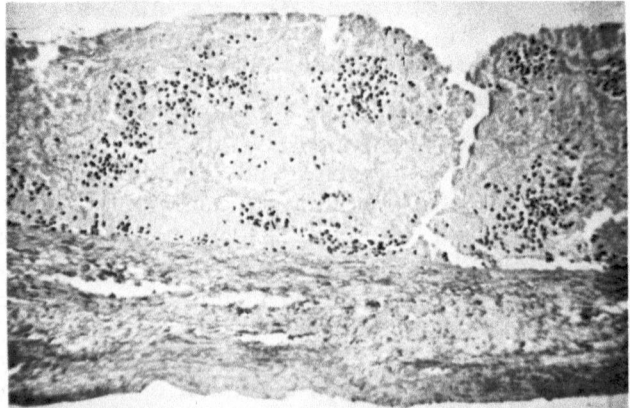

Figure 37.3 Aortic xenograft eight months after implantation

the elastic and collagen fibre structure was perfectly intact, there was no cellular infiltration, there was no endothelium and only a thin layer of fibrin covered the aortic surface of the cusps (Figure 37.3).

Eight patients have been recatheterised; six of them were those with insufficiency murmurs. Except in the case with the diastolic murmur grade III due to a perivalvular leak, the other patients had no haemodinamically significant insufficiencies and were minimal on angiocardiography (Figure 37.4). Therefore the insufficiency murmurs that are

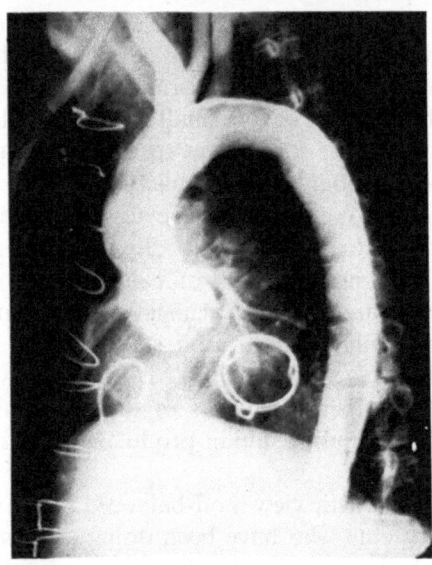

Figure 37.4 Aortic and mitral xenograft. Carpentier annuloplasty in tricuspid

presented in the patients with bioprosthesis, if they appear immediately after surgery, could be due to a perivalvular leak or to a malposition of the cusps due to the rigid valvular stent. The latter is probably only important when of late appearance.

However, there have been three valve failures (6·5% incidence) at 11, 24 and 27 months after surgery. One aortic and one mitral valve was calcified. The aortic patient had a pseudomona bacterial endocarditis induced at a check-up catheter study because of his aortic diastolic murmur. The mitral patient had been reoperated on for bleeding in the immediate postoperative period and had to be resutured twice making a low grade infection a possible causative factor. The third valve failure was a completely destroyed aortic xenograft with no special features in the case history. Two of them were reoperated and their valve replaced by a prosthesis Histologically besides the presence of the massive calcification, the valve cusp tends to be acellular except for the presence of the occasional histiocyte near its surface. In the destroyed xenograft recovered after 27 months in the aortic position, fragmentation of the surface of the cusp, which gave a festooned appearance, and the presence of calcium at the base of the valve were observed. In addition another patient was reoperated on seven months after surgery for an angiographic diagnosis of perivalvular leak. The first operation had been performed during the acute phase of SBE. Surgery did not reveal any faults but the valve was replaced by a prosthesis. The valve was normal anatomically and functionally when tested in the pulse duplicator. However, on microscopic examination the presence of histiocytes near the surface of the cusp substance and the existence of very small spicules of calcium were revealed.

Therefore, out of these four valves recovered at surgery, two at seven and eight months, although normal macroscopically, histologically have shown the patchy presence of histiocytes near their surface. One at 27 months was found to be macroscopically destroyed and microscopically had a torn surface and spicules of calcium and one at 24 months revealed histiocytes and massive calcification. It is tempting to think that the very discrete cellular infiltration starts at the level of the mural thrombus adherent to the aortic aspect of the valve. This infiltration might rupture the superficial layers of the valve cusps permitting the inflow of the surrounding fluid, producing oedema and eventually calcification.

This slightly pessimistic view is off-balanced by the symptom-free, non-anticoagulant patients who have been doing very well for a maximum follow-up period of 44 months. The latest compound statistic on another glutaraldehyde valve mounted on a flexible stent – the Hancock Laboratories valve – was recently presented in Los Angeles by Dr Zuhdi. It shows 711 xenografts without any valve failure except for two cusp perforations related to SBE and no degenerative changes in 10 valves recovered. Long-term results between three and four and one half years show no valve failures in 29 patients of Dr Zuhdi's personal series. The valve failures in the author's own series are in some cases, and could be in others, related to infection. The author certainly does not intend to use them again in cases of active bacterial endocarditis but feels that if it is shown that these bioprostheses last for over six years with an attrition rate inferior to 5%, he would not hesitate to use them systematically, since when they fail there is ample time for their elective replacement.

An entirely different approach would be to use fresh heterografts. The possibility of reducing their already poor antigenic capacity but at the same time maintaining their viability has been studied. Initially the antigenic pattern of the fresh pig aortic valve was studied using Ouchterlonys immunodiffusion technique and immunoelectrophoresis. Nine distinct bands were detected, seven of them common with the dog aortic valve.

The valves were then cultured at 37 °C in a growth medium for five days with one change of medium at three days. An antigenic simplification was found to have occurred since only six antigens could be detected. The fresh and cultured valves were then transplanted into the abdominal muscles and the descending aorta of the dog and a further antigenic

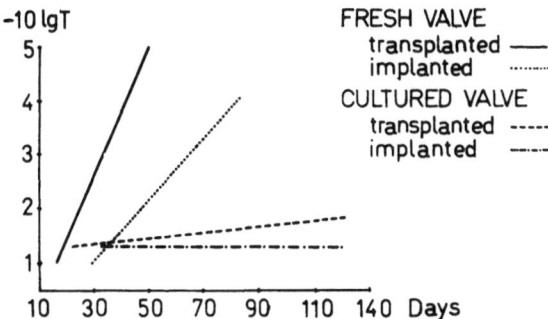

Figure 37.5 Titre of circulating antibiodies in the recipient dogs after fresh and cultured aortic valve transplantation. Note the different responses to the graft

simplification occurred in the cultured valves. Pyronin positive cells could not be found in the transplanted valves up to 142 days. The titre of circulating antibodies in the recipient animal was studied with Boyden's passive haemagglutination (Figure 37.5). A very striking difference could be detected between the fresh and the cultured valve recipients and the antibody response was significantly lower in the animals with the cultured valve transplants.

The author therefore concluded that culturing the valve graft reduces its antigenicity. Although a chronic low grade rejection might be present it could be hoped that the process of destruction would be compensated by that of repair since it is a living tissue and durability might be achieved. However, further extensive studies are obviously required to clarify this point.

References
1. Duran, C. M. G. and Gunning, A. J. (1962). A method for placing a total homologous aortic valve in the subcoronary position. *Lancet*, **2,** 488
2. Duran, C. M. G., Manley, G. and Gunning, A. J. (1965). The behaviour of homo-transplanted aortic valves in the dog. *Year Book of Cardiov. and Renal Dis.* (Chicago: Year Book Med. Publishers Inc.)
3. Duran, C. M. G. and Gunning, A. J. (1965). Heterologous aortic valve transplantation in the dog. *Lancet*, **2,** 114
4. Duran, C. M. G., Whitehead, R. and Gunning, A. J. (1969). Implantation of homo-logous and heterologous aortic valves in prosthetic vascular tubes. *Thorax*, **24,** 142

5. Binet, J. P., Duran, C. M. G., Carpentier, A. and Langlois, J. (1965). Heterologous aortic valve transplantation. *Lancet*, **2**, 1275
6. Carpentier, A., Chanard, J., Briotet, J. M., Harada, S., Archundia, J., Salamagne, J. C., Vigano, M., Laurens, P., Laurent, D. and Dubost, C. (1967). Remplacement de l'appareil valvulaire mitral par des heterogreffes heterotopiques. *Presse Med.*, **75**, 1603

38
Homograft replacement of the mitral valve
M. H. Yacoub

Valve replacement has favourably altered the natural history of patients with advanced mitral valve disease whose valves are not suitable for reconstructive procedures. The choice of a valve substitute, however, remains a problem. Homograft valves offer the advantages of ideal flow characteristics and freedom from thromboembolic complications; their main disadvantages are infection and mechanical failure. Long-term function of the grafts depends on preserving their physical and biological properties as well as guaranteeing ideal functional conditions at the time of insertion.

PHYSICAL PROPERTIES

In order to test the effect of antibiotic sterilisation on the physical properties of the valves, the tensile strength and secant modulus of elasticity have been measured using an Instron universal testing machine. This study showed that neither of these parameters changed significantly following sterilisation.

BIOLOGICAL PROPERTIES

To test 'viability' of homografts following sterilisation and storage three methods have been used.
1. Conventional tissue culture techniques.
2. Testing for intracellular reductase systems.
3. Establishing the cytotoxicity of each antibiotic using established tissue culture cells (mainly Chang's human liver cells).

The results of these investigations showed that although 'viability' as defined by the first two methods was retained for 28 days when the valves were kept at 4 °C, using the third method it was found that each antibiotic had a different degree of cytotoxicity, which was directly proportional to the time of contact with the tissues. Because of this the valves are transferred after 24 h from the strong antibiotic solution to tissue culture medium containing small amounts of penicillin and strepto-mycin.

TECHNIQUE OF INSERTION

This should provide optimal functional conditions – these include:

1. Preservation of all functional components of the valve homograft, including the sinuses of Valsalva, which are an integral part of any semilunar valve mechanism.
2. Preservation of the ability of the valve to alter its shape during the different parts of the cardiac cycle. This is rendered impossible if

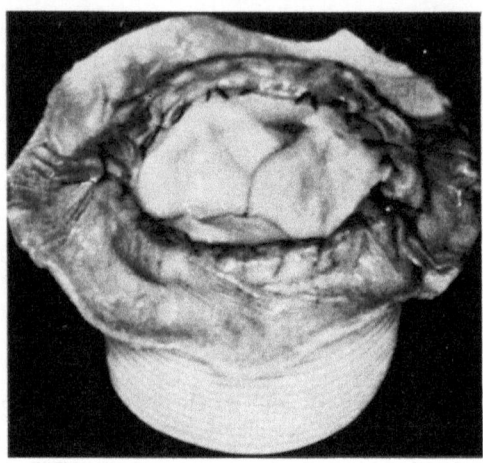

Figure 38.1 Aortic valve homograft prepared for insertion into the mitral position by fixation inside a Dacron tube. A collar of Dacron covered by autogenous pericardium is attached to the atrial side of the tube

the valve is fixed to a rigid stent, which appreciably increases the strain on all the cusps.

3. Preservation of the normal anatomical relations of the different components of the valve mechanism. This can be altered if the valve is fixed to a stent consisting of a ring and three equidistant prongs, as we have found that the height and distance between the commissures of an aortic valve vary from one homograft to another and are not equal in any one valve.

The technique used in the author's series consists of fixing an aortic homograft inside a 35 mm Dacron tube to the top of which a patch of two-way stretch Dacron is sutured, the latter then being covered by autogenous pericardium (Figure 38.1). The valve is then inserted by two suture lines. The first suture line consists of a series of interrupted everting mattress sutures, which fix the homograft and surrounding Dacron tube to the mitral annulus after excising the diseased valve; the second suture line fixes the pericardium to the surrounding atrial wall, thus covering all prosthetic material, the knots of the first suture line and the left atrial appendage (Figures 38.2a & b).

This technique, apart from satisfying the three conditions which help

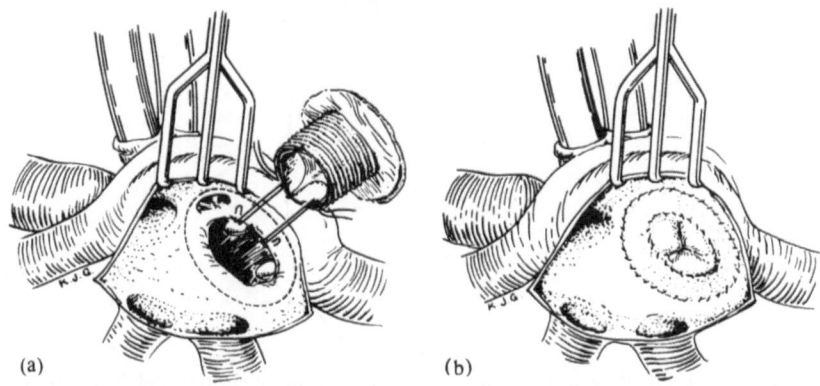

(a)   (b)

Figure 38.2 Diagrams illustrating the stages of insertion of the valve homograft in the mitral position

to guarantee optimal functional conditions of the graft, has the additional advantages of:

1. Covering all prosthetic material by homograft autogenous pericardium.
2. Excluding the left atrial appendage from circulation.
3. Allowing smooth flow of blood from the pulmonary veins into the homograft without stasis or turbulence (Figure 38.3).
4. Preservation of mobility of the mitral annulus.
5. Absence of any protrusion into the left ventricular cavity or outflow tract.

PATIENTS AND RESULTS

Between August 1969 and March 1974, 428 patients underwent mitral valve replacement using this technique. The aortic valve was replaced at the same time in 100 patients. The operative mortality (defined as all deaths occurring within the first four weeks after operation) was 6·7% for patients' mitral valve replacement, with or without replacement of the tricuspid valve and 9% for those undergoing homograft replacement of the aortic and mitral valve. The late mortality was 6·1% for mitral valve replacement and 9% for double valve replacement (aortic and mitral) (Table 38.1).

Expressed in the form of an actuarial survival curve, including operative

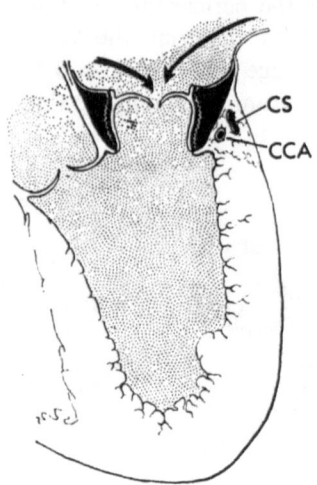

Figure 38.3 Diagram showing the aortic homograft in the mitral position and demonstrating the absence of any protrusion into the ventricular cavity

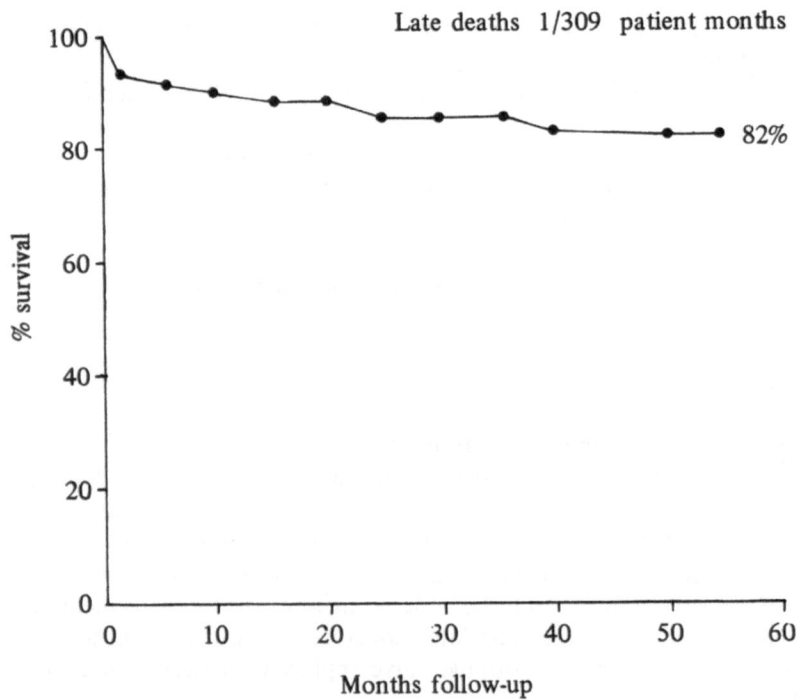

Figure 38.4 Aortic homograft replacement of the mitral valve in 328 patients

and late death, the results are shown in Figure 38.4. This shows that survival at 55 months was 82%. The curve shows a slow, continuous drop with time. Figure 38.5 shows actuarial survival of patients undergoing homograft replacement of aortic and mitral valves. Table 38.2 shows the

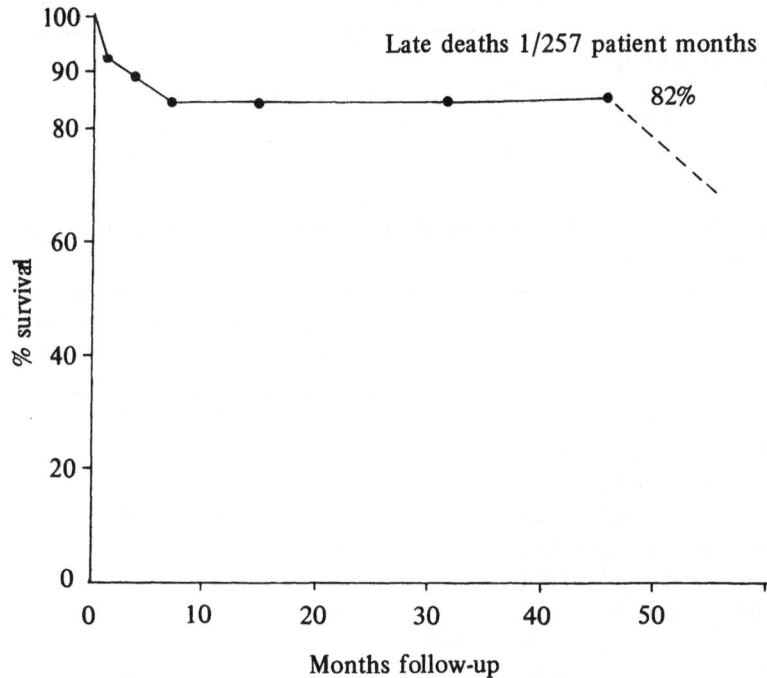

Figure 38.5 Double valve replacement using aortic homografts in 100 patients

causes of late deaths after single and double valve replacement. Table 38.3 summarises incidence of complications, which could be related to this type of valve substitute. Thromboembolism occurred in two patients (6·6%), both of whom had a massive clot removed from the left atrium. Anticoagulants were not used postoperatively, unless there was a specific indication like deep-vein thrombosis. Fungus endocarditis has been a problem, particularly after double valve replacement. This complication has not been encountered since using Nystatin in the tissue culture medium, which was started six months ago. However, it is too soon to be sure whether this dangerous complication has been eliminated.

The haemodynamic response to this form of valve replacement has been good (Figure 38.6).

In conclusion, experience with the use of aortic valve homografts

Table 38.1 The late mortality for mitral valve and double valve replacements. August 1969–March 1974. 428 patients

	Patients	Early deaths	Patients	Late deaths	Total
MVR (including TVR)	6·7%	20	6·1%	12·8%	
MVR and AVR	9	9 %	9	9 %	18 %
TOTAL	31	7·2%	29	6·8%	14 %

Table 38.2 Causes of late deaths after single and double valve replacement. August 1968–March 1974

	Patients	MVR (%)	Patients	DVR (%)
1. Fungus endocarditis	3	0·9	2	2
2. Detached upper suture line or prolapsing cusp	2	0·6	0	
3. Coronary artery disease	3	0·9	0	
4. Arrhythmia (sudden death)	1	0·3	2	2
5. Congestive failure (valve functioning well)	4	1·2	0	
6. Non-cardiac causes (Ca. colon, Tb., gastrectomy, CVA)	4	1·2	3	3
7. Unknown	3	0·9	2	2
Total	20	6	9	9

Table 38.3 Late complications related to single and double valve replacements

	Patients	MVR (%)	Patients	DVR (%)
1. Thromboembolism	2	0·6	0	
2. Transient haemolysis	1	0·3	0	
3. Fungus endocarditis	4	1·2	4	4
4. Miliary Tb.	1	0·3	1	1
5. Mitral regurgitation	2	0·6	1	1
Total	10	3	6	6

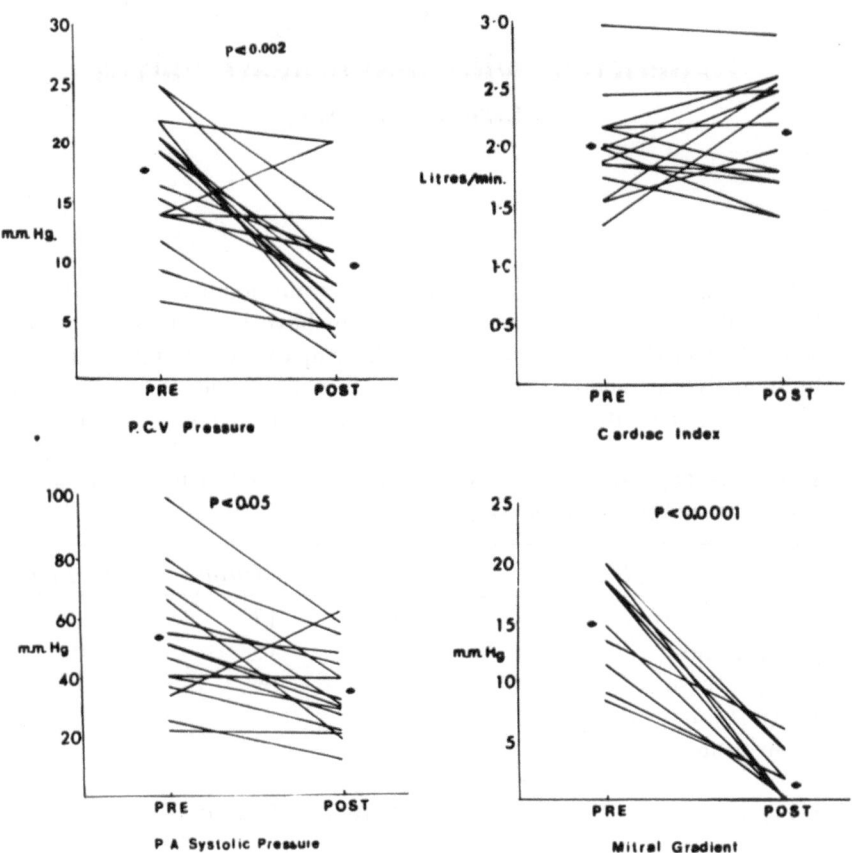

Figure 38.6 Haemodynamic changes following homograft replacement of the mitral valve

(without rigid stents) for mitral valve replacement over the past four and a half years has been encouraging. Currently the author continues to use this form of valve replacement as the method of choice.

39
Experience with tissue heart valves

Marian I. Ionescu

Since April of 1969 valves made of either autologous or homologous fascia lata or of heterologous pericardium have been used[1]. A homogeneous group of 241 patients with a follow-up of seven to 62 months has been analysed. There were 131 patients with single aortic valve replacement, 103 with single mitral valve replacement and seven patients

Table 39.1 Type of valve lesions in 241 patients – 143 men and 98 women, 9–69 years old (median age 47·5)

Valve Lesion	Aortic	Mitral*	Tricuspid
Predominant stenosis	38	17	–
Regurgitation	36	15	6
Mixed disease	50	66	1
Malfunction of previous valve substitute	7	5	–
TOTAL	131 (67)	103 (40)	7

* – 37 patients had one or two previous closed mitral valvotomies (35·9%)
+ – 3 aortic heterografts, 2 Starr prostheses and 2 fascial valves (one unstented valve and one valve damaged by infection)
+ + – 4 aortic heterografts and one Alvarez prosthesis
( ) – Figures in parentheses represent number of patients with valve calcification

with tricuspid replacement either alone or in combination with other cardiac surgical procedures. Details of valve lesions, age and sex of the patients are shown in Table 39.1.

Frame mounted, three-cusp tissue valves were used throughout the series[2]. The type of tissue, the number of valves and the period of time of their use are shown in Table 39.2.

RESULTS

Mortality. The main causes of early and late deaths were heart failure and infective endocarditis in both aortic and mitral groups (Table 39.3).

Table 39.2 Types of tissue valves and the period of time of clinical use

Type of valve	Time of use	Valves replaced Aortic*	Mitral*	Tricuspid**	Total
Autologous fascia lata	April 1969 – September 1970	25	50	3	78
Homologous fascia lata †	April 1969 – February 1971	43	21	1	65
Heterologous pericardium + +	March 1971 – November 1973	63	32	3	98
Total		131	103	7	241

* – Single valve replacement
** – Tricuspid valve replacement single or in combination with other cardiac surgical procedures
+ – Valves preserved with either 4% buffered formaldehyde or with 0·2% glutaraldehyde
+ + – Valves preserved with either 0·2% glutaraldehyde or with 0·6% stabilised glutaraldehyde

Table 39.3 Early and late deaths in 241 patients

Cause of death	Aortic replacement Early	Late	Mitral replacement Early	Late	Total Early	Late
Heart failure	8	5	10	5	18	10
Infective endocarditis	2	4	2	4	4	8
Other causes	2	2	3	3	5	5
Cerebral infarction	1				1	
Respiratory failure		1	1	1	1	2
Ileal gangrene	1	1			1	1
Gastro-intestinal bleeding			1		1	
Status epilepticus			1		1	
Serum hepatitis				1		1
Oesophageal rupture				1		1
Total	12	11	15	12	27	23

Infective endocarditis occurred in 18 patients (11 with aortic and seven with mitral replacement). Six patients survived, four after reoperation and two after antibiotic treatment alone. Table 39.4 shows the distribution of infective endocarditis over the years.

Thromboembolism. The incidence of thromboembolism has been very low although anticoagulants were not used. In the aortic series there have been 0·6 episodes of embolism per 1000 patient-months. In the mitral series there have been 1·5 episodes of thromboembolism per 1000 patient-months. All episodes in mitral patients occurred during the first postoperative month.

Table 39.4 Incidence of infective endocarditis

	Year of operation	1969	1970	1971	1972	1973
Early occurrence,	Aortic replacement	0/10	4/28	2/38	1/28	0/27
first 6 months	Mitral replacement	0/37	2/31	2/11	0/16	0/8
postoperatively						
	Total	0/47	6/59	4/49	1/44	0/35

Late occurrence (7–62 postoperative months)
4 patients with aortic and 3 with mitral replacement

Postoperative regurgitation. The assessment of valve function was made by aortic root angiography[3] and clinical examination for patients with aortic valve replacement. In the mitral group clinical examination and phonocardiography were used for defining the presence and degree of mitral regurgitation. Only a limited number of patients had left ventriculography.

Aortic diastolic murmurs appeared in 18 out of 119 operative survivors (15·1%). Of 61 patients with fascial valves (autologous and homologous) 13 (21·3%) had diastolic murmurs at three years and 15 (24·6%) at five years postoperatively (nine patients grade I, two patients grade II and four patients grade III[3]). In contrast, of the 58 patients with pericardial valves, three (5·2%) had diastolic murmurs at three years postoperatively (two patients grade I and one patient grade II).

Mitral systolic murmurs developed in 40 out of 88 operative survivors (40·4%). Of 59 patients with fascial valves (autologous and homologous) 32 (54·1%) had apical systolic murmurs at three years and 34 (57·6%) at five years postoperatively (23 patients had static and 11 patients progressive murmurs). In contrast with the fascial group, of the 29 patients with pericardial valves six (20·7%) had apical systolic murmurs at three years postoperatively (five patients had static and one patient progressive murmurs) (Figure 39.1).

Haemolysis. None of the patients with tissue valves have shown clinical signs of haemolysis. A specific investigation for red cell destruction demonstrated that laboratory evidence of haemolysis was present only in patients with aortic regurgitation[4].

Tissue valve failure and dysfunction. There has not been any instance of valve failure in the aortic replacement series. However, two valves, both made of autologous fascia have been removed from the aortic position

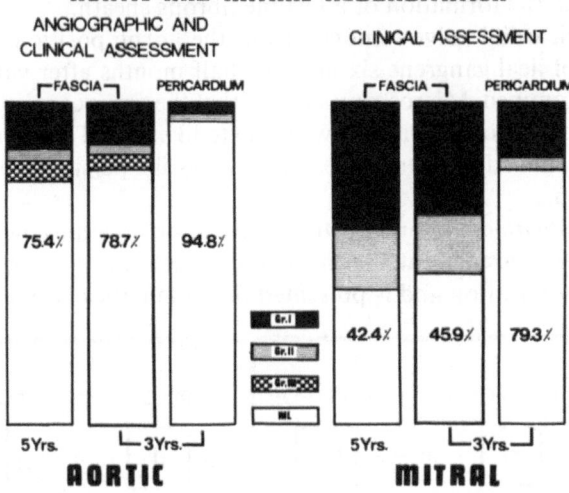

Figure 39.1 Diagrammatic presentation of the incidence and degree of regurgitation in patients with aortic and mitral valve replacement. For the fascial group the incidence of regurgitation is shown both at five and three years follow-up in order to facilitate comparison with the pericardial valve groups. In the aortic series the regurgitation was graded by angiographic and clinical criteria. The mitral regurgitation was graded as static (Grade I) or progressive (Grade II)

at eight and 37 months after operation respectively. The first one was incorrectly constructed and regurgitation developed immediately after insertion while the second valve became damaged by infective endocarditis in the early postoperative period and developed progressive regurgitation.

In the mitral replacement group there have been six valve failures (all six valves were made of autologous fascia). The mitral systolic murmur appeared in all six cases during the first six months after operation. These valves were removed at between 10 and 38 months postoperatively. All showed retraction and severe thickening of one of the cusps and moderate thickening of the other two cusps. There was no relationship between the retracted cusp and the circumferential position of that cusp as regards the left ventricular outlet. Two other valves, both made of homologous fascia, were removed from the mitral position at six and 18 months after insertion. Both were incorrectly constructed. One had a central leak while the second one became incompetent due to acute detachment of a cusp from the frame at a suture line.

Histologic examination. All the failed valves (made of autologous fascia) were examined microscopically[5]. The severely retracted cusps showed a central band of fragmented and necrotic looking connective tissue and thick marginal bands of fibrous tissue. The thickening of the cusps seemed to be due to the formation of a hyaline fibrous sheath.

One pericardial valve removed from the aortic position of a patient who died of ileal gangrene six and one half months after valve insertion was also examined. Microscopy showed that the tissue consisted of hyaline collagen bundles containing a few fibrocyte-like cells. The collagen seemed to have retained its structure. Elastic fibrils persisted in a regular distribution.

Clinical evaluation. Pre and postoperative effort tolerance with respect to dyspnoea was graded, at the most recent assessment, according to the NYHA classification and is presented diagrammatically in Figure 39.2.

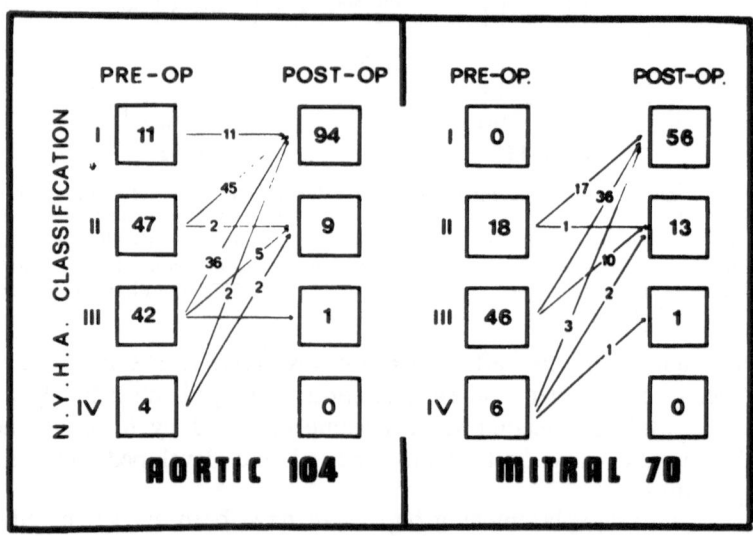

Figure 39.2 Diagrammatic presentation of pre and postoperative effort tolerance graded according to the N.Y.H.A. classification in patients with aortic and with mitral valve replacement followed-up for a period of from seven to 62 months postoperatively

The suboptimal results are explained by valve related complications in seven patients (two with aortic and five with mitral replacement). In the remaining eight aortic and nine mitral patients the persisting disability is due to factors unrelated to the tissue valves.

Electrocardiographic changes. In the majority of patients with aortic valve replacement there was a statistically significant reduction ($P < 0.001$) in the summation of voltage of R in V_6 and S in V_1 following operation. In patients with mitral valve replacement the electrocardiographic changes were not statistically significant.

Radiologic changes. There was a variable decrease in the cardio-thoracic ratio (CTR) in the majority of patients with aortic valve replacement. The mean reduction was statistically significant ($P < 0.001$) in all patients. When present, the reduction in CTR took place mainly during the first six postoperative months. In patients with mitral replacement the mean reduction in CTR was not statistically significant.

Calcification of the tissue valves has not been seen in any patient.

Haemodynamic investigations. From the aortic replacement group 10 patients with fascial valves and 12 with pericardial valves had haemodynamic studies performed at a mean interval of nine and 10 months respectively after valve replacement. All these patients had competent valves as demonstrated by angiography.

Table 39.5 Data concerning patients with tricuspid valve replacement

No.	Age	Sex	Previous operations	Aetiology and type of tricuspid lesion	Additional surgery at time of tricuspid replacement	Type of valve used	Follow-up months	Present condition NYHA Grade
1.	40	F	CMV M replacement	Rheumatic regurgitation	—	AFL	60	I
2.	43	M	None	Rheumatic regurgitation	M replacement	AFL AFL	59	I
3.	32	M	Repair VSD	SBE regurgitation	Closure VSD	AFL	51	I
4.	49	M	CMV M replacement	Rheumatic regurgitation	—	HFL	48	II
5.	30	M	None	Traumatic** regurgitation	—	HP	29	I
6.	35	F	CMV	Rheumatic stenosis and regurgitation	M annuloplasty	HP	28	I
7.	38	F	CMV M replacement	Rheumatic regurgitation	—	HP	26	I

* – SBE – Subacute bacterial endocarditis on residual VSD and tricuspid valve
** – Penetrating injury to the tricuspid valve
CMV – Closed mitral valvotomy
VSD – Ventricular septal defect
AFL – Autologous fascia lata
HFL – Homologous fascia lata
HP – Heterologous pericardium
M – Mitral
NYHA – New York Heart Association

The peak systolic gradient across the aortic fascial and pericardial valves at rest was 14 ± 3 mmHg and 7 ± 1 mmHg respectively and during exercise 17 ± 3 mmHg and 15 ± 2 SEM mmHg respectively.

There was no statistically significant change in cardiac output as compared with the preoperative values. The pulmonary wedge pressure (PWP) and pulmonary artery pressure (PAP) showed a significant reduction both at rest and during exercise.

From the mitral replacement group, 10 patients with competent fascial valves had haemodynamic studies performed at mean intervals of six and 38 months after operation, at rest and during exercise.

The cardiac output did not change significantly from the preoperative values, and cardiac output response, in relation to oxygen uptake during exercise remained impaired.

The mean PWP and PAP showed a significant reduction at the first postoperative study at rest and during exercise. At the second postoperative study there was further significant decrease in PWP and PAP. The end diastolic gradient across the mitral valve was 6 ± 1 mmHg at rest and 20 ± 4 mmHg during exercise.

Similar haemodynamic studies were performed in five patients with pericardial valves at a mean interval of 14 months after operation. The results, at rest and during exercise, were similar to those obtained in the fascia lata group.

Tricuspid valve replacement. The results of tricuspid replacement were not analysed because of the very small number of patients, the different types of tissue used and the differing periods of follow-up. Table 39.5 gives details of the pre and postoperative status of these patients. In the tricuspid group there have not been any early or late deaths, infective endocarditis, thromboembolism, valve failure, valve dysfunction or regurgitant murmurs. Only one patient has a 2/6 tricuspid diastolic murmur.

DISCUSSION

The early mortality rate compares favourably with results obtained with other types of valve substitutes. The main causes of late death in this series were the advanced cardiac condition preoperatively and postoperative infective endocarditis.

Since 1971 the prevention and treatment of infection have been changed. Prophylactic antibiotics are given only for 48 h after surgery. Pre and postoperative bacteriologic screening is performed and the diagnosed infections are treated electively[6]. Since this policy was adopted, there has been a progressive and significant reduction in the incidence of infective endocarditis.

The incidence of thromboembolism in the entire series has been very low (0·7/1000 patient-months), although anticoagulants were not used.

Haemodynamic studies in patients with aortic replacement have demonstrated acceptable pressure gradients across the aortic valve.

Following mitral valve replacement there was a significant haemodynamic improvement which was maintained at least up to three years postoperatively. As with other types of mitral replacement the cardiac index did not increase significantly after tissue valve replacement.

The most important criterion in the evaluation of tissue valves is their durability.

In this series there have been significant differences in valve function with regard to both the site of valve insertion and the type of tissue used.

When the results of aortic replacement at a similar follow-up of three years were compared, the fascial valves (autologous and homologous) have shown an incidence of 21·3% regurgitation as opposed to 5·2% in the pericardial valve group.

The time of appearance of aortic diastolic murmurs in the fascial series was distributed over the entire follow-up period, while in the pericardial series the three diastolic murmurs appeared all in the immediate postoperative period. None of the patients with diastolic murmurs, whether with fascial or pericardial valves have significant aortic regurgitation. The incidence of aortic regurgitation seems to be related both to previous aortic valve replacement (where perivalvular leaks are strongly suspected) and to the use of autologous fascial valves.

In the mitral position, the difference in function between fascial and pericardial valves, was even more evident. At three years postoperatively 54·1% of patients with fascial valves (autologous and homologous) had systolic murmurs as compared with 20·7% of patients with pericardial valves. Murmurs with progressive loudness were encountered only in patients with autologous fascial valves.

The six valve failures in this series occurred with autologous fascia in the mitral position. The degree of pathological changes in these valves was very similar although the time of their removal varied from 10 to 38 months after insertion. The fact that there was no relationship between the circumferential position of the severely altered cusp and the left ventricular outlet, supports the view that the flow characteristics in the left ventricle cannot explain entirely the mechanism of valve failure in the mitral position.

On the other hand, biological factors alone cannot be responsible for the different behaviour of fascial valves in the mitral as compared with the aortic position.

Technical factors in valve construction and haemodynamic differences between the mitral and aortic areas may play a certain role.

In vitro hydrodynamic studies concerning the opening mechanism of three-cusp valves have elucidated some aspects of the mechanism of function of tissue valves[7].

One observation was that virtually all three-cusp valves open in a sequential manner and the order in which the cusps of a particular valve open is maintained irrespective of the circumferential position of the cusps as regards the left ventricular outlet. Irregularities in the shape and size of the cusps or in the physical properties of the material accentuate this phenomenon.

The pressure gradient across the valve increases rapidly as the diameter of the valve is reduced and with reduction in valve diameter complete opening of all three cusps can be obtained by a smaller flow rate.

It is postulated that in patients with low cardiac output post-operatively, large size three-cusp valves in the mitral position may not open fully and that the cusp with little or no mobility may undergo structural changes leading to fibrosis and atrophy. This may occur when the valve is made of biologically active tissue such as autologous fascia lata.

Under the haemodynamic conditions prevailing in the aortic area, complete opening of every cusp of the valve is facilitated by the forceful left ventricular ejection through an orifice comparatively smaller than the mitral valve. The maintenance of full mobility of all cusps may prevent the occurrence, delay the onset, or lessen the extent of structural alterations of the living autologous tissue.

Table 39.6 Percent incidence of major complications in patients with tissue valves

Complication	Aortic replacement		Mitral replacement	
	Fascial valves	Pericardial valves	Fascial valves	Pericardial valves
Infective endocarditis:				
early	8·8	1·6	4·2	3·1
late	5·9	0	2·8	3·1
Regurgitant murmurs	24·6	5·2	57·6	20·7
Valve failure	0	0	17·2	0
Valve dysfunction	1·6	0	3·4	0

In order to avoid sequential opening the three cusps of the valve must be absolutely identical in thickness, pliability and shape[8,9].

In the present series, autologous fascia was replaced with homologous fascia for two reasons. Firstly, the viability of the transplanted

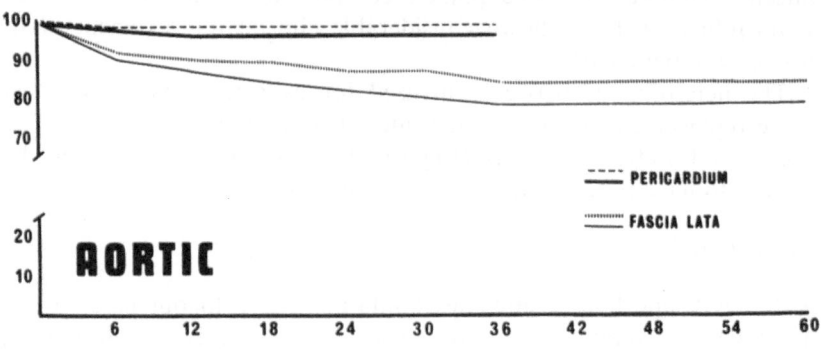

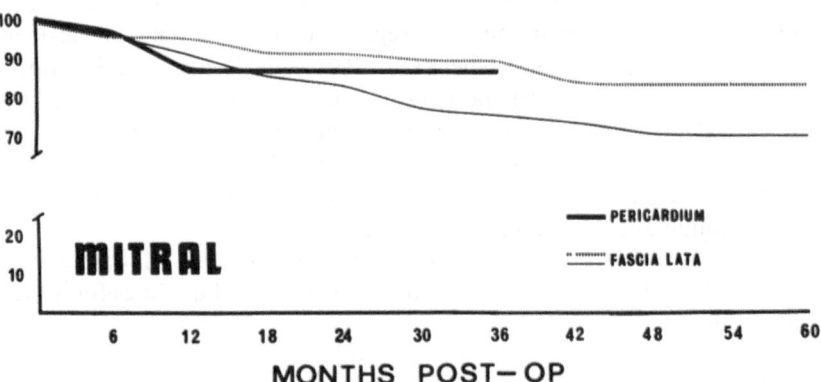

MONTHS POST–OP

Figure 39.3 Actuarial analysis of survival rates of patients discharged from hospital. There were 119 patients with aortic valve replacement (61 fascial and 58 pericardial valves) and 88 patients with mitral replacement (59 fascial and 29 pericardial valves). The upper dotted lines, when present, represent survival rate while the solid lines represent survivors with tissue valves. The follow-up period is 62 months for patients with fascial valves and 38 months for patients with pericardial valves

tissue is uncertain[10] and secondly the conditions for valve construction during the operation are far from ideal.

Since 1971 preserved heterologus pericardium has been used because of the high incidence of systolic murmurs in the mitral fascia lata valve series on the one hand and because of the thinness, pliability and availability of animal pericardium on the other.

The chemical treatment used for heterologous pericardium seems to attenuate the antigenic potential and to preclude denaturation of the collagen by creating permanent intermolecular cross-linkages.

Although autologous fascia lata valves in the mitral position have produced a number of valve related complications, the results at five years follow-up have shown considerable clinical improvement in the majority of patients[11].

The heterologous pericardium used for over three years for heart valve replacement has performed much better than fascia lata in both aortic and mitral positions (Figure 39.3 and Table 39.6) and has proved to have potential qualities for a heart valve substitute.

SUMMARY

Autologous and homologous fascia lata and heterologous pericardium, mounted on a support frame, were used for heart valve replacement in 241 patients (131 aortic, 103 mitral and seven tricuspid).

The follow-up for the fascia lata group was 40 to 62 months and for the pericardial group seven to 39 months. There have been significant differences in valve function with regard to both the site of valve insertion and the type of tissue used. Pericardial valves in the aortic position have produced the best results and autologous fascial valves in the mitral position the worst. Valve failure has occurred only in six patients, all with autologous fascia in the mitral position.

The incidence of thromboembolism in the entire series has been very low although anticoagulants were not used.

The analysis of clinical and haemodynamic results has shown that preserved heterologous pericardium has the potential qualities for a heart valve substitute.

References

1. Ionescu, M. I. and Ross, D. N. (1969). Heart valve replacement with autologous fascia lata. *Lancet*, **21**, 335
2. Bartek, I. T., Holden, M. P. and Ionescu, M. I. (1974). Frame-mounted tissue heart valves: Technique of construction. *Thorax*, **291**, 51
3. Brandt, P. W. T., Roche, A. H. G., Barratt-Boyes, B. G. and Lowe, J. B. (1969). Radiology of homograft aortic valves. *Thorax*, **241**, 129
4. Dave, K. S., Madan, C. K., Pakrashi, B. C., Roberts, B. E. and Ionescu, M. I. (1972). Chronic haemolysis following fascia lata and Starr–Edwards aortic valve replacement. *Circulation*, **461**, 240
5. Prioleau, N. H., Sutherland, T. W. and Ionescu, M. I. (1975). Pathology of failed autologous fascia lata mitral valves. *Thorax*, (in press)
6. Freeman, R. (1975). Microbiological aspects of open heart surgery; Diagnosis and Management. In: *Current Techniques in Extracorporeal Circulation* (M. I. Ionescu and G. H. Wooler, editors) (London: Butterworths)

7. Swales, P. B., Holden, M. P., Dowson, D. and Ionescu, M. I. (1973). Opening characteristics of three cusp tissue valves. *Thorax*, **28**, 286
8. Ionescu, M. I., Deac, R. C., Whitaker, W., Wooler, G. H., Holden, M. P. and Petrila, P.A. (1972). Fascia lata heart valves. In: *Biological Tissue in Heart Valve Replacement* (M. I. Ionescu, D. N. Ross and G. H. Wooler, editors) (London: Butterworths)
9. Ionescu, M. I., Pakrashi, B. C., Mary, D. A. S., Bartek, I. T. and Wooler, G. H. (1974). Long term evaluation of tissue valves. *J. Thorac. Cardiovasc. Surg.* **68**, 361
10. Silver, M. D. and Trimble, A. S. (1972). Structure of autologous fascia lata heart valve prostheses. *Arch. Pathol.*, **93**, 109
11. Mary, D. A. S., Pakrashi, B. C., Catchpole, R. W. and Ionescu, M. I. (1975). Tissue valves in the mitral position; Five years experience. *Brit. Heart J.* (in press)

40
Late results of cardiac valve replacement with autologous fascia lata
D. J. Parker

From April 1969 to December 1970 autologous fascia lata was used at the National Heart Hospital for the majority of aortic and mitral valve replacements. It was also used for a small number of tricuspid valve replacements and right ventricular outflow tract reconstructions.

Fascia lata was used following the encouraging reports of its use, unsupported, in aortic valve replacements by Senning.[1] It was believed to offer the advantages of an autologous and viable tissue without the risks of thromboembolism or anticoagulants. Being autologous and viable it was hoped that it would remain durable. The ready availability of tissue allows construction of a variety of sizes of valves.

This report is concerned with the late follow-up of single valve surgery in the aortic, mitral, tricuspid and right ventricular outflow tract positions. Multiple valve replacements have not been analysed as there is no way of knowing from which valve certain complications arise, for example, systemic embolism.

CLINICAL MATERIAL

Frame-mounted fascia lata valves for insertion in the aortic, mitral and tricuspid positions were prepared from fascia lata removed from the thigh at the beginning of the operation. The details of construction of the trileaflet valves have been described.[2, 3] Although the majority of valves used in the aortic position were frame-mounted in the latter part of this series, free unsupported fascia lata was used making use of the work of Yates.[4] This showed that the aortic valve is a frustrum or a horizontal section of a cone. Accordingly, a strip of fascia lata was made into a cone of appropriate size (Figure 40.1) and sutured into the aortic root.[5] The base of the frustrum was sutured horizontally into the aortic root and the top edge was sutured to the aortic wall in three places to produce a three-cusp valve. In the right ventricular outflow tract the fascia lata was formed into a tube containing a trileaflet valve,[6] similar to that described by Ionescu and Deac.[7]

This report is concerned with the following valves:

1. Frame-mounted aortic valves   77 patients
2. Unsupported aortic valves   22 patients
3. Frame-mounted mitral valves   41 patients
4. Frame-mounted tricuspid valves   5 patients
5. Right ventricular outflow reconstructions   9 patients

TOTAL   154 patients

The hospital mortality and morbidity was no greater or less than that associated with the use of other valves at a similar time. Immediate valve dysfunction was not a significant problem.

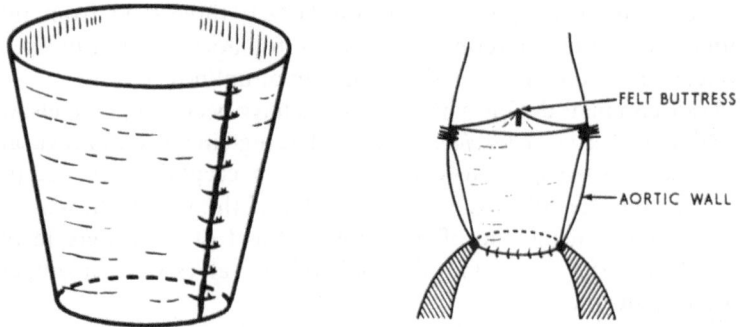

Figure 40.1 On the left the frustrum formed from fascia lata removed from the thigh. On the right the valve sutured into the aortic roof and attached at three points to the aortic wall.

The late mortality and morbidity of these valves is detailed below. The follow-up period ranges from three to four years. Follow up has been on a six-monthly routine and a variable proportion of the valves in the different positions have been investigated late after surgery. Most patients had anticoagulants for the first three months.

1. Aortic frame-mounted fascia lata valves. Five of the 77 patients developed important regurgitation within three months and reoperation was soon required. All were due to peripheral leaks between the valve ring and aortic wall and represented technical failures. A further 6 patients left hospital after operation with evidence of mild aortic regurgitation and this has not been progressive. Thus 11 patients (14%) had early regurgitation.

A further 15 patients (21%) developed late regurgitation and of these seven have required reoperation. In six of these patients the fascia had fractured from the frame at the site of the strut of the frame.

Thus at three years after aortic frame-mounted fascia lata valve replacement, 51 of 77 valves (66%) are clinically competent and 12 (15%) have required reoperation. In the valves removed the fascia was always thickened and shortened to some degree.

Bacterial endocarditis occurred in three patients (4%) at five, six and 34 months after operation. All three patients died although only one was referred back for reoperation.

Nine patients (12%) have developed visual or neurological symptoms. In six of these there was transient visual disturbance which could have been caused by microemboli, perhaps coming from the site of the fractured fascia close to the struts. Three patients developed hemiplegias and in two significant neurological defects have persisted. These embolic episodes have occurred scattered throughout the follow-up period.

There have been eight late deaths (10%); three died from infective endocarditis, four at reoperation either for aortic regurgitation or for associated disease and one died suddenly of unknown cause.

More complete details of these patients have been published elsewhere.[8]

2. Unsupported aortic fascia lata valves. The high incidence of regurgitation through this valve made its continued use unacceptable. Only 22 patients are available for follow-up. Overall, 50% of the valves showed signs of incompetence at the end of one month. Most of these were in the first half of the series. By 16 months 100% of the valves were incompetent to a varying degree.

Sixteen patients (73%) have been investigated at varying stages after operation and in only three patients investigated early was the valve competent. A central regurgitant jet was the usual finding. Eleven patients (50%) have now required reoperation. In three requiring early reoperation technical factors had caused failure. However, all the valves removed later showed thickening and contracture of the fascia producing a wide central orifice. Only three patients remain with signs of trivial aortic incompetence and a good clinical result.

Thus this experience with free unsupported fascia lata in the aortic position is less favourable than that of Senning.[1] It is also less favourable than frame-mounted fascia lata in the aortic position. The reasons for these differences are not clear. There have been no embolic or infective episodes associated with this small series of valves.

3. Frame-mounted mitral fascia lata valves. Forty-one frame-mounted mitral fascia lata valves are available for long-term follow-up. Four patients (10%) had evidence of mitral incompetence within one month of operation. By one year 38% of patients had evidence of regurgitation and at three years only two valves remained competent. The mitral incompetence has been progressive in most patients but the rate of deterioration in individual patients has varied considerably.

By three years 16% had required reoperation for mitral regurgitation and the rate of reoperation is rising rapidly at the present time. Figure 40.2 shows the typical findings in a valve removed for progressive mitral regurgitation. Although all three cusps are shortened and thickened, and

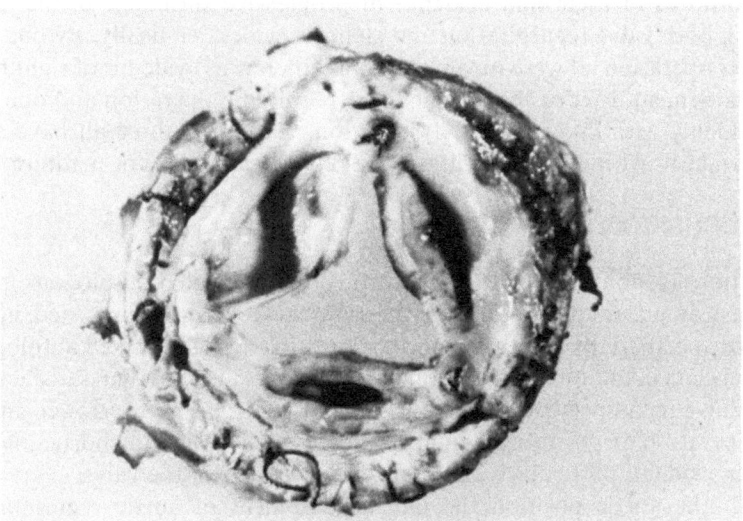

Figure 40.2 The ventricular aspect of a frame-mounted mitral fascia lata valve removed fourteen months after insertion. All three cusps are thickened and shortened with the changes being most marked in the posterior cusp.

this has been the usual finding, the changes are most marked in the posterior cusps. The cusp sitting in the outflow tract of the left ventricular is similar in position to the anterior leaflet of the mitral valve and has shown less thickening and shortening. These findings have also been shown in another series of mitral fascia lata valves.[9]

There have been no episodes of infective endocarditis in the follow-up of these valves. Two embolic episodes occurred: one early at three weeks and one late at three years.

Seven late deaths have occurred (16%). Two of these were due to pulmonary embolism at seven and 21 months after surgery. One died from hepatitis and two have died suddenly without known cause. One patient died at reoperation and the seventh from congestive cardiac failure with trivial mitral regurgitation. This was considered to be due to ischaemic damage occurring at the time of surgery.

The full details of this series of patients have been published elsewhere.[10]

4. Frame-mounted tricuspid fascia lata valves. This valve was inserted in five patients and all became markedly incompetent within three months and early reoperation was required.

5. Right ventricular outflow tract reconstruction. Although these valves functioned well initially in the nine patients followed-up, by six months two-thirds of them had evidence of progressive shrinkage of the fascia with both valve regurgitation and stenosis evident clinically. By one year after operation all were incompetent and there was evidence of right heart enlargement. Five of the patients have required reoperation and one died suddenly with known valve dysfunction. The other three all have signs of right heart failure and will require reoperation in the near future.

DISCUSSION

Within six months of operation it was very evident that autologous fascia lata was unsuitable for use in the right heart and unsupported in the aortic position. By three years the results using frame-mounted autologous fascia lata in the aortic and mitral positions were also less than satisfactory.

Valve incompetence in the mitral position has been progressive and at reoperation or postmortem marked valve thickening and shortening has been evident, particularly in the posterior leaflets of the valve.

In the aortic position the late development of aortic regurgitation which may be severe appears to be on the basis of late fragmentation of the fascia close to the point of attachment of the fascia to the strut of the valve cage.

Thus fascia lata has failed at differing rates in the different positions. Shortening and thickening of the fascia has occurred in all valves. Superficially at least, the evidence suggests that the less mechanical stress placed on the valve, the earlier the failure. This appears to be true for the different leaflets in the different positions of the mitral valve.

It was hoped that fascia lata would provide a viable autologous valve substitute. The histological findings of valves removed shows varying degrees of fragmentation of collagen, loss of nuclei, and deposition of fibrin on its surface. The viability of the fascial cells is not maintained.[11] In 17 fascia lata valves removed the viability has generally been about the 20% level of that at the time of insertion.

Thus autologous fascia lata has disappointed us as to competency, embolic complications and viability. This experience of 'man-made tissue valves' has shown many problems and any further use of such valves requires much more experimental work to ascertain that the tissue will function satisfactorily in the mechanical environment in which it is to be placed. It appears that the free edge of fascia lata was persistently prone to shrink and thicken. Fixation of the tissue prior to insertion may reduce this problem. However, this would exclude the possibility of a viable valve which one would hope may be able to replace and service its own tissue from its viable cells.

Since the end of 1970 the only tissue valves used at the National Heart Hospital have been homograft valves with the majority of these being viable and preserved in a nutrient antibiotic solution.

SUMMARY

The late follow-up of 154 patients having autologous fascia lata valve replacement at the National Heart Hospital in 1969 and 1970 is reported. Early on in the follow-up these valves were unsatisfactory in the right heart. In the left heart the unsupported aortic valves were unsatisfactory early on, and with time the frame-mounted mitral and aortic valves have shown unacceptable levels of incompetency. In the frame-mounted aortic valves a significant (12%) embolic rate has occurred. Autologous fascia data does not retain its viability or histological integrity when used as a valve substitute and its use cannot be recommended. Any other attempts to use man-made tissue valves must take cognisance of the reasons for failure in this series of patients.

Acknowledgment

The vast majority of the follow-up work on the fascia lata valves has been undertaken under grants from the British Heart Foundation and the Clinical Research Committee of the National Heart and Chest Hospitals to Dr Jane Somerville; she kindly provided access to her data.

References
1. Senning, A. (1967). Fascia lata replacement of aortic valves. *J. Thorac. Cardiovasc. Surg.*, **54**, 465
2. Ionescu, M. I. and Ross, D. N. (1969). Heart valve replacement with autologous fascia lata. *Lancet*, **ii**, 335
3. Ionescu, M. I., Ross, D. N., Wooler, G. H., Deac, R. and Ray, D. (1970). Replacement of heart valves with autologous fascia lata. *Surgical Technique, Brit. J. Surg.*, **57**, 437
4. Yates, A. K. (1971). A fascial frustrum valve for aortic valve replacement. *Thorax*, **26**, 184
5. Hearn, K., Somerville, J., Sutton, R., Wright, J. and Ross, D. (1973). Aortic valve replacement with unsupported fascia lata. *Thorax*, **28**, 603
6. Somerville, J. and Ross, D. N. (1971). Fascia lata reconstruction of the right ventricular outflow tract. *Lancet*, **1**, 941
7. Ionescu, M. I. and Deac, R. C. (1970). Fascia lata composite graft for right ventricular outflow tract and pulmonary artery reconstruction. *Thorax*, **25**, 427

8. Joseph, S., Somerville, J., Emanuel, R., Ross, D. and Ross, K. (1974). Aortic valve replacement with frame-mounted autologous fascia lata: long-term results. *Brit. Heart. J.*

9. McEnany, M. T., Ross, D. N. and Yates, A. K. (1972). Cusp degeneration in frame-supported autologous fascia lata mitral valves. *Thorax*, **27,** 13

10. Petch, M., Somerville, J., Ross, D., Ross, K., Emanuel, R. and McDonald, L. (1974). Replacement of the mitral valve with autologous fascia lata. *Brit. Heart. J.*, **36,** 177

11. Al-Janabi, N. (1974). Personal communication

41
Reconstructive valve surgery
A. Carpentier, J. Relland and Ch. Dubost

Opinions continue to differ as to which is the best valve substitute. General agreement should be easily reached on the theoretical superiority of conservative valve surgery. The only limitation of this technique is the difficulty in repairing the valve in such a way that a predictable and stable result can be obtained.

There have been several techniques of mitral valvuloplasty described in the last 20 years, many of which have been forgotten; others are still in use. The most common is the postero-medial annuloplasty to which the names of Kay,[1] Wooler and Reed are linked. This technique was associated with an unacceptably high incidence of recurrent mitral insufficiency, due either to the process of dilatation of the annulus continuing unchecked or the possibility of tears at the commissures. This in addition to the unpredictability of the repair explained the progressive disenchantment of the surgeon with conservative techniques.

In an effort to develop a technique of valvuloplasty which might be an answer to these criticisms, the use of prosthetic rings to reshape the mitral valve annulus on a more precise and physiologic basis was proposed in 1968.[2] Analysis of pure mitral insufficiency reveals three major lesions (Figure 41.1):

 – annulus dilatation,
 – commissure enlargement,
 – modification of the shape of the orifice resulting particularly in an increase in its antero-posterior diameter.

Figure 41.1 shows how the use of a suitably shaped and sized prosthetic ring sewn to the mitral annulus corrects all three abnormalities. The main advantages of this repair are its predictability, the restoration of a physiologic orifice area, the preservation of normal valve function in particular at the commissures and finally the prevention of recurrent dilatation of the annulus.

It must be emphasised however that this technique is only appropriate for the correction of annulus dilatation, which may be only one of the lesions responsible for mitral valve insufficiency. Lesions of the valvular or subvalvular structures must be treated as well and this is possible because the ring does not reduce the orifice area or impair valve function. In order to clarify the different techniques we have separated them into: repair of annulus lesions, repair of the valvular lesions and repair of the subvalvular lesions. It is important to keep in mind that the various lesions are usually associated.

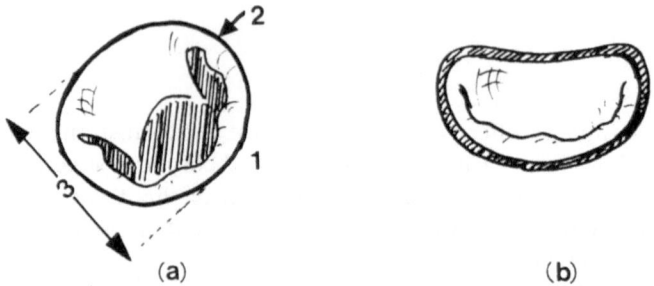

(a)   (b)

Figure 41.1 Concept of mitral valve ring valvuloplasty (a) Pathology: 1 – annular dilatation 2 – commissural enlargement 3 – increase in antero-posterior diameter (b) Reconstructed valve with prosthetic ring in place

REPAIR OF ANNULAR LESIONS

Dilatation of the annulus fibrosus is generally considered to be responsible for insufficiency, an assumption that supports the concept of correction˙ by the narrowing of the annulus. In point of fact, a careful analysis of the lesions shows that many factors play a part in insufficiency.

1. Dilatation of the annulus fibrosus certainly is one of the main factors involved. It is important to emphasise that this dilatation affects only two-thirds of the annulus, that section corresponding to the posterior leaflet. In contrast, the anterior leaflet portion of the annulus is not affected in the same way because of its continuity with the aortic root.

2. Commissural enlargement (asymetrical dilatation localised at the commissure) may exist with only a slight degree of annulus dilatation. Modification of the normal shape of the orifice may result from the two previous abnormalities but may also be due to a posterior displacement of the aortic leaflet and a change in the axis of the orifice: the antero-posterior diameter becoming superior in dimension to the transverse diameter.

These findings permitted a statement of the conditions of an anatomic and physiologic reconstruction of the mitral valve: not only must the annulus be reduced to its physiologic dimensions but the commissures must be remodelled as well in order to restore their physiologic curvature and the aortic leaflet must be repositioned in order to correct its displacement and shortening if any. The use of suitably shaped and sized prosthetic rings makes it possible to accurately and permanently accomplish each of these corrections.

The size of the rings and their corresponding interior areas are as follows: 26 mm (3·05 cm²), 28 mm (4·09 cm²), 30 mm (4·85 cm²) 32 mm (5·19 cm²), 34 mm (5·50 cm²), 36 mm (5·78 cm²). Each ring is made of stainless steel and covered with a fine Rhodergon* fabric which favours the incorporation of the prosthesis.

The approach to the mitral valve is made by either a direct atrial incision or by the biatrial trans-septal incision when the left atrium is small.

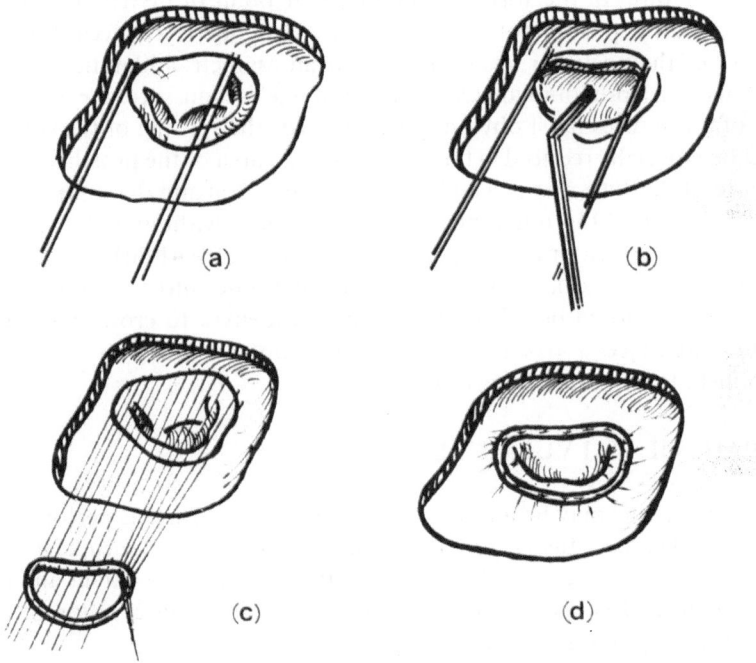

Figure 41.2 Technique of ring insertion (a) Pilot sutures placed at each commissure (b) Measurement by obturators of distance between commissures (c) Spacing of sutures on prosthetic ring: parallel for aortic leaflet sutures, reduced for sutures of the remainder of the annulus (d) Sutures tied, ring in place

The mitral valve is viewed directly and it is necessary to determine the feasibility of the operation according to the lesions observed. The most favourable condition for remodelling of the valve is a dilated mitral valve ring with an aortic leaflet which remains flexible and which is of sufficient size.

*Registered Trademark Rhone Poulenc France

The choice of the ring is based on the measurement at the base of the aortic leaflet which is not affected by the annulus dilatation and therefore can be used as a guide for the determination of the physiologic dimensions of the mitral orifice. In order to facilitate this measurement two pilot sutures are placed at each commissure (Figure 41.2a). The distance between these two points is measured with the obturators (Figure 41.2b).

Fifteen sutures are placed through the annulus along the whole periphery of the mitral ring. These sutures are then passed through the sewing ring of the prosthesis. The same space interval must be maintained between sutures of the aortic leaflet and their point of insertion into the corresponding portion of the prosthesis. Spacing is reduced for the sutures of the posterior leaflet. If there is an asymetric dilatation of the annulus with a predominant enlargement of one commissure, the distribution of the sutures must obviously be adapted: the spacing of the sutures must be especially reduced in the corresponding area of the prosthetic ring (Figure 41.2c). The ring is then brought into position and the sutures tied. This repositions the different annular structures without reducing the normal orifice area or affecting leaflet motion (Figure 41.2d).

The repair is verified by the injection of saline into the ventricular cavity. Care should be taken during this manoeuvre to cross-clamp the aorta and place a trochar in the aortic root in order to avoid air embolism to the coronary arteries.

REPAIR OF VALVULAR LESIONS

The leaflet tissue may be affected by different lesions such as perforation, cleft, thickening, fusion of the commissures, valve shrinkage, or calcifications. A careful analysis of the nature, the site, the extent and the severity of the lesions leads to a judgment regarding conservation of the valve rather than replacement.

Perforation may be treated by resection. Perforations of the mural leaflet may be treated by cuneiform resection of the leaflet and subsequent suture of the remaining edges. Only small perforations (< 5 mm) of the anterior leaflet may be treated by resection and subsequent suture.

Valve thickening, a consequence of rheumatic valve disease generally does not overly affect the pliability of the leaflet. It may be localised, taking the aspect of a fibrous nodule or a fibrous band, which should be either resected or thinned. If the pliability of the valve is affected by the fibrous process, the valve should be replaced.

Calcification of the valvular orifice usually leads to prosthetic replacement.

This can be avoided if the calcification is localised and can be treated by a limited resection.

Fusion of the commissures must be treated by commissurotomy taking care that the incision is made between two chordae and extends to within no more than 2 mm from the annulus.

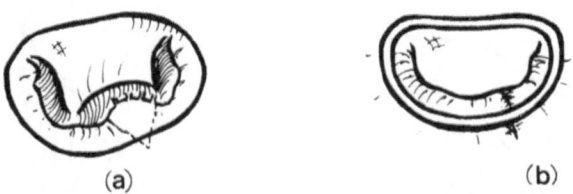

(a)   (b)

Figure 41.3 Resection of prolapsed portion of posterior leaflet secondary to ruptured chordae tendinae (a) Portion to be resected (b) Repair completed with prosthetic ring in place

REPAIR OF SUBVALVULAR LESIONS

The subvalvular apparatus may present different lesions of various aetiologies:
- ruptured papillary muscle, or fibrosis of a papillary muscle secondary to myocardial infarction,
- ruptured chordae due to either bacterial endocarditis, degeneration of the chordae or rheumatic valve disease,
- elongated chordae due to chordae dysplasia or the rheumatic process,
- fusion and retraction of the chordae.

In most instances, the three latter types of lesions can be treated by conservative procedures.

Ruptured chordae are treated by resection of the prolapsed part of the valve and suturing of the remaining edges (Figure 41.3). Valvular replacement may be necessary if the rupture affects the main chordae of the aortic leaflet, that is those arising from the free edge of this leaflet.

Elongation of chordae are treated by the following technique: the extremity of the corresponding papillary muscle is longitudinally incised. In this trench the extra length of the chordae is firmly attached by closing the papillary muscle around the buried portion of the chordae (Figure 41.4).

Fused chordae are treated by incision of the chordae or by resection of a triangular portion of the scarred tissue in order to completely release the subvalvular stenosis. Those hypertrophic and shortened chordae arising from the inferior surface of the leaflets and not from their free margins are resected (Figure 41.5).

These different techniques are the result of the evolution of the authors' experience in mitral valve surgery during the past six years. In the beginning, attention was concentrated on pure mitral insufficiency due to annular lesions which could accurately be treated by the ring valvuloplasty. This group represents only 4% of open-heart mitral valve surgery. Since remodelling of the valve appeared not to reduce the normal orifice area, valvular reconstruction could be extended to the treatment of more complex lesions. These include combined mitral insufficiency and stenosis which

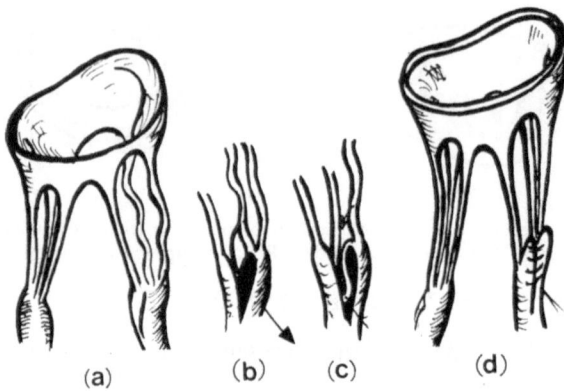

(a)   (b)   (c)   (d)

Figure 41.4 Shortening of elongation of chordae tendinae (a) Elongated chorda (b) Incision of papillary muscle (c) Shortening of chorda (d) Closure of papillary muscle

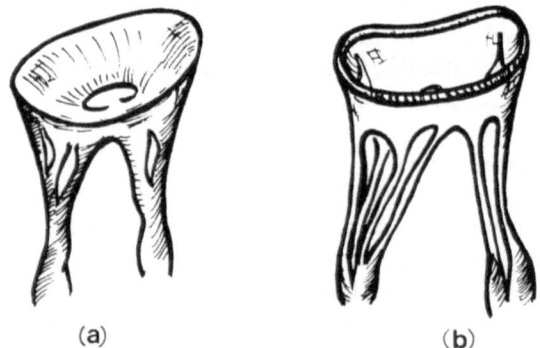

(a)   (b)

Figure 41.5 Fenestration of fused chordae tendinae (a) Fused chordae (b) Liberated chordae after fenestration

was heretofore considered to be a contraindication to reconstructive procedures. Thus, most of the non-calcified mitral valve disease, that is 40% of the open-mitral valve surgery has been treated by such conservative procedures in the past two years. This resulted in a significant reduction in morbidity and mortality in mitral valve surgery.

Experience at the Broussais Hospital consists of 186 patients operated on for isolated mitral valvuloplasty. Pure mitral insufficiency corrected by the ring valvuloplasty represents 56 cases, less than one-third of the patients. In most cases, the placement of the ring was associated with treatment of valvular or subvalvular stenosis (62 patients), ruptured chordae (32 patients) and elongation of the chordae (24 patients). Operative mortality was 6·5%. The late mortality was 2% and not related to valve malfunction. There were no reoperations in this series and good results were obtained in 92% of the cases. in 20% of the cases, a residual murmur persisted but with the exception of one case had no haemodynamic significance.[3]

One late death occurred in a patient who died from cancer, allowing examination of the repair after three years. The ring was completely incorporated and the valve perfectly competent.

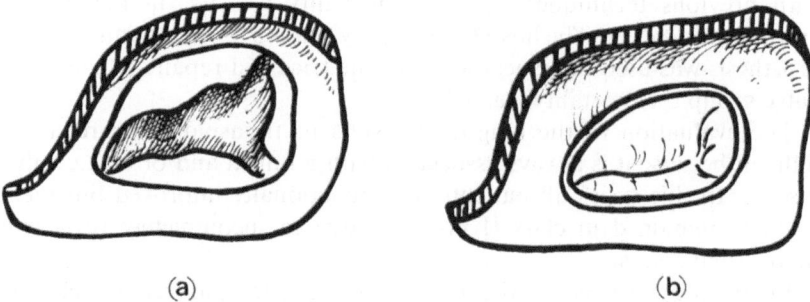

(a) (b)

Figure 41.6 Tricuspid valve ring valvuloplasty (a) Tricuspid insufficiency due to annular dilation (b) Reconstructed valve with prosthetic ring in place

Tricuspid valvuloplasty
The same concept was extended to the treatment of tricuspid valve disease. In 85% of the cases tricuspid insufficiency is the result of an annulus dilatation which may be treated by a prosthetic ring. The shape of the ring is adapted to the tricuspid configuration and is chosen according to the measurement of the septal leaflet which is not affected by the process of dilatation because of its attachment to the septum. As for the mitral valve, mattress sutures are placed around the annulus and then in the prosthetic ring keeping the same intervals for the sutures placed along the septal leaflet and reducing the interval between sutures for the rest of the annulus. The annulus is thus fixed in a definite shape and size preserving normal valve function and preventing recurrent dilatation (Figure 41.6).

Most patients with combined tricuspid stenosis and insufficiency can be treated by the same technique, since the orifice area is not reduced by the prosthetic ring. Commissurotomy is performed under direct vision with division of fused chordae, if necessary. When the posterior leaflet is severely injured and shrunken, only a double commissurotomy should be performed. This is done at the anteroseptal commissure and at the middle of the posterior leaflet, thus assuring a bicuspid appearance. Normal cusp apposition is then obtained by the insertion of a prosthetic ring. The ring is selected both by measurement of the septal leaflet and evaluation of the surface of the anterior leaflet. When the surface of this leaflet is slightly smaller than that of the obturator a smaller ring must be chosen.

A series of 269 patients have been operated on for associated tricuspid valve disease. In most cases (85%) the insufficiency was only due to the dilatation of the annulus. In 50 cases, the insufficiency was associated with a stenosis. The operative and late mortalities were improved in comparison with previous techniques. Hospital mortality was 9% in the double valvuloplasty series. The hospital mortality was 9·5% when a mitral valve prosthesis was used in association with the tricuspid repair. In the triple valve group the mortality was 16%.

The evaluation of the long-term results of tricuspid valve repair is difficult because it is always associated with a mitral and/or aortic valve disease. In this series all patients were functionally improved but most of them remained in class II probably due to incompletely reversible myocardial disease.

In an effort to assess the results of the tricuspid repairs clearly, intracardiac investigations have been performed on a series of 25 patients, i.e. catheterisation, intracardiac phonocardiogram and dilution curves with ascorbic acid and angiography. These results indicated perfect valvular competence and the absence of a gradient across the valve.[4]

Finally, the authors would like to discuss the problem of the clinical indications for a surgical repair of the tricuspid valve. This is difficult because tricuspid insufficiency is mainly the result of pulmonary hypertension. It is true that the valvular incompetence may disappear after mitral valve correction, but this is unpredictable. The systematic surgical abstention in tricuspid insufficiency as advised by Braunwald[5] is a dangerous policy resulting in a higher hospital mortality rate and a significant incidence of residual insufficiency.

Unlike many authors, we consider that digital exploration of the tricuspid valve has little place in the evaluation of tricuspid insufficiency. Moreover, it may convey false information because of the particular haemodynamic conditions under anaesthesia. Irreversible tricuspid regurgitation may apparently disappear in such circumstances, leading the surgeon not to explore a valve which should be corrected.

More confidence is placed in the evolution of the clinical and haemodynamic symptoms under preoperative optimal medical treatment for heart failure. This permits a clear distinction between totally reversible, irreversible and partially reversible insufficiency. Totally reversible tricuspid insufficiency, whatever the severity of the symptoms before medical treatment, does not require correction. Irreversible insufficiency always requires surgical correction. In partially reversible insufficiency, the valve must be explored by direct vision during operation. If there is no valve lesion and the annulus is smaller than three fingerbreadths, the insufficiency should not be corrected. If there are lesions of the valve or if the annulus admits more than three fingers, correction should be undertaken (Table 41.1).

CONCLUSION

Based on experience of more than 600 valvular repairs, it is believed that there is, at present, a definite place in valve surgery for valvular reconstructive procedures. Recent technical advances have made results predictable. Significant advantages of valve reconstruction over prosthetic replacement are: a decrease in thromboembolic risks, avoidance of anti-coagulants and the progressive nature of the occasional failures.

Those who oppose reconstructive surgery cite the unpredictable results, the ease and security of valve replacement and the small number of cases susceptible to being corrected by conservative techniques. These arguments are no longer valid. Remodelling of the annulus associated with a plastic repair of the other lesions have led to a high level of predictability of the results as shown by the authors' own experience. The slightly increased complexity and difficulty of these techniques for the surgeon should not outweigh the added benefits to the patient. The statements are made in the light of a hospital mortality which is the same as that for valve replacement.

Lastly, while it is true that calcified valvular disease is being seen with increasing frequency, this is largely due to advances in medical therapy which allow carrying the patient for a longer time before submitting him to operation. This is done of course at the expense of the myocardium which has sustained relatively greater damage during this period. An earlier reconstructive procedure prior to the advent of valvular calcification and irreversible myocardial damage might be advanced as a viable alternative.

Calcified valvular disease notwithstanding, there still remains a sufficiently large number of cases affected by endocarditis, elongated chordae and tricuspid insufficiency to warrant the development of reconstructive valvular surgery, which while it undoubtedly requires additional effort on the part of surgeon will by the same token assure him

Table 41.1 Flow chart showing pathways to correction or non-correction of tricuspid insufficiency

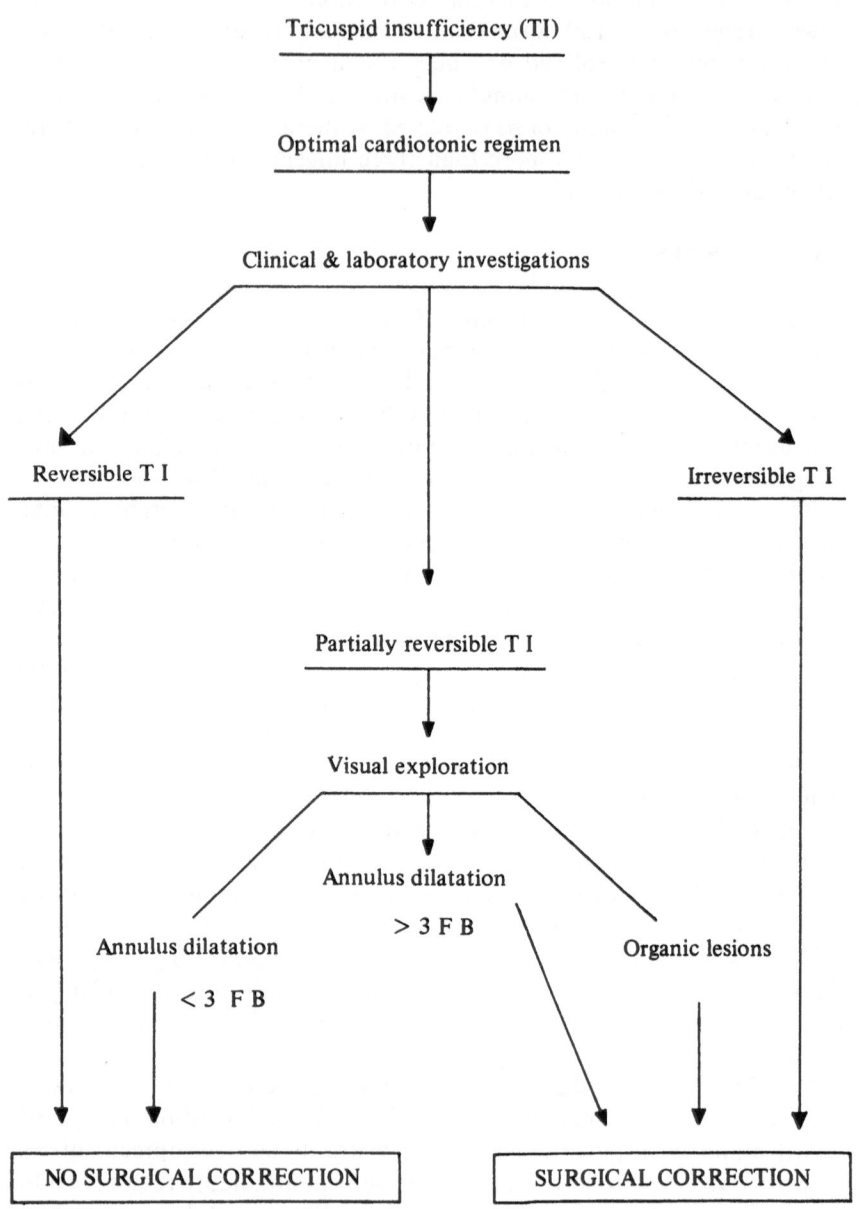

of the satisfaction of being able to offer his patients a superior quality of life following operation.

References

1. Kay, J. H., Maselli Campagna, C. and Tsuji, H. K. (1965). Surgical treatment of tricuspid insufficiency (1965). *Ann. Surg.*, **53**, 162
2. Carpentier, A. (1969). La valvuloplastie reconstitutive. *Presse Méd.*, **77**, 7
3. Carpentier, A., Deloche, A., Dauptain, J., Soyer, R., Prigent, C., Blondeau, P., Piwnica, A. and Dubost, C. (1971). A new reconstructive operation for correction of mitral and tricuspid insufficiency. *J. Thorac. Cardiovasc. Surg.*, **61**, 1
4. Carpentier, A., Deloche, A., Hanania, J., Forman, J., Sellier, P., Piwnica, A. and Dubost, C. (1974). Surgical management of acquired tricuspid valve disease. *J. Thorac. Cardiovasc. Surg.*, **67**, 1
5. Braunwald, N. S., Ross, J. and Morrow, A. G. (1967). Conservative management of tricuspid regurgitation in patients undergoing mitral valve replacement. *Circulation*, **35, Suppl. 1**, 63

Part 5

Open-Heart Surgery under One Year of Age

42
Open-heart surgery in the first year of life
J. Stark

Open-heart surgery may be required very early in life in two main groups of patients. In the first, operation is performed as a life-saving, often emergency, procedure for severe hypoxaemia, intractable heart failure or for a combination of both. Typical of this emergency group are infants with total anomalous pulmonary venous drainage (TAPVD) for whom the mortality rate without treatment is 85% during the first years of life. In the second group, operation is performed early in life because the prognosis without treatment, or even after palliative treatment, is unfavourable. The best example of the second group are infants with transposition of the great arteries (TGA). Balloon septostomy or surgical septectomy improved an otherwise unfavourable prognosis but thromboembolic episodes and the early development of pulmonary vascular disease present life-threatening complications.

The Hospital for Sick Children believe that operation should be performed early in infancy, if the risk of such operation is lower than the combined risk of waiting, palliation and subsequent correction. This would vary according to the lesion and to the experience of the team of physicians and surgeons. A high survival rate can be achieved only if the preoperative diagnosis is complete, operation accurate and expert intensive care is given before, during and after the operation. The facilities for investigation and surgery should therefore be available on a 24 h basis.

Important advances have been made in the techniques of open-heart surgery in small infants in the last ten years. Increasing numbers of infants with congenital heart disease are operated each year and the mortality rate steadily decreases. This trend can be seen in Figure 42.1 which summarises the ten year experience of this Unit. In the early years only patients for whom palliative operation was not available were submitted for open-heart surgery and the mortality rate was high. When more occurred the results started to improve. For example in 1972, 50 infants had open-heart operation and 41 (82%) survived (Figure 42.1).

Some patients were corrected using conventional cardiopulmonary bypass and moderate hypothermia, others were operated on using circulatory arrest under deep hypothermia (Table 42.1). The question of

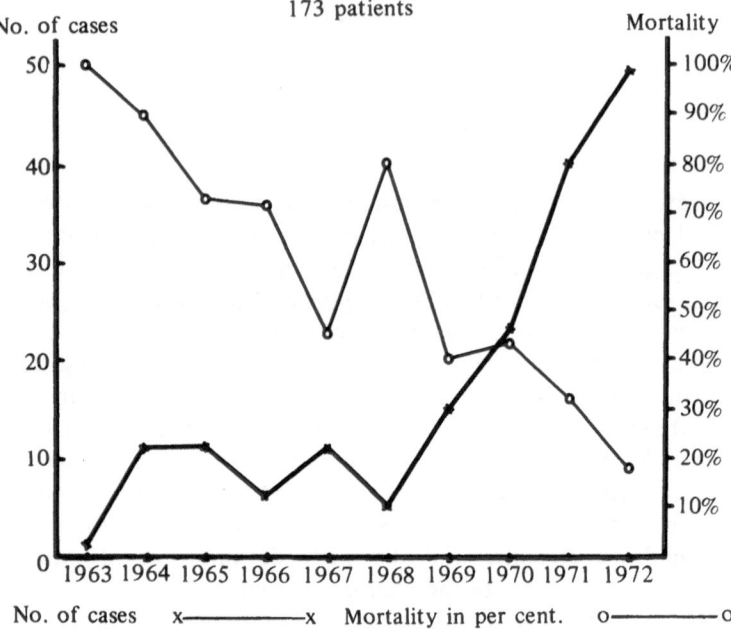

OPEN-HEART SURGERY IN THE FIRST YEAR OF LIFE

173 patients

No. of cases ... Mortality

No. of cases   x————x   Mortality in per cent.   o————o

Figure 42.1 The results of open-heart surgery in small infants at the Hospital for Sick Children (1963–1972)

Table 42.1 Operative techniques in open-heart surgery in infants in the first year of life

	114 INFANT BYPASSES		May 1971—October 1973	
Diagnosis	*Bypass + moderate hypothermia*	*Died*	*Circulatory arrest + deep hypothermia*	*Died*
TGA	31	0	8	1
TAPVD	6	2	20	8
VSD	12	0	9	0
Aortic stenosis	4	2	4	1
Miscellaneous	11	4	9	6
Total	64	8	50	16

(includes 6 patients operated twice)

whether to use one or other technique remains open. The Hospital for Sick Children believes that a technique which suits the whole team and gives good results for that particular lesion should be used. Currently a 'compromise' technique is being used. Small, sick infants are surface cooled with ice bags after the introduction of anaesthesia. Arterial and venous monitoring lines are inserted and patients cooled to a nasopharyngeal temperature of 28 °C. At this temperature the chest is opened and it is decided whether the patient will be operated on cardiopulmonary bypass or whether further cooling and circulatory arrest at 20 °C. will be employed. The advantage of this approach is the extra time gained should cardiac arrest occur when opening the chest. Surface cooling is more even and the heart is very stable at this temperature. If bypass at a lower temperature is used, perfusion rates can be decreased or circulatory arrest introduced for shorter periods.

Postoperative care is an integral part of the surgical treatment of congenital heart disease. Careful clinical observation as well as monitoring is necessary. Systemic, central venous and left atrial pressures, heart rate and temperature are recorded continuously. Circulatory volume is kept at its optimal level by transfusion of blood or plasma, depending on the left

Table 42.2 Results of 108 infant bypass operations at the Hospital for Sick Children between May 1971 and October 1973

Diagnosis	No.	Died
TGA	36	0
TAPVD	26	10
VSD	20	0
Aortic stenosis	8	3
Pulmonary atresia	2	2
Pulmonary stenosis	2	1
Triatrial heart	2	0
Mitral incompetence	2	0
Mitral stenosis	1	1
MI + AS + ASD + PDA	1	1
Primum ASD	1	0
Common atrium	1	1
Complete AV canal	1	1
AP window	1	0
Hemi truncus	1	0
Fallot	1	1
Ao-LV tunnel	1	1
Cardiac tumour	1	1
Total	108	23

atrial pressure and haematocrit. Contractility can be improved by a catecholamine infusion. Digoxin is given to patients who develop postoperative heart failure or supraventricular tachyarrhythmias. Epicardial pacemaker wires are inserted in all patients so that the heart can be paced if necessary.

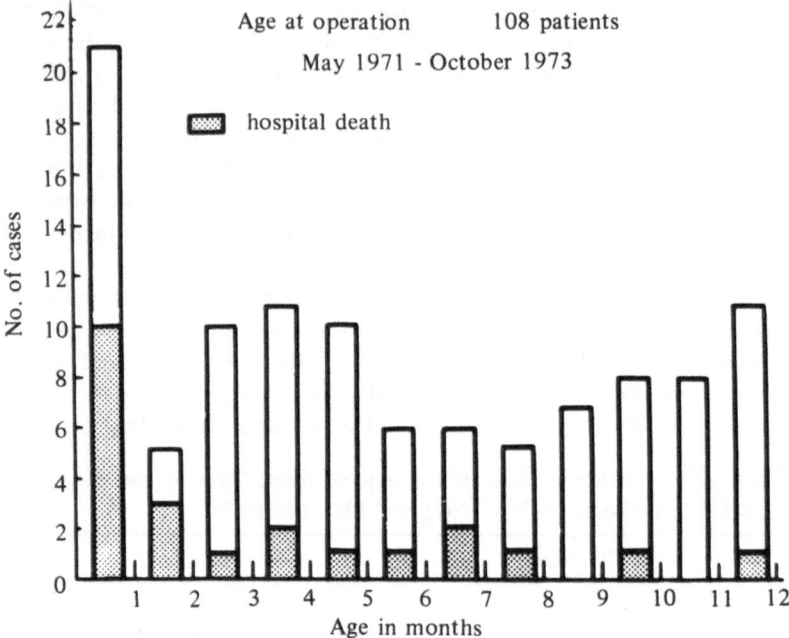

Figure 42.2 The age of infant patients treated with open-heart surgery at the Hospital for Sick Children between May 1971 and October 1973

Every infant is intubated with a nasotracheal tube and ventilated on a volume controlled respirator (Engstrom) for 24–48 h. Arterial blood gases are measured at frequent intervals and ventilation adjusted accordingly. Sedation with morphine (0·2 mg/kg body weight) is used. Gastric distension is avoided by free drainage via nasogastric tube. The patient is turned at hourly intervals and physiotherapy given two to four hourly. Fluid intake and output must be carefully measured. 5% dextrose is administered intravenously, 20, 30, 40 cc/m²/h during the first, second and third postoperative day. Potassium chloride is given intravenously (10 mEq/m² on the day of operation and 20 mEq/m² the following day. Oral fluids are usually started after 24 h.

More recent results from the Hospital for Sick Children are given in Table 42.2. 108 infants were operated between May 1971 and October 1973. There were three major groups in the series, infants with TGA,

TAPVD and ventricular septal defect (VSD). These three groups of patients will be discussed in detail later.

The age of the patients is shown in Figure 42.2. In the neonatal period, i.e. under four weeks of age, 11 out of 21 infants survived the operation.

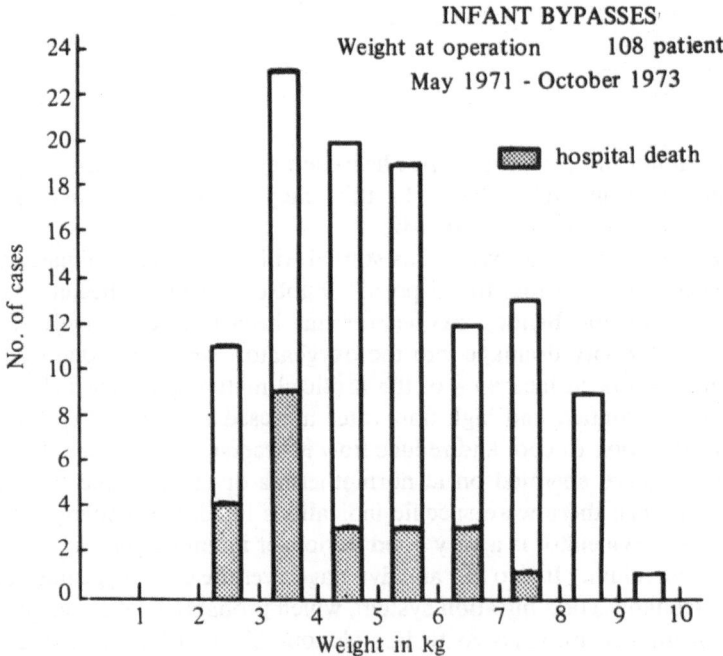

Figure 42.3 The weight of infants treated with open-heart surgery in the first year of life at the Hospital for Sick Children between May 1971 and October 1973

The higher risk in the first two months is caused by natural selection. Only patients with complex anomalies or severe forms of a single lesion have severe symptoms and require treatment.

The patients' weight is illustrated in Figure 42.3. All were under 10 kg. This demonstrates that age and weight in themselves are not significant risk factors. For the team using miniaturised equipment and dealing with small infants regularly, young age and low weight are not a contra-indication for surgery. Previously open-heart surgery has been considered too risky in children smaller than 10–15 kg. It is now felt that small, sick infants with congenital heart disease need operation because without it, survival is often unlikely.

43
Experience with infant perfusions
A. Starr

The author has performed open-heart surgery in infancy almost exclusively using conventional bypass. In this chapter, the experience with that technique will be briefly reviewed.

In the early 1960s, work was started with the use of a miniaturised disc oxygenator, i.e. before the disposable bubble oxygenator became available. Since 1968 the Bentley oxygenator has been used exclusively for infant bypass. Gravity drainage into the oxygenator, very small diameter tubing to reduce the surface area of the artificial materials with which the blood comes in contact and high flow rates are used under most circumstances but the option to cool and reduce flow if necessary is retained. Most of the patients were operated on at normothermia or at very mild hypothermia, except when there were specific indications for deeper cooling. The infant Bentley oxygenator is a very good device for infant surgery with a very low priming volume. It also has an advantage over the disc oxygenator , namely a reasonably good filtration system, which probably is of some importance when infants are exposed to homologous blood, which can undoubtedly contain foreign elements which result in microembolisation.

The preoperative treatment of patients coming to infant perfusion is quite simple in that after the diagnostic studies are made, the author does not hesitate to use respiratory support prior to operation if necessary. If the child is in a bad condition after study, intubation is performed in the patient's incubator and the infant is taken to the operating room while artificial ventilation is maintained. One of the problems with infant perfusion is not so much the perfusion but the problems of anaesthesia. Halothane was used in the past, but currently ketamine anaesthesia is used. The patients have an uncuffed nasotrachial tube in place and the arteries are not cannulated for arterial pressure, a Doppler ultrasonic probe on the skin being used instead. However, all the patients have a jugular venous catheter placed for central venous pressure measurements. The priming volume of the perfusion system is about 500 cm^3. Heparinised blood was used in the past but because of operational problems, ordinary blood-bank blood which is buffered with sodium bicarbonate is now used. 10% mannitol is added to the perfusate in the hope of diminishing the possibility of renal injury by improving renal blood flow during cardiopulmonary bypass. This blood is filtered through a swinnex filter to remove any of the usual debris which occurs in bank blood. Additional blood is added as required, ordinary ACD blood which is filtered through a swank filter being used. No filters are used in the system except for filtering the blood which is added to the system and the priming blood. An attempt has been made to reduce the surface area of the extra corporeal circuit as much as possible and there is evidence that the increased surface area of the surface-acting filters such as the swinnex filter, removes platelets from the circulation producing a clotting defect, which is sometimes difficult to manage.

The operative approach in almost all cases has been a median sternotomy. The cannulation of the ascending aorta rather than the iliac or femoral artery has greatly facilitated infant surgery. Separate venous cannulation through two separate purse strings for the inferior and superior vena cava is used with some special catheters for cannulation in the transposition group, since exposure of these cannulation sites at the entrance of the inferior and superior vena cava may be diffucult. Of course, the patient is always explored for ductus of left cava which can easily be missed on study and which can make perfusion difficult.

In the first 100 cases of infant perfusion using the standard perfusion technique we found that there was, almost always, metabolic acidosis which may be present in the infant prior to bypass can be reversed without medication by maintaining a high flow of normothermic perfusion. The amount of red cell damage is relatively small, the mean free haemoglobin in the first 100 cases being 78 mg % at its peak. It has been noticed that almost all the infants have a marked thrombocytopenia and that very meticulous haemostasis is required at the end of bypass. This is more important than with adult patients. It has also been noticed, that when proper attention is paid to postoperative care, he incidence of pulmonary deaths in a series of patients such as this is quite small. Therefore it can be said that the infant perfusion *per se* does not result in a high incidence of pulmonary injury. Postoperative care is important in obtaining good results with infant perfusion and perhaps the most important in this list of items, is the prophylactic direct vision suction of the patient after extubation. This is done frequently, even though the patient has no physical signs of retained secretions and of course frequent arterial blood gas determinations are made to indicate how to proceed.

These results are similar to those described by J. Stark (Chapter 42) in terms of showing the relative safety of cardiopulmonary bypass with the conventional approach in older infants. Bypass still represents a relatively high risk in younger patients. For example, in those patients under three

Table 43.1 INTRACARDIAC SURGERY WITH CARDIOPULMONARY BYPASS IN
108 INFANTS, UNIVERSITY OF OREGON MEDICAL SCHOOL

Lesion	No. of Patients	Deaths No.	Deaths %	Causes of Death (No.)
Tetralogy of Fallot				
Correction	34	3	9	Error in case selection (2); technical error (1)
Infundibulectomy	2	0	0	
Transposition (simple)	10	2	20	Arrhythmia (1); technical error (1)
Transposition (complex)	8	4	50	Arrhythmia (1); bleeding (1) respiratory (1); uncorrectable (1)
Total anomalous pulmonary venous return	7	4	57	High pulmonary vascular resistance (1); arrhythmia (1); left ventricular failure (1); anastomotic structure (1)
Ventricular septal defect (simple)	11	1	9	Respiratory (1)
Ventricular septal defect (complex)	10	5	50	Uncorrectable (2); high pulmonary vascular resistance (2); arrhythmia (1)
Single ventricle (PA banding)	2	1	50	Uncorrectable
Atrial septal defect (secundum)	6	1	17	Inadequate left ventricle
Atrial septal defect (primum)	1	0	0	
Atrioventricular canal	1	1	100	Left ventricular failure
Cor triatriatum	1	0	0	
Aortic stenosis	6	1	17	Technical error
Hypoplastic left ventricle	3	3	100	Uncorrectable (3)
Pulmonic stenosis	4	1	25	Arrhythmia
Double-outlet right ventricle	2	2	100	Arrhythmia (1); anaesthesia (1)
Total	108	29	27*	
No. correctable	100	21	21	

*Average.

months, there has been a 60% mortality. In those patients between three and six months there has been a 50% mortality. However, there is a significant change at the six months' level and in any of the infants over six months, there is a relatively low risk of conventional cardiopulmonary bypass. This holds true when considering the weights of the patients as well. For example, there have been problems with patients under four kilos. with a 66% mortality, and there have even been significant problems in patients under six kilos with a 47% mortality. There certainly is room for improvement here. However, in patients over six kilos, the mortality for conventional bypass and total correction is quite small.

In Table 43.1 the first 108 cases are listed according to diagnosis. In patients with obstructive lesions 11 correctable lesions), there were two deaths—a mortality of 18%. One patient showed a spectacular result following correction of cortriatriatum valve, at six weeks of age. With regard to left to right shunts, in 23 correctable lesions there were five deaths—a mortality of 22%. One of two patients survived with a single ventricle. This is an interesting group of patients with secundum type ASD who present in the first six months of life with severe congestive heart failure, due to a massive shunt. All these patients survived operation. Finally, with right to left shunt groups, there were 61 such patients in the first 100, with a mortality rate of 23%. The mortality in the tetralogy group was 10% and there was also a significant mortality in transposition of 30%. With TAPVD, mortality was 43%

Table 43.1 lists causes of death in these first 108 cases. Very few of the patients died as a direct result of the use of cardiopulmonary bypass, as compared with scme other method of obtaining access for open-heart surgery. Only one patient died of pericardial tamponade as a result of a clotting defect, perhaps induced by cardiopulmonary injury relating to the bypass.

The author's experience very closely parallels the experience at Great Ormond Street, except that there are more problems in the group between three and six months of age. The use of cardiopulmonary bypass has many advantages not the least being that there are no pressures of time in this operation as there are in conditions of circulatory arrest.

44
Management of ventricular septal defects in infants
A. J. Furst

Ventricular septal defects are one of the most common forms of congenital heart disease and only a small number of patients with ventricular septal defects are symptomatic during the first few months of life. If congestive heart failure is present it can usually be treated adequately in most cases with Digoxin and diuretics. However if death occurs from a ventricular septal defect in the first fifteen years of life it is usually within the first six to twelve months. In a minority of cases medical therapy is ineffective and surgical intervention is indicated.

During the past few years, as more experience and greater safety in infant perfusion has been achieved, the trend has been shifted from palliative to corrective procedures.

Prior to 1971, at the Hospital for Sick Children, surgical therapy for ventricular septal defects in infancy was pulmonary artery banding followed by elective closure of the defect and debanding before school age. At present banding is reserved only for some complex cases; complete A-V canal, single ventricle and multiple ventricular septal defects. In cases where a patent ductus arteriosus is felt to be a major factor responsible for heart failure, it is ligated. If the pulmonary artery pressure does not drop and failure persists following duct ligation, early correction is performed.

Table 44.1 Indications for closure of VSD in the first year of life

Indications	No.
Inadequate banding	5
Persistent heart failure despite maximum medical treatment	15

Since 1971 all infants with ventricular septal defects refractory to maximal medical therapy have undergone primary closure during the first year of life (Table 44.1). Five patients in the group had previously undergone pulmonary artery banding.

There have been 21 operations in 20 patients under the age of one year. It is of importance that associated malformations contributing to the severity of heart failure were present in eight (Table 44.2). In each case of operated VSD, cardiac catherisation data was consistent (Table 44.3).

Table 44.2 Ventricular septal defect closure in infancy May 1971–October 1973

Diagnosis	No.
VSD	6
VSD + PFO	5
Gerbode VSD	1
VSD + PFO + Coarctation	1
Multiple VSD + PDA + Coarctation	1
VSD + ASD	3
+ PDA	2
+ PAPVD	1
TOTAL	20

Table 44.3 Cardiac catheterisation data in cases of operated VSD

Haemodynamic data	
Qp/Qs	> 2
Pp/Ps	> 0·6
Rp/Rs	< 0·2

Initial results of operated VSD cardiac catheterisation data was consistent (Table 44.3). Initial results of medical therapy in many cases eventually requiring operation were encouraging. However as pulmonary vascular resistance decreased, heart failure could not be controlled and surgical intervention was indicated. The age distribution was between three and nine months (Figure 44.1). Ten patients were between three and five months of age. The average weight in our series was 4·9 kg ranging between 2·8 and 6·2 kg (Figure 44.2).

OPERATIVE TECHNIQUE

Surface cooling is used in the smaller and severely ill patients. The nasopharyngeal temperature is monitored and as surface cooling pro-

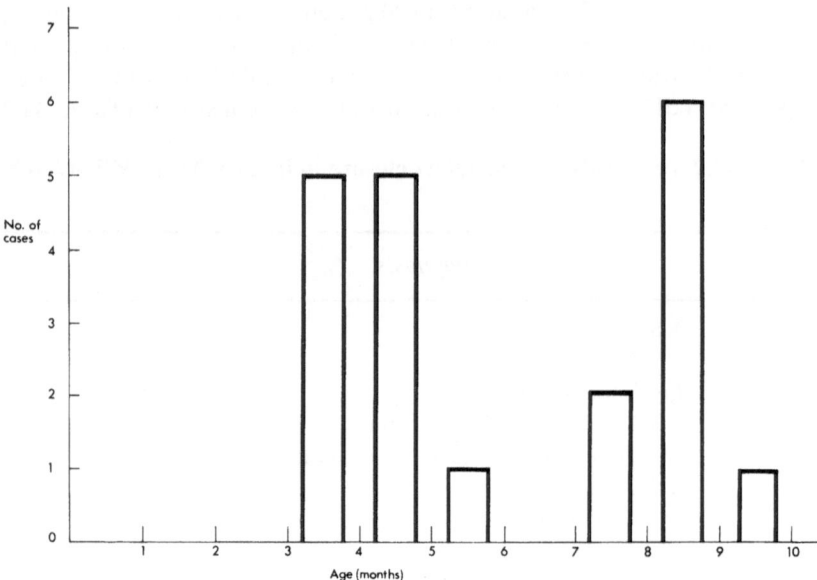

Figures 44.1 Illustrates the relationship between the number of patients and their age in months

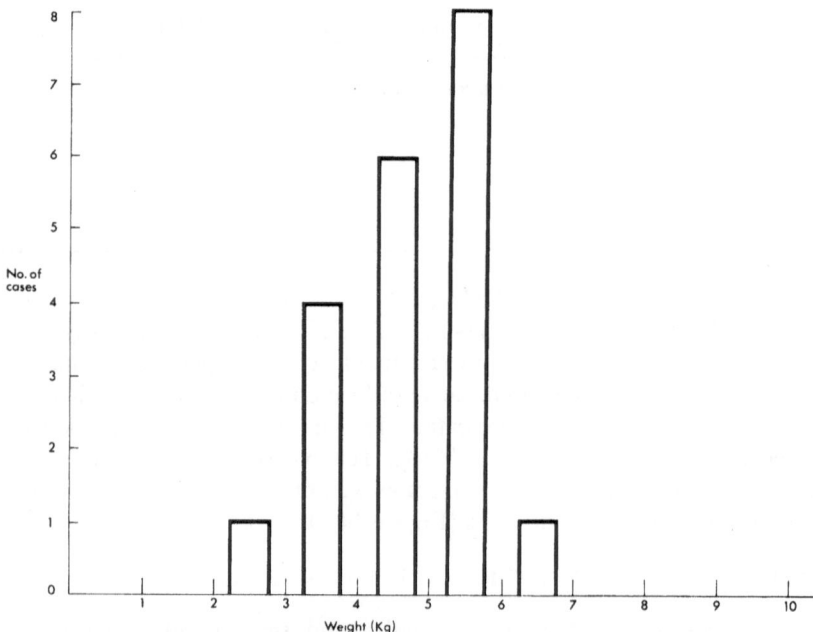

Figure 44.2 Shows the relationship between the weight in kg and the age in months

gresses, arterial and SVC monitoring lines are placed. When a naso-pharyngeal temperature of 27 °C is reached the ice bags are removed and the patient prepared and draped. Perfusion lines are divided and the defibrillator made ready prior to the surgical incision.

A median sternotomy incision is used and only after assessing the anatomy is the decision for circulatory arrest or conventional cardio-pulmonary bypass made. If the right atrium appears large enough for cannulation and adequate exposure, bypass is selected. Right-angled Rygg cannulae are used to facilitate the exposure in small infants. If how-ever, favourable anatomy is not present, core cooling by partial bypass with a single large venous cannula in the right atrium is used. When a nasopharyngeal temperature of 19 °C is reached, perfusion is stopped and the procedure done with circulatory arrest. The length of operation is somewhat increased with the circulatory arrest. However, perfusion time is virtually the same in both methods. Bypass was utilised in 12 cases and circulatory arrest in nine (Table 44.4).

Table 44.4 Operative technique in cases of VSD in infants

Surgical technique			
Right atriotomy	8	Conventional bypass	12
Right ventriculotomy	13	Circulatory arrest	9

Initially the approach to the VSD was by a right ventriculotomy, however we now visualise the defect through the tricuspid valve and if exposure is adequate the defect is repaired through the valve, otherwise right ventriculotomy is utilised. The atrial approach has been used in eight operations and the right ventricle in 13. In the later cases the atrial approach has been used more frequently. Great care must be exercised when dealing with the tricuspid valve. The tissue is extremely fragile and the chordae can be easily entrapped. Although the defects may be small, suture placement can be difficult. At present we are using a special small needle with 3–0 silk to allow safe suture placement especially near chordae and conducting tissue. Teflon patches were used in the majority of cases. Direct suture was accomplished only three times. In each case postoperative RV pressure was less than half the systemic pressure.

POSTOPERATIVE CARE

Surprisingly the postoperative course in most infants has been re-markably smooth. In each case nasotracheal intubation and ventilation has been utilised. Extubation is frequently possible in 16–24 h. Blood gases, left atrial and arterial pressures, electrolytes and osmolality of plasma and urine are monitored. Fluid and respiratory therapy are carefully adjusted with regard to the parameters. Digoxin and diuretics are continued if indicated.

Table 44.5 Results in 20 cases operated on for VSD

Results	*No. of Cases*
Mortality	0
Complications:	
Temporary complete A-V dissociation	1
Postoperative infection and reopening	
of VSD	1

RESULTS (Table 44.5)

Fortunately there has been no mortality in the 20 operated patients. Complications included temporary A-V dissociation which reverted to sinus rhythm after 14 days. Another patient had a severe mediastinitis and sternal dehiscence reopened the VSD. This was closed at a second operation. At last follow-up all patients were well.

In summary, the presented data suggest that primary closure of ventricular septal defects in infancy is a relatively safe procedure. When indicated it is possible to offer a one-stage procedure with its medical, social and psychological advantages for both the child and family.

45
Total surgical correction of total anomalous pulmonary venous drainage in infancy
F. Midgley

While total anomalous pulmonary venous drainage (TAPVD) represents a relatively rare abnormality in the total picture of congenital heart disease (about 1·5%), it does constitute a significant proportion of infant bypass procedures. At the Hospital for Sick Children, Great Ormond Street, in the time period 1963–1971, TAPVD represented 44% (55/124) infant bypass procedures, while in recent years it has ranged between 20 and 30%.

In the three years ending March 1974 there have been 27 infants that have undergone bypass at this hospital for TAPVD, the methods of treatment and results of which are presented here.

ANATOMY

TAPVD presents in four anatomical patterns of drainage. Most commonly in the 'supracardiac' type, pulmonary venous drainage is to the innominate vein or SVC via an anomalous communicating vertical vein. In the 'cardiac' type, pulmonary venous drainage is to the right atrium or coronary sinus, while in the 'infradiaphragmatic' type, the pulmonary veins drain via an anomalous descending trunk through the diaphragm to connect either with the portal vein or the inferior vena cava. The fourth type is termed 'mixed' and consists of any combination of the foregoing types.

PHYSIOLOGY

The physiological derangements associated with TAPVD are somewhat variable and are related to the size of the atrial patency, the degree of pulmonary venous obstruction and the presence of pulmonary hypertension. Those patients with a restrictive atrial patency or obstructed anomalous vein often present early in infancy in severe congestive heart failure. This is due to volume overload of the right ventricle and the pulmonary circuit, arterial desaturation and the frequent occurrence of obstruction to pulmonary venous flow from a restrictive ASD or restrictive communicating vein or system. At the other end of the pathophysiologic spectrum, those patients with non-restrictive pulmonary venous drainage and no pulmonary hypertension often do not present until later in life, much as a patient with a large ASD.

The indications for operation are clear once a definitive diagnosis has been made. Any infant with the diagnosis of TAPVD with symptoms, with pulmonary hypertension or with pulmonary venous obstruction should undergo urgent total correction.

OPERATIVE TECHNIQUE

The operative approach as we presently employ it at Great Ormond Street, begins when necessary with intensive preoperative care with endotracheal intubation, ventilation, and arterial and venous pressure lines. In those patients not requiring these before operation, they are placed after the administration of anaesthesia, while the patient is undergoing a preliminary period of surface cooling as the initial stage of the technique of profound hypothermia with limited cardiopulmonary bypass and circulatory arrest as employed in many centres today. After surface cooling to 27 °C. has been achieved, a midline sternotomy is made with subsequent placement of the ascending aortic arterial cannula and a single venous cannula with cooling on bypass to 19 °C. The anomalous vein is dissected as is the common trunk and its relation to the left atrium carefully assessed. With circulatory arrest the anastomosis between the common trunk and the left atrium is made. We presently prefer the 'open' technique of anastomosis. The anomalous communicating vein is occluded as the common trunk is opened. At the completion of the side-to-side anastomosis the anomalous vein is ligated and the atrial patency closed. With the cardiac type of TAPVD to the right atrium or coronary sinus, patch diversion of pulmonary venous blood to the left atrium is accomplished by the usual techniques. At the completion of the procedure the patient is rewarmed on bypass.

RESULTS

The overall operative results for our group of 27 patients treated and operated by this method are presented here (Table 45.1). The patients ranged in age from four days to 11 months. Of the 27 patients operated on, 17 survived (63%). When analysed by types (Table 45.2), we see that there is a definitive relationship between the pattern of drainage and mortality. In the more common supracardiac type the mortality was 29% while for the other types grouped together it was 46%.

These numbers, while high, represent a significant improvement over figures from this institution for an earlier time period as shown in Table 45.3. This is especially true for the group under three months (Table 45.4). While one would assume mortality would be age-related in

Table 45.1 The overall operative results for 27 infant perfusions for TAPVD at the Hospital for Sick Children, Great Ormond Street, March 1971–March 1974

No. of Operations	No. of Survivors	Age range
27	17 (63%)	4 days–11 months

Table 45.2 The relationship between the pattern of draining and mortality in infants with TAPVD

	No. of Cases	No. of Deaths
To innom. vein	14	4 (28%)
Other	13	6 (46%)

Table 45.3 Operative results for infant perfusions for TAPVD at the Hospital for Sick Children, Great Ormond Street

	No. of cases	No. of survivors
Feb. 1963–April 1971	47	15 (32%)
May 1971–Oct. 1973	26	16 (62%)

Table 45.4 Operative results at the Hospital for Sick Children, Great Ormond Street, for infants of less than 3 months

	No. of cases	No. of survivors
1963–1971	21	0
1971–1973	16	10 (63%)

this infant group, as several previous reports have suggested, by looking at Table 45.5 we see that this is not so. Nor is it related to the presence of pulmonary hypertension or pulmonary venous obstruction in our series.

Table 45.5 The relationship between age and mortality in infants with TAPVD

	No. of cases	No. of deaths
< 1 month	9	4
1–3 months	8	2
3–6 months	6	2
6–12 months	4	2

Complications of surgery have included two cases of stomal stenosis, congestive failure, atelectasis, seizures, bleeding, metabolic acid-base and electrolyte abnormalities, as well as cardiac arrest.

It is a generally accepted statistic that the mortality without surgery for TAPVD in the first year of life approaches 80%. Certainly the results of the definitive operative therapy of TAPVD have improved dramatically in recent years. This is true not only at Great Ormond Street, but is evidenced in reports from many other Units as well. There are many reasons for this improvement, and certainly high on the list are the technique of profound hypothermia and circulatory arrest, the method of 'open' anastomosis and improved early and complete diagnosis and treatment.

The technique of profound hypothermia and circulatory arrest, as we use it today greatly facilitates the actual mechanics of the operation, but equally successful and improved results have been reported utilising standard perfusion techniques. Certainly more sophisticated equipment and perfusion techniques in general for infant bypass have played their role.

The 'open' method of anastomosis that we have utilised in this series for the supra and infracardiac types was reported in the literature by Gersony *et al.* in 1971, as a modification of the method originally reported by Shumaker and King in 1961. It has proved extremely valuable in accomplishing a larger, more accurately placed and well-overted anastomosis between the common pulmonary venous trunk and the left atrium. It has the additional element that some volume may be 'borrowed' from the right atrium for the left atrium simply by shifting the point where the septum is reattached.

Thus, in summary, we report the recent Great Ormond Street experience of 27 infant perfusions for TAPVD with a mortality of 37%. This represents a significant improvement over previous years' results. This has occurred in a setting of a new perfusion technique and a new anastomotic technique. We feel that an aggressive surgical policy is justified by the improved results obtained by current methods.

46
Operative treatment of patients with transposition of the great arteries in infancy

J. Stark

Transposition of the great arteries (TGA) is one of the most common cyanotic congenital heart lesions presenting in infancy. The natural history of patients with TGA is very unfavourable. Without treatment 85–90% of children with TGA die during the first year of life. Balloon septostomy[1] has markedly improved the chances of survival of an infant born with TGA. Anatomic correction has not been achieved in patients with un-complicated TGA. However, physiological correction by redirecting the systemic and pulmonary venous returns has succeeded. The principle of this operation was established by Albert[2] in 1955. Mustard[3] described his modification in 1964 and since then Mustard's operation has been success-fully used in a great number of patients[4-8]. The optimum age for correction remains controversial. If corrective surgery is delayed too long, many infants will die. The probability of surviving to two and a half years without corrective surgery is no more than 50%[9]. The major causes of death are cerebrovascualr accidents and other thromboembolic episodes and this is the first argument for an early correction. The second argument is the failure of palliative treatment. The size of the atrial septal defect is not the sole determinant of mixing between the pulmonary and systemic circulations. Some infants do not mix adequately despite a good-sized atrial septal defect. In these patients only early correction can give a chance for survival.

Mustard's operation can be performed on cardiopulmonary bypass and moderate hypothermia, or the Kyoto technique of circulatory arrest under deep hypothermia can be used. The heart is exposed through a median sternotomy and the ascending aorta cannulated for arterial return. Venous cannulation is facilitated by the use of a right-angled Rygg cannula with a semirigid tip (Figure 46.1). This method of cannulation is easy even in small infants and the cannula will not obstruct the operative field. The right (systemic) ventricle is vented. Fresh heparinised blood is used whenever possible. pH of the perfusate is corrected with sodium bicarbonate and haemodilution to a PCV of 30% achieved by adding Ringer's lactate. Operation is performed at mild hypothermia, 28–30 °C, at a flow of 2–2·4 l/min/m².

At the present time a pericardial patch, tailored into a trouser shape is used (Figure 46.2), as suggested by Professor Brom. The coronary sinus is left to drain with the pulmonary venous blood. A shunt caused by coronary sinus blood has not been detected at postoperative investigations. The advantage of this approach is the absence of stitching

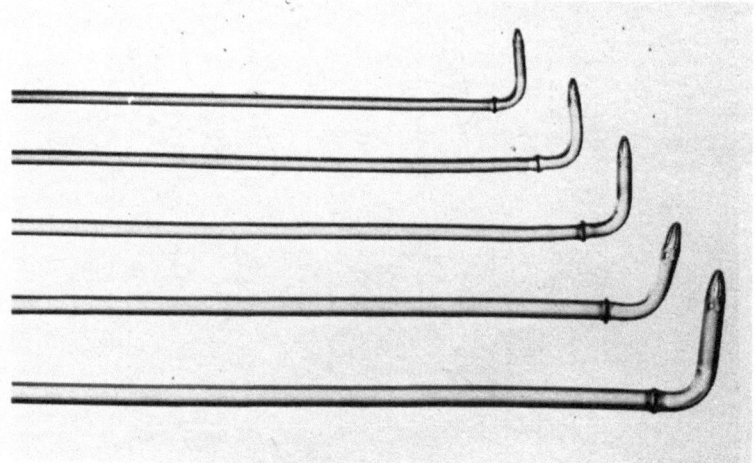

Figure 46.1 Right-angled Rygg cannulae with semirigid tips

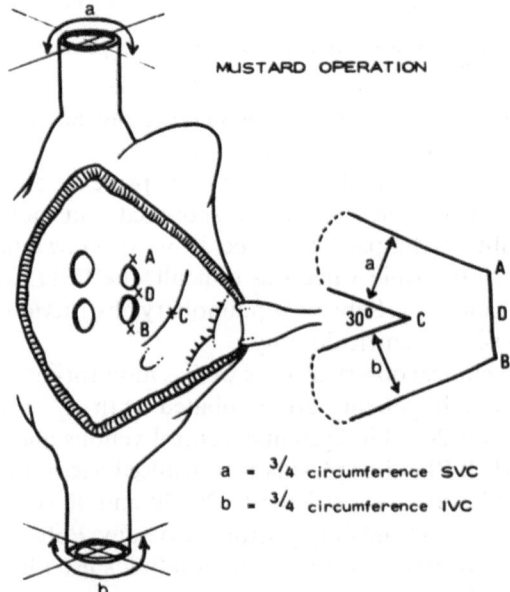

MUSTARD OPERATION

30°

a = ³/₄ circumference SVC
b = ³/₄ circumference IVC

Figure 46.2 Mustard's operation using a pericardial patch tailored into a trouser shape

anterior to the coronary sinus and possible injury to the A-V node or bundle of His. Care is taken not to bring the upper and lower suture lines too close together on the lateral atrial wall (Figure 46.3). If this happens a constricting ring may be formed and may contribute to the development of pulmonary venous obstruction. If the size of the pulmonary

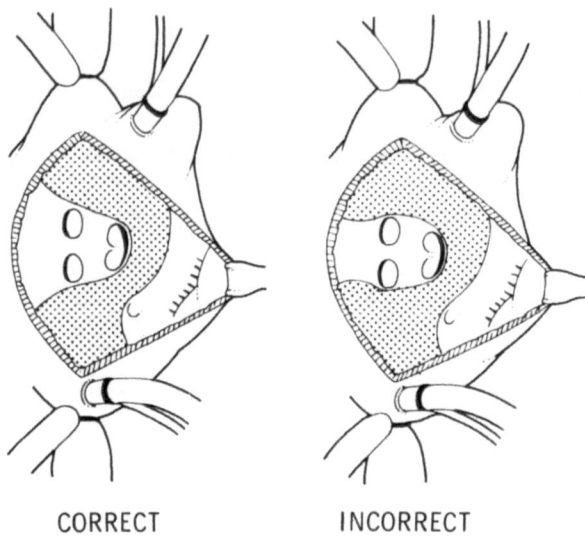

CORRECT   INCORRECT

Figure 46.3 Correct and incorrect positions of the upper and lower suture lines on the lateral atrial wall

venous atrium seems to be inadequate it can be enlarged with a patch, but this technique is not used routinely.

If a ventricular septal defect (VSD) is present, it is closed through the tricuspid valve which is gently retracted but not detached. Anoxic arrest facilitates this part of the operation. In a few infants in whom access through the tricuspid valve was difficult, the VSD was closed through a left ventriculotomy. Subvalvar pulmonary obstruction can also be relieved through the left ventriculotomy.

Careful clinical observation as well as monitoring after the operation is obligatory. All patients are intubated with a nasotracheal tube and ventilated for 24–48 h. Systemic, central venous and left atrial pressures are recorded. Blood or plasma is transfused according to PCV and atrial pressures. Fluids are restricted to 20, 30 and 40 cc of 5% dextrose/h/m^2 on the first, second and third postoperative day. Potassium chloride is given intravenously in small doses[10] and oral fluids usually restarted after 24 h. All patients have two pacemaker wires inserted. Catecholamines, Digoxin and diuretics are used on the usual indications.

Since 1967, 63 infants have had Mustard's operation in their first year of life (Table 46.1). Age, weight and their relationship to the mortality rate in patients with TGA + ASD is shown in Figures 46.4 and 46.5. Table 46.2 emphasises that early correction is preferable and that the risk compares favourably in the group of patients corrected in the first year of life to those corrected later. The two youngest patients in this group were only three weeks old and both survived the operation. There was no hospital death in the last 37 operated infants.

The group of patients with TGA + VSD presents a more difficult problem. Correction has been attempted in 10 infants with four survivors.

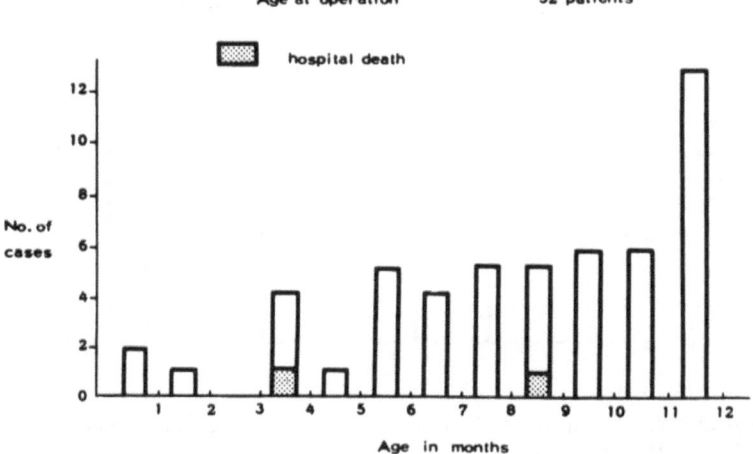

Figure 46.4 The age of infants undergoing Mustard's operation within the first year of life at the Hospital for Sick Children

Table 46.1 The number of infant patients on whom Mustard's operation was performed at the Hospital for Sick Children between 1965 and October 1973

Diagnosis	Age at operation	
	1 year	1 year
TGA + ASD	52	143
TGA + VSD	10	52
TGA + VSD + LVOTO	—	15
TGA + LVOTO	1	5
TGA other	—	2
Total	63	217

It has been emphasised in the literature that operation for TGA + VSD carries a higher risk even in older children. Pulmonary vascular disease can develop very early, therefore operation should probably be done before the age of four to six months. The problem of whether pulmonary artery banding followed by 'early correction' at the age of 12 to 18 months, or whether early primary correction with closure of the VSD should be performed, has not yet been solved.

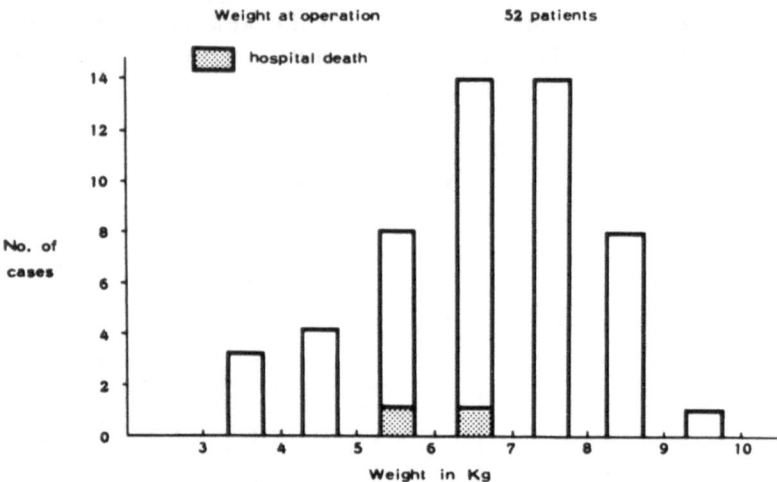

Figure 46.5 The weight of infants undergoing Mustard's operation within the first year of life at the Hospital for Sick Children

Table 46.2 Hospital mortality in infants operated on for correction of TGA and ASD (1965–October 1973)

	< 1 year			> 1 year	
Cases	Died	Per cent	Cases	Died	Per cent
52	2	4	143	14	10

Table 46.3 Complications of Mustard's operation

1. Arrhythmias
2. Pulmonary venous obstruction
3. Systemic venous obstruction
4. Detachment of the Baffle
5. Tricuspid incompetence

316

Infants with TGA + VSD + left ventricular outflow tract obstruction (LVOTO) are best treated by an aorto-pulmonary shunt when they become too cyanosed. A Rastelli-type repair is then performed at the age of five to six years. Currently the risk of this corrective procedure is under 20%.

The most difficult combination of lesions is TGA + VSD + preductal coarctation of the aorta. The operative risk used to be very high. Recently three out of four patients survived the resection of the coarctation and banding of the pulmonary artery. They are now awaiting correction.

Several complications can develop following Mustard's operation. They are listed in Table 46.3. The incidence of arrhythmias was greatly reduced by two changes in the operative technique; the suture line was kept behind the coronary sinus and the superior vena cava cannulation site was removed far from the sinus node. There were 24 atrial flutters and 14 A-V dissociations in the first group of 50 survivors of Mustard's operation. In the last 94 survivors, there were three patients with atrial flutter and two with A-V dissociation.

The incidence of systemic venous obstruction was related to the use of a Dacron patch and to the size of the patient. Of 172 patients surviving Mustard's operation with a pericardial baffle, eight developed systemic venous obstruction, while in the group of 84 survivors in whom a Dacron baffle was used 26 developed obstruction (Table 46.4).

Table 46.4 Systemic venous obstruction after Mustard's operation

Site of obstruction	Baffle	
	Pericardium (172 survivors)	Dacron (84 survivors)
SVC	8	16
IVC	–	4
SVC and IVC	–	6
Total	8	26

Pulmonary venous obstruction[11] and tricuspid incompetence[12] are rare but possibly serious complications. In order to avoid the obstructive complications a pericardial baffle cut into a trouser shape is now being used. The pressures in the systemic venous atrium, superior and inferior vena cava at the completion of the operation are carefully measured and biplane SVC cineangiography is performed 48–72 h after operation. The short-term results in the last 52 patients are encouraging but only several years' follow-up will prove or disprove this policy.

The late results (minimum follow-up of three years) were studied in a group of 113 survivors of Mustard's operation (all ages). Forty-nine patients (44%) were found in excellent health, attending normal school and taking part in sports. They were not receiving medication and were pink and the heart size was normal on X-ray. Fifty-seven patients (50%) were considered satisfactory. They still attended normal school but some of them showed slight fatigue on exertion, some suffered from arrhythmias and the heart size was enlarged on X-ray in others. Only seven patients (6%) were handicapped. In this group there were patients attending special schools, patients in chronic heart failure and patients in complete A-V dissociation.

The data presented demonstrates that Mustard's operation is a highly successful treatment for patients with TGA. It can be performed safely in the first year of life. Long-term results are satisfactory but more effort is needed to avoid late complications such as arrhythmias and systemic and pulmonary venous obstruction.

References

1. Rashkind, W. J. and Miller, W. W. (1966). Creation of an atrial septal defect without thoracotomy. A palliative approach to complete transposition of the great arteries. *JAMA*, **1961**, 991

2. Albert, H. M. (1954). Surgical correction of transposition of the great vessels. *Surg. Forum*, **51**, 74

3. Mustard, W. T. (1964). Successful two-stage correction of transposition of the great vessels. *Surgery*, **55**, 469

4. Danielson, G. K., Mair, D. D., Ongley, P. A., Wallace, R. B. and McGoon, D. C. (1971). Repair of transposition of the great arteries by transposition of venous return. *J. Thorac. Cardiovasc. Surg.*, **61**, 96

5. Breckenridge, I. M., Oelert, H., Stark, J., Graham, G. R., Bonham-Carter, R. E. and Waterston, D. J. (1972). Mustard's operation for transposition of the great arteries. *Lancet*, **1**, 1140

6. Clarkson, P. M., Barratt-Boyes, B. G., Neutze, J. M. and Lowe, J. B. (1972). Results over a ten-year period of palliation followed by corrective surgery for complete transposition of the great arteries. *Circulation*, **45**, 1251

7. Stark, J., de Leval, M., Waterston, D. J., Graham, G. R. and Boham-Carter, R. E. (1974). Corrective surgery of transposition of the great arteries in the first year of life. *J. Thorac. Cardiovasc. Surg.*, **67**, 673

8. Trusler, G. A. and Mustard W. T. (1974). Palliative and reparative procedures for transposition of the great arteries. *Ann. Thorac. Surg.*, **17**, 410

9. Tynan, M. (1971). Survival of infants with transposition of great arteries after balloon atrial septostomy. *Lancet*, **1**, 621

10. Breckenridge, I. M., Deverall, P. B., Kirklin, J. W. and Digerness, S. B. (1972). Potassium intake and balance after open intracardiac operations. *J. Thorac. Cardiovasc. Surg.*, **63**, 305

11. Stark, J., Tynan, M. Ashcroft, K. W., Aberdeen, E. and Waterston, D. J. (1972). Obstruction of pulmonary veins and superior vena cava after the Mustard operation for transposition of the great arteries. *Circulation*, **45 & 46 (Suppl. 1)**, 1–116

12. Tynan, M., Aberdeen, E. and Stark, J. (1972). Tricuspid incompetence after the Mustard operation for transposition of the great arteries. *Circulation*. **45 & 46 (Suppl. 1)**, 1–111

47

Treatment of valvar stenosis

A. Rees

The purpose of this report is to present the results of two groups of infants, one with a critical pulmonary stenosis, and the other with aortic stenosis. There are 19 in the pulmonary group, and 8 in the aortic group, all under 1 year. 8 of the infants with pulmonary stenosis were female, whereas all the children with aortic stenosis were male. I would like to deal with the pulmonary group first.

All the infants had a systolic murmur, with a single second sound which was usually heard soon after birth and the present symptoms in the majority of patients was cyanosis. This developed at a varying time after birth, ranging from the first day to 6 months. Feeding difficulties were not generally a problem and tachypnoea occurred in only 7 patients and these were all neonates. A significantly enlarged liver was seen in 8, but oedema occurred in only 1 infant. The X-ray finding showed cardiomegaly in all but 1 and pulmonary oligaemia in all but 2.

The ECG usually showed right ventricular hypertrophy, with a newborn RS pattern in the neonates. The axis varied more in the neo-natal group from $+60$ to $+150$, with a mean of 110, whereas those aged from 1 month to 1 year, the right axis was more pronounced varying from 120 to 180 with a mean of 140. 2 patients had secundum type ASD's whereas all the rest had a patent foramen (ovale) and 7 had evidence of tricuspid regurgitation. The first 3 infants who were operated on between 1961 and 1966, all underwent closed pulmonary valvotomy through a left anterior thoracotomy. Graduated sounds were passed through a right ventriculotomy, through the valve which was felt to split. The first of these infants died, but in fact she was in a moribund condition prior to operation and post mortem showed a satisfactory split of the valve.

Several years then passed before another one appeared in the Brompton and two patients were seen in 1966. Both underwent closed pulmonary valvotomy and one is still doing well on his original operation, whereas the other had a subsequent open valvotomy two years later and is now asymptomatic. From 1966 onwards, cardiopulmonary bypass was consistently used in preference to the closed technique and also in preference to the inflow occlusion method, which was at that time reported by Mustard, Jane and Trusla. It was thought that the greater control of the circulation, with a correction of hypoxia and acidosis, and the added time allowed to make a careful commissurotomy that also closed the associated interatrial communication, was more important than the disadvantage with the more complicated operative technique. On bypass, the infants were cooled universally to 25 °C and the circulation was then arrested for a time required to correct the defect, which averaged 20 minutes in all the patients.

There were 9 children in the neo-natal group, of which 3 died. 1 died on the table in irreversible asystole, another had an initially good result but died following a septicaemia 3 weeks post operatively consequent on an infected sternotomy. The third died 16 hours post operatively after initially good progress and the cause of this child's death is obscure. There were 10 children aged 1 month to 1 year, and of these 2 died, giving an overall mortality of 5 or 26%. Post mortem findings of 1 showed the right ventricle to be severely hypertrophied and with a thickened opaque endocardium and the other was the first case which I previously mentioned who was moribund pre-operatively.

Following up these children, 1 had open valvotomy subsequently, 2 have been lost to follow up because they emigrated and the remainder all are asymptomatic but all have rejection systolic murmur in the pulmonary area. 4 have a diastolic murmur, 5 have cardiomegaly which is not increasing, only 2 have recognisable pulmonary oligaemia and the right ventricular hypertrophy which has persisted in 7, has not progressed.

In contrast to the pulmonary stenotics, the infants with aortic stenosis all presented with symptoms in the first two months of life and the oldest to undergo valvotomy was in fact 4 months of age. 4 of the 8 were neonates, and the other 4 were aged 6, 8, 9 and 12 weeks respectively. Dyspnoea was the earliest symptom, with the association of rejection systolic murmur heard at the right sternal border. All of them presented with congestive failure, with hepatomegaly, although only 1 had generalised oedema. There was-evidence of cardiomegaly in 7 out of 8 X-rays, pulmonary plethora in 4 and frank pulmonary oedema in 2. The ECG showed left ventricular hypertrophy in 7 and bi-ventricular hypertrophy in 1. The mean axis was of +30 with a close range of 70 to 95.

All the infants underwent cardiac catheterisation, and the gradient across the aortic valve ranged from 40 to 120 mm of mercury. All except one showed moderate elevation of the pulmonary artery pressure and the weight of these infants ranged from 2.9 to 5 kilos. For the correction of aortic stenosis, cardiopulmonary bypass was used but with a variety of techniques. Normothermia was used in 3, continuous perfusion but cooling to 31 °C in 1 and cooling to 25 °C with circulatory arrest in 4. And of these 8 patients, 3 died, 1 having definite fibro-elastosis of the left ventricle on post mortem. 1 died on the table in irreversible asystole and the third died two hours after returning to intensive care in apparently good condition and again the cause of this death is unknown but was probably respiratory.

Of the 5 survivors, all are asymptomatic, but all 5 have moderate systolic murmurs in the aortic area and one has a diastolic murmur. One continues to have cardiomegaly which is not progressive. Describing the valves themselves, 7 of the pulmonary valves were composed mainly of mixomatus masses, which were converted into a bicuspid structure with excision of some of the mixomatus tissue. 4 of the valves were tricuspid with fusion of the commissures and these were treated by dividing each of the commissures converting the valve into a tricuspid opening. 5 appeared to be membraneous structures with a pinhole orifice and these were converted into a bicuspid valve by transverse division. Bougies were then passed through the valve into the ventricle and on occasion a small dilator was opened to stretch the ring. Of the aortic valves, 5 were bicuspid and the commissures were open to the ring, whereas three comprised mixomatus masses without recognisable cusps. These were all converted into bicuspid structures by incision of the mass forming apparently adequate orifices. The type of valve had no bearing on mortality but in the aortic group further surgery will no doubt be required in the future, especially in the mixomatus types. Longest follow up so far is 7 years in the pulmonary group, and 5 years in the aortic group.

Part 6

Post-operative Care following Cardiothoracic Surgery

48
Osmolar balance after open-intracardiac operation in children

P. B. Deverall

Body compositional changes after open-intracardiac operations include an increase in extracellular fluid, an increase in total exchangeable sodium and a decrease in total exchangeable potassium[1,2]. Despite the sodium increase, plasma hyponatraemia is common in the postoperative period.

A low plasma sodium may arise because of a shift of sodium ions from the extracellular to the intracellular compartment or because the extracellular sodium is diluted by a disproportionate increase in extracellular water, i.e. dilutional hyponatraemia. The former ionic shift is part of what is called the sick-cell syndrome.

The author has studied osmolar balance in children and tried to answer these questions:

1. What is the normal pattern of osmolar change after open-intracardiac operations?
2. Is this influenced by perfusate composition?
3. Do the findings support the ionic shift or dilutional basis of plasma hyponatraemia?

DETAILS OF INVESTIGATION

Three groups of eight children undergoing elective open-intracardiac operations were studied. All had uncomplicated progress. Group I were perfused with a perfusate of diluted acid citrate dextrose blood. Postoperatively blood or plasma was given as required plus 5% Dextrose in water, 500 ml m^{-2} on day 0 and 750 ml m^{-2} on days 1 and 2. No sodium was added. 10 mEq m^{-2} potassium was added on day 0 and 20 mEq m^{-2} on days 1 and 2. Group II were perfused with whole heparinised blood but had the same postoperative management as Group I. Group III had the same perfusate as Group I but a severely restricted postoperative third intake, i.e. 100 ml 5% Dextrose m^{-2} on day 0 and 200 ml m^{-2} on day 1.

RESULTS

Changes in plasma osmolality in the three Groups are shown in

Figures 48.1, 48.2 and 48.3. Intraoperative changes are influenced by perfusate composition but postoperative changes are similar in all three groups. The hypo-osmolar state paralleled observed changes in plasma sodium in that hypo-osmolality and hyponatraemia occurred simultaneously. This suggests that the hyponatraemia in these children, who were doing well, was dilutional in origin.

Perfusate composition does not influence the postoperative osmolar trends if these results are added to those already published by other workers[3], who used perfusates of different composition to those used

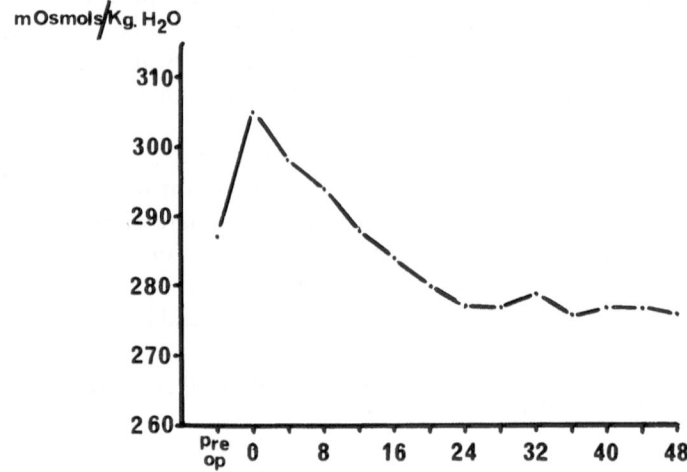

Figure 48.1 Plasma osmolality in cases with an ACD Ringers prime

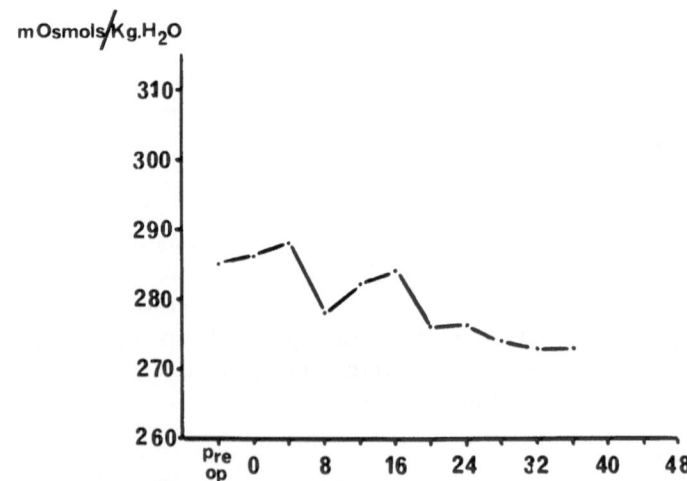

Figure 48.2 Plasma osmolality using heparinised blood prime

in our study but noted similar postoperative plasma hypo-osmolality.

Total fluid balance, urinary output, urinary osmolality, osmolar clearance and free osmolar output were measured and calculated in these

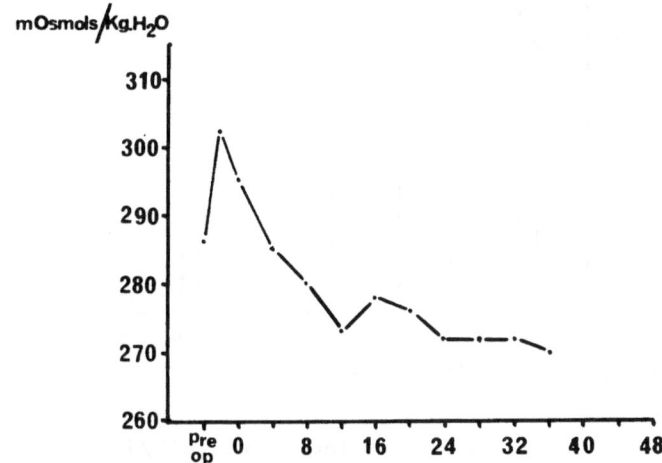

Figure 48.3 Plasma osmolality with ACD Ringers prime

Groups. The following conclusions have been drawn:

1. Urinary output in the early postperfusion period is determined by perfusate composition (Figures 48.4 and 48.5).
2. Total osmolar output in the three groups over the 48 h study period was similar and thus the demands on renal concentrating mechanisms were influenced by perfusate composition.
3. However there was evidence of excellent concentration with a normal renal response to a solute load.
4. Free osmolal output, which is a measure of the body's ability to excrete a relative water or solute load always remained positive, i.e. excess water was not excreted even in the presence of plasma hypo-osmolality.
5. This implies, in this postoperative period, that there is an abnormal response to a water load.
6. The overall findings support the use of moderate haemodilution perfusion.

Since severe water restriction did not influence plasma osmolar changes postoperatively and only produced a fall in urinary output and marked thirst (despite plasma hypo-osmolality) one must support a policy of moderate postoperative fluid intake.

The data suggest but do not prove that excessive fluid intake may be

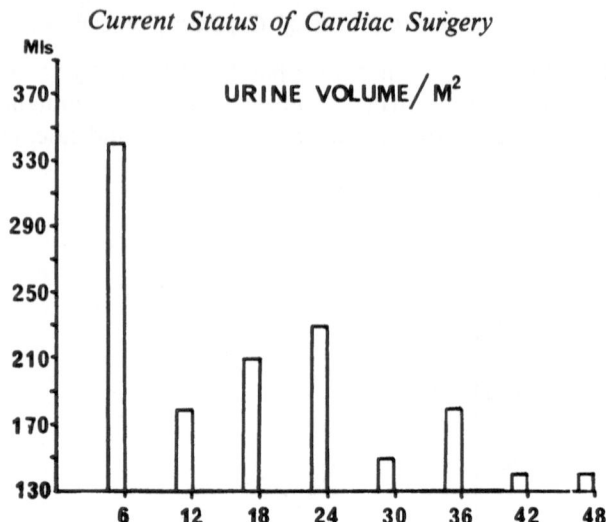

Figure 48.4 Urinary volume with ACD Ringers prime

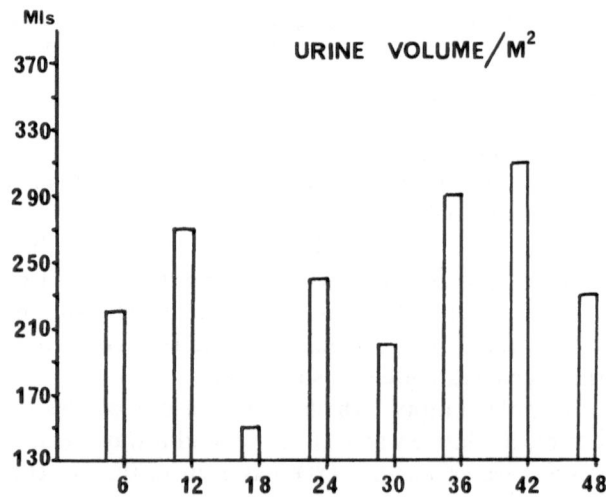

Figure 48.5 Urinary volume with heparinised blood prime

accompanied by more severe plasma hypo-osmolality. We have in the past observed this in patients with otherwise unexplained cerebral dysfunction and not only in cardiac patients, e.g. postburn encephalopathy.

References

1. Pacifico, A. D., Digerness, S. B. and Kirklin, J. W. (1970). Acute alterations of body composition after open intracardiac operations. *Circulation*, **41**, 331
2. Breckenridge, I. M., Deverall, P. B., Digerness, S. B. and Kirklin, J. W. (1972).

Potassium intake and balance after open intracardiac operations. *J. Thorac. Cardiov. Surg.*, **63,** 305

3.   Moffitt, E. A., Rosevear, J. W. and McGoon, D. C. (1970). Myocardial metabolism in children having open heart surgery. *JAMA*, **211,** 1518

4.   Deverall, P. B., Muss, D. C., Macartney, F. J. and Settle, J. D. (1973). Osmolal balance after open intracardiac operations in children. *Thorax*, **28,** 756

49
Peripheral temperature measurement as an aid to postoperative care
H. R. Matthews

The principal concern of those responsible for the postoperative care of the cardiac patient is to ensure that the flow of blood through the vital organs is sufficient to sustain normal metabolism. Using this criterion it is pertinent to examine the relevance of existing methods of monitoring the circulation (Table 49.1).

Table 49.1 Current methods of monitoring the circulation

Non-flow parameters	Flow parameters
pulse rate/form	urine output
blood pressure	arterio-venous O_2 difference
venous pressure	acid-base balance
left atrial pressure	cardiac output
electrocardiogram	peripheral temperature

The first point to observe is that a great deal of nursing and medical activity is devoted to recordings of parameters that give no information about flow whatsoever. Pressures and pulse waves can exist in entirely static systems and a fair representation of the arterial wave form could be obtained by hitting an inflated balloon with a rolled up newspaper; even the passage of an electrocardiographic wave of depolarisation across the ventricles does not guarantee subsequent myocardial contraction. These parameters do, of course, have great clinical value, but this derives from the fact that they are maintained within fairly well-defined limits in health and not because they give any indication of flow.

FLOW PARAMETERS

What measures of flow are currently available to the clinician? There are five (Table 49.1) and their advantages and limitations need to be briefly reviewed. Urine output is simple to monitor and gives an indirect index of renal blood flow. Its value after open-heart surgery is, however, diminished in two ways. Firstly by actual renal damage in patients with long-standing heart disease, who may thus be oliguric even when the cardiac output is perfectly adequate and secondly by the administration of any diuretic (whether fluid load, osmotic agent or cellular inhibitor) which may mask the renal response to an inadequate circulation.

Measurements of arterio-venous O_2 difference and acid-base balance are relatively simple to perform. Theoretically both these methods should reflect tissue metabolism and blood flow, but if arteriovenous shunts are open and tissues are being bypassed (as is often the case in shock) then entirely normal values may be obtained. In fact both these parameters often show greater change when a patient is recovering from a period of low perfusion than when he is entering one. Their clinical value is correspondingly limited.

Cardiac output can now be monitored postoperatively either continuously (q.v.) or by repeated determinations. Existing methods are relatively expensive and invasive but do quantitate blood flow directly in 1 min^{-1} – though with varying degrees of accuracy. This is useful in assessing improvement or deterioration, but the absolute value does not necessarily indicate whether the output is sufficient for a particular patient at a particular moment in his recovery. One patient may be in trouble with an output of $3 \text{ } 1 \text{ min}^{-1}$ while that flow may be sufficient for the metabolic requirements of another.

The only other available parameter that gives any indication of blood flow is the peripheral or surface temperature. The theory of the method is simple. If there is a vigorous flow of blood through the skin then it will be warm and conversely if there is cutaneous vasoconstriction the skin will be cold. Recordings of the surface temperature therefore quantitate the state of the peripheral circulation. The necessary apparatus is cheap, simple to operate and entirely non-invasive. Recordings are made from the digits, where there is no local heat production and those reported here have been obtained from the plantar surface of the great toe (which is clinically the most convenient and sensitive site) using an electrical resistance thermometer. It is the application of this method to postoperative care that forms the basis of this report.

THE NORMAL PERIPHERAL WARM-UP PATTERN

Figure 49.1 shows a typical sequence of changes in toe temperature after operation in a patient who made a normal recovery from aortic valve replacement. The initial vasoconstriction, with a toe temperature of 26 °C, lasts for three hours but is followed by a rapid opening-up of the peripheral circulation so that a toe temperature of 34 °C is reached within four hours. Subsequently the toe temperature stabilises at a level approximately 2 °C lower than that of the core.

From an analysis of over 150 such warm-up patterns[1] it became clear

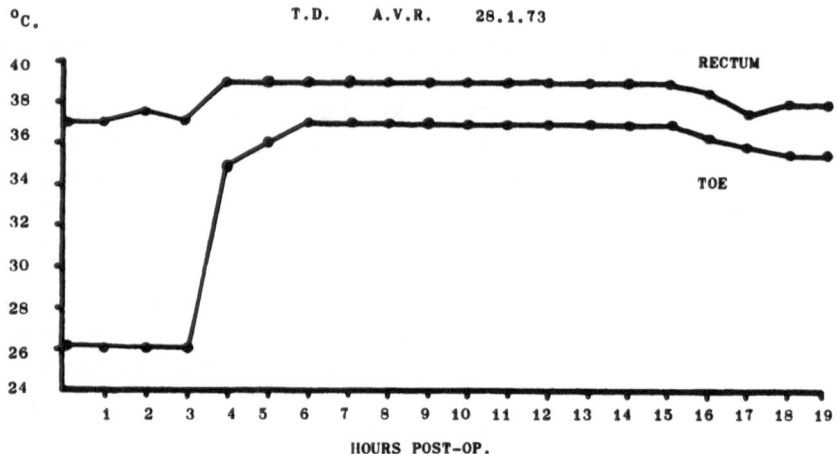

Figure 49.1 Typical toe and rectal temperatures after open-heart surgery

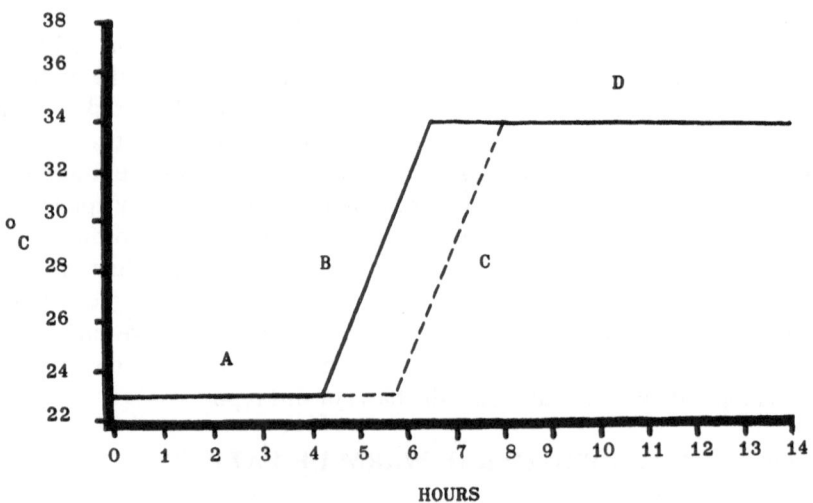

Figure 49.2 Graph defining the normal limits of toe temperature after open-heart surgery for patients breathing spontaneously (ABD) or on a ventilator (ACD)

that the above sequence does not occur at random. Patients with a normal circulation are found to warm peripherally (i.e. to 34 °C) within well-defined time limits, while those with circulatory impairment show abnormally prolonged peripheral vasoconstriction. For cases operated on in our Unit these time limits are represented by a graph (Figure 49.2). This indicates that the toe temperature of any patient with a normal circulation after operation should remain to the left of, or above, the line ABD if he is breathing spontaneously, or the line ACD if he is on a ventilator.

Since January 1973 all open-heart surgery patients in our Unit have been monitored prospectively against this standard. Figure 49.3 shows the clinical record of a normal warm-up pattern in a patient who was on a ventilator after mitral valve replacement.

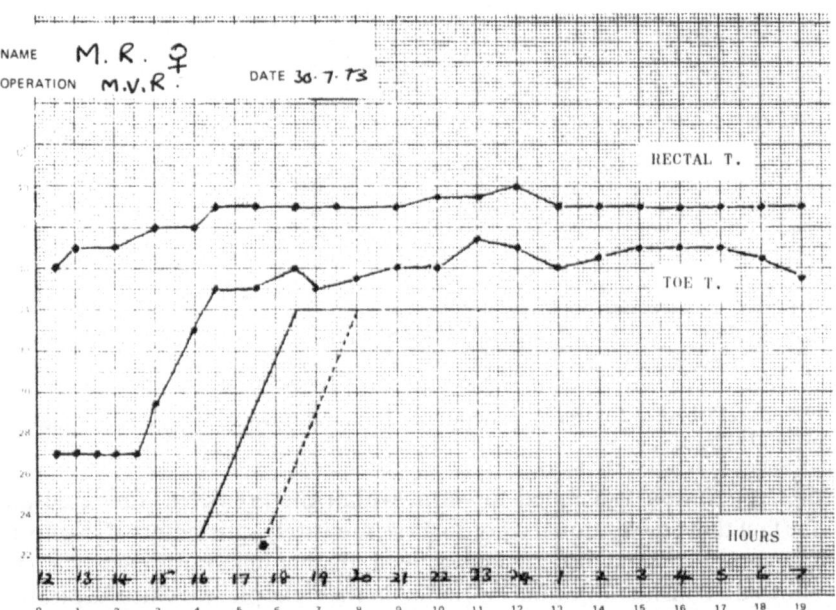

Figure 49.3 Clinical record of a normal warm-up pattern after mitral valve replacement, plotted against the nomogram

ABNORMAL WARM-UP PATTERNS

Two principal abnormalities are seen in the toe temperature curves of patients with circulatory impairment after open-heart surgery. The first is a prolongation of the initial period of vasoconstriction, so that the curve crosses the sloped limits of the nomogram, and the second is a late decline in toe temperature below 34 °C irrespective of the initial warm-up pattern.

Figure 49.4 is the record of a patient aged 65 after aortic valve replacement in whom prolonged vasoconstriction led to the discovery of concealed haemorrhage. He was breathing spontaneously but six hours

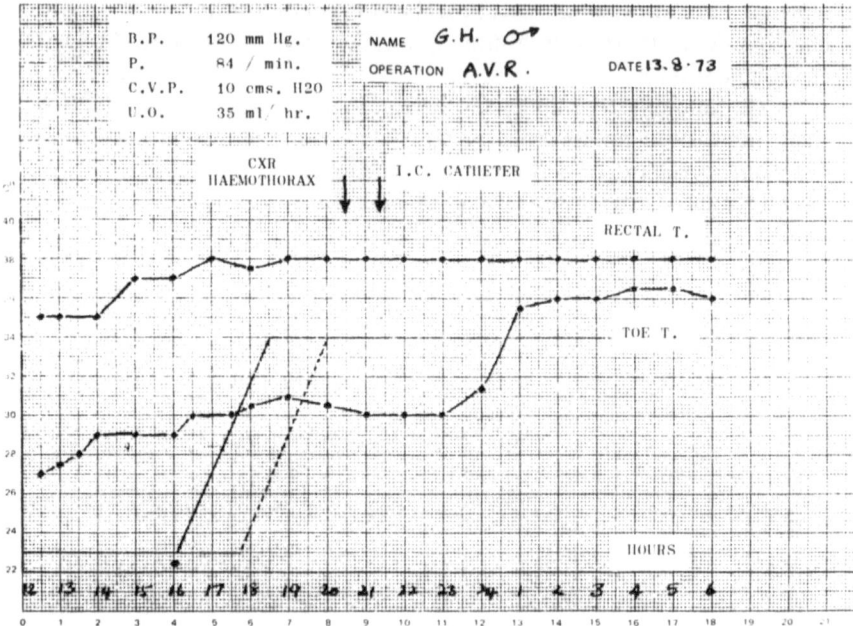

Figure 49.4 Abnormal warm-up pattern after aortic valve replacement, due to concealed haemorrhage

after operation had failed to warm within the predicted limits, despite the fact that conventional recordings were entirely satisfactory. Diagnostic measures were instituted, including a further chest radiograph. This showed a considerable fluid collection in the right pleura. Chest aspiration revealed liquid blood and an intercostal tube was inserted. Over the next two hours 1·5 l of blood were drained and the patient then warmed peripherally to 36 °C.

Figure 49.5 shows the second type of abnormality in a patient aged 42 who was on a ventilator after double valve replacement. During the early postoperative period there was excessive blood loss from the drains, but this was replaced by transfusion and her initial warm-up and other cardiovascular parameters were quite satisfactory. From the eleventh hour the chest drainage was considerably reduced, but from the seventeenth hour the toe temperature started to drop, eventually reaching 27 °C. In the absence of any other detectable cause this indicated that the apparent cessation of drainage might be spurious and pericardial tamponade was suspected. Operation was performed before further deterioration occurred. A large quantity of clot and fluid was evacuated from the pericardium, following which a normal peripheral temperature was rapidly restored.

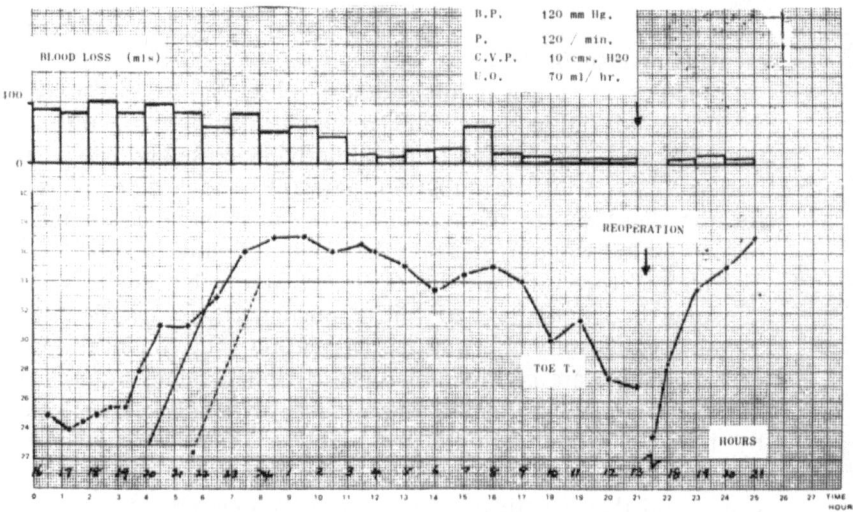

Figure 49.5 Normal initial warm-up pattern but late cooling after double valve replacement, due to pericardial tamponade

CONCLUSIONS

Using a toe thermometer and a nomogram it has been a simple matter to recognise abnormal peripheral vasoconstriction after open-heart surgery. A detailed report of experiences with the method has already appeared[2], but only the principal conclusions will be stated here:

1. Abnormal peripheral vasoconstriction is prognostically very serious. 53% of patients with an initial abnormal warm-up pattern died in hospital compared to 6% of patients having a normal warm-up ($p < 0.001$). Using the nomogram the prognosis can be assessed within 8 h of operation at the latest.

2. Abnormal vasoconstriction always has a pathological cause. Ross *et al.*[3] first showed that it could result from hypovolaemia, but in

our experience many other causes can be responsible, including an important group of patients with myocardial failure.

3. Abnormal vasoconstriction is often the first or only evidence of a circulatory disorder. In low cardiac output states, the blood pressure and urine output are frequently maintained simply by the operation of peripheral vasoconstrictive mechanisms. It is the activation of these that is detected so readily by peripheral temperature measurement.

4. Abnormal vasoconstriction requires prompt diagnosis and treatment. Diagnosis of the cause will be based on evidence from conventional sources, including clinical observations, laboratory analysis and radiography, and sometimes only by therapeutic trial. Treatment is directed to the underlying cause and should be initiated early while the situation may still be reversible. Waiting for the development of hypotension, acidaemia and secondary organ damage will only increase the likelihood of death.

5. Toe temperature will only detect abnormalities that are adversely affecting the circulation and will be unchanged by disorders that are not significantly affecting the circulation. The practical applications of this are considerable. The peripheral temperature will indicate whether a patient is tolerating or being adversely affected by blood gas abnormalities or changes in heart rhythm. A temperature above 34 °C will indicate that oliguria is renal in origin and that a patient with a central venous pressure of 3 cm H_2O is not hypovolaemic.

Toe temperature monitoring is simple, cheap and extremely informative. Moreover it is one of the few parameters we have that tells us anything about blood flow. It is not a replacement for existing methods; it should be added to them. It does not attempt to quantitate cardiac output but will indicate whether a patient has a normal circulation at any given time or not. The value of this information to all those concerned in the management of shock and the cardiac surgeon in particular should be self-evident.

References
1. Matthews, H. R., Meade, J. B. and Evans, C. C. (1974). *Thorax* **29,** 338
2. Matthews, H. R., Meade, J. B. and Evans, C. C. (1974). *Thorax* **29,** 343
3. Ross, B. A., Brock and Aynsley-Green, A. (1969). *Brit. J. Surg.*, **56,** 877

50
Atrial pressure measurement after open-heart surgery

R.D. Bradley

Before operating on a patient, physicians expend considerable effort squeezing water out of him and having operated they then fill him with fluid again. This procedure is not as illogical as it appears at first sight and it is worthwhile looking into the relationship between the atrial pressures after bypass to discover why this procedure is necessary.

The useful work produced by the left and right heart can be related to the filling pressure of the two sides of the heart, and the equations that have been obtained representing the activity of the right and left heart in these terms appear to lie in two fan-shaped arcs.

The stroke volume produced by each side of the heart will be the resultant of the stroke work generated by the ventricle and the impedance into which it is discharging its load. The stroke volume pumped into the pulmonary or systemic impedances will vary as the stroke work alters and so can in turn, be related to the filling pressure. The stroke volume produced by the two sides of the heart must be equal in a stable state. If the volumes pumped are unequal, this will cause a transfer of blood between systemic and pulmonary systems which will alter the atrial pressures until the stroke volumes generated on the two sides are again equal.

The variables which determine the relation between the atrial pressures are the equations of stroke work related to filling pressure and the impedance to which the work is matched. Thus poor performance in terms of stroke work on the part of the left ventricle, or an increase in the systemic impedance, will cause wider than normal separation of the atrial pressures. Poor right ventricular performance or an increase in pulmonary impedance will cause them to come together or may even cause them to be laterally reversed, so that the right atrial pressures are higher than the left.

Following cardiopulmonary bypass the most common configuration is a relatively small separation of the atrial pressures. Demonstrably poor right ventricular function in these cases is the most probable cause, although the effect would also be seen with a rise in pulmonary vascular resistance, or a relatively greater increase in left than right ventricular performance which is of course unlikely, following mitral or aortic valve

337

replacement. It would also be possible to produce the observed approximation of the left- and right-sided filling pressures with a diminution of left-sided afterload if there were no reduction in left ventricular stroke work; this did not appear to be the mechanism in the patients observed.

The practical application of these observations is that it is extremely unusual after cardiopulmonary bypass for the left atrial pressure to rise to levels which will generate pulmonary oedema providing that the right atrial pressure is not allowed to exceed 10 mmHg above the sternal angle.

Patients with moderate cardiac performance will of course have greater stroke volumes at high filling pressures. However, those with bad myocardial function who give the most cause for concern post-operatively, show only the most marginal increase in stroke output as the filling pressures are raised.

51
Assessment of left ventricular function and simultaneous measurements of pressure and dimension

D. G. Gibson

Simultaneous measurement of left ventricular pressure and dimension have been reported by a number of authors in the experimental animal[1,2] and have proved a sensitive method of studying left ventricular function. These techniques can be adapted for use in man, by measuring left 'ventricular dimension by echocardiography and pressure by micromanometer[3,4]. Initially, this information was processed manually, but as this proved very laborious, a digitising technique was substituted, which greatly facilitates the method. Observations can either be made at cardiac catheterisation, when the micromanometer is inserted into the left ventricle by the retrograde arterial route, or since it is mounted on a number 5

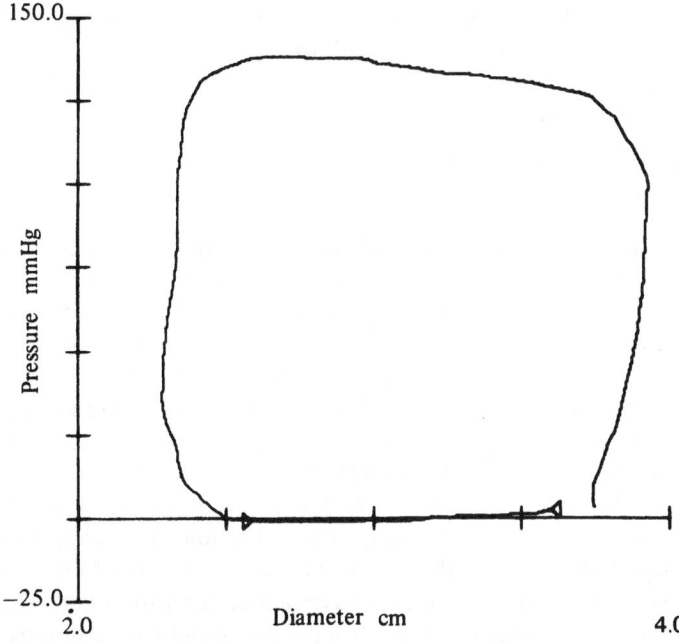

Figure 51.1 Pressure–dimension loop from a patient with mild mitral stenosis. Its configuration is normal

catheter, it can be left *in situ* at the time of surgery, passing either through the ventricular vent wound or via the left atrium. Measurements can most conveniently be presented as a pressure–dimension loop,

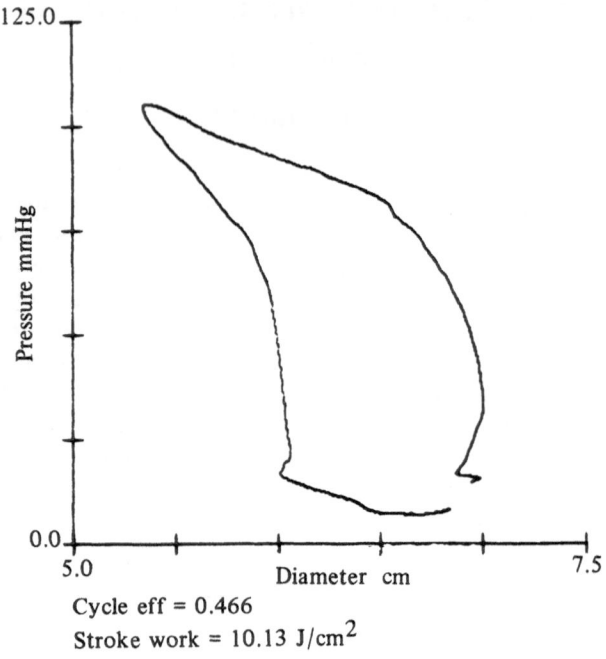

Cycle eff = 0.466
Stroke work = 10.13 J/cm^2

Figure 51.2 Pressure–dimension loop from a patient with aortic regurgitation and severe left ventricular disease

an example from a patient with mild mitral stenosis and normal ventricular function being given in Figure 51.1. It is apparent that the pressure pulse reflects the overall performance of the ventricle, while the dimension represents localised behaviour in a region immediately below the mitral valve. When ventricular function is normal, the loop is approximately rectangular, with an area corresponding to the useful work done in the circulation by the beat in question. In the presence of ventricular disease, the loop becomes distorted (Figure 51.2) so that its area becomes reduced with corresponding loss of efficiency of energy transfer from myocardium to blood and may even become negative, reflecting aneurysmal behaviour of the region studied. Starling's Law would be associated with an increase in loop area associated with a corresponding rise in end-diastolic dimension, while a positive inoptropic stimulus would increase the loop area at constant end-diastolic dimension. It is apparent, therefore that this method might be used to dissociate the effects of these two mechanisms from those of inco-ordinate contraction. In a series of 24 patients with valvular heart disease or cardiomyopathy, cycle efficiency, defined as loop area divided by the product of maximum pressure and dimension change occurring in the beat in question, was found to be closely related to peak left ventricular dP/dt, a sensitive

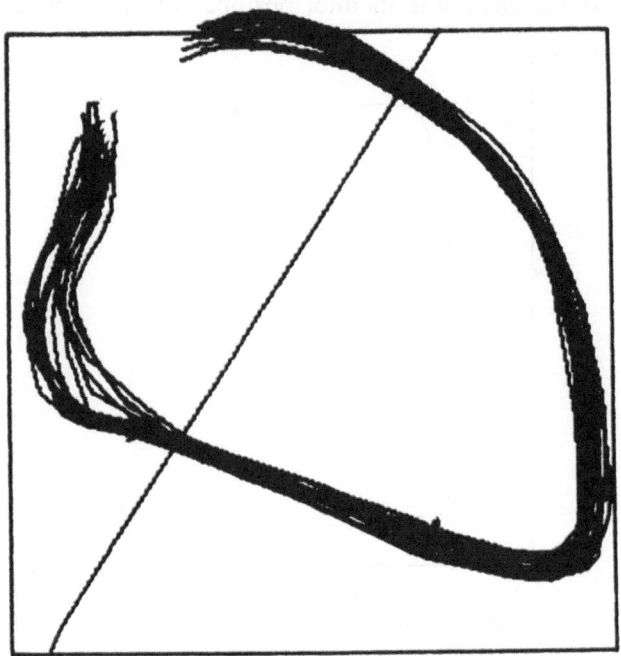

Figure 51.3 Digitised systolic cineangiogram frames from a patient with mitral stenosis. Ejection fraction is strikingly reduced

but non-specific index of cardiac function[4]. These results suggest that inco-ordinate contraction may be a significant cause of depressed ventricular function in valvular heart disease and cardiomyopathy, as well as in ischaemic heart disease where its effects are well-recognised. The effect of valvular regurgitation on the loop configuration was small in patients in whom left ventricular function was judged to be good, haemodynamically and angiographically. The presence of a distorted loop, however, even in the presence of valvular heart disease, indicates impaired function, an example from a patient with aortic regurgitation who died of myocardial failure after valve replacement being given in Figure 51.2. Conversely, Figure 51.3 represents the digitised systolic frames from the cineangiogram of a patient with rheumatic mitral valve disease, showing an ejection fraction of 30%. In spite of this, the loop configuration was normal (Figure 51.4), so that mitral valve replacement was undertaken, with successful results. Since then four similar patients, three with rheumatic mitral valve disease and one with a stenosed mitral homograft have undergone successful valve replacement.

The use of the method to monitor postoperative progress is shown in

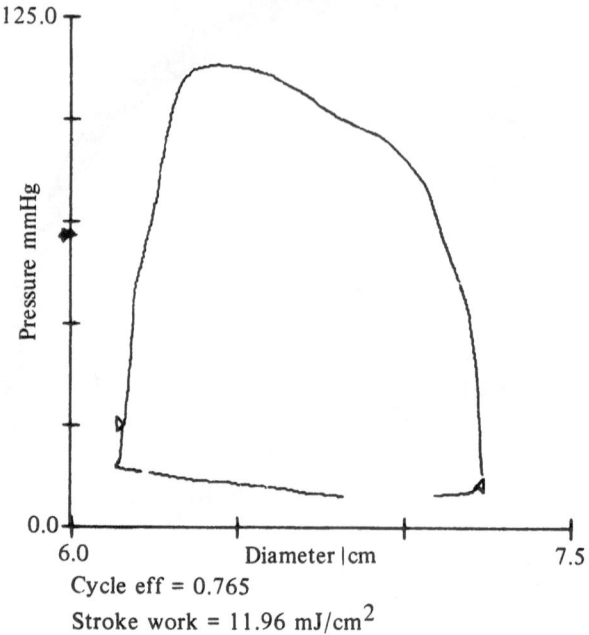

Cycle eff = 0.765

Stroke work = 11.96 mJ/cm^2

Figure 51.4 Pressure–dimension loop from the patient whose cineangiogram' is shown in Figure 51.3

Figure 51.5 from a patient who underwent aortic, mitral and tricuspid valve replacement. The right-hand pair of loops represent left ventricular function on return to the recovery Unit and show a somewhat distorted configuration with a peak dP/dt reduced at 1140 mmHg s^{-1}. Fourteen hours later, there had been a considerable increase in loop area and peak dP/dt, in spite of a reduction in end-diastolic dimension, which was reflected in an improved clinical state.

Simultaneous measurement of left ventricular pressure and dimension thus provides a sensitive method of studying cardiac function which does not require angiography. It is thus applicable in the postoperative situation as well as the catheter room, where it may allow more comprehensive monitoring of the cardiac state.

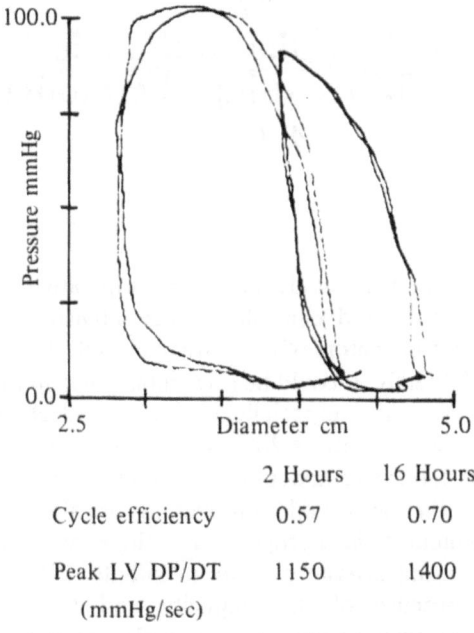

	2 Hours	16 Hours
Cycle efficiency	0.57	0.70
Peak LV DP/DT (mmHg/sec)	1150	1400

Figure 51.5 Pressure–dimension loops showing postoperative progress after triple valve replacement. The right-hand pair of loops were recorded 2 h after discontinuation of bypass and the left-hand pair were recorded 16 h after discontinuation of bypass

References

1. Rushmer, R. F. (1956). Pressure–circumference relations of the left ventricle. *Amer. J. Physiol.*, **115**
2. Horwitz, L. D. and Bishop, V. S. (1972). Left ventricular pressure–dimension relations in the conscious dog. *Cardiovasc. Res.*, **6,** 163
3. Gibson, D. G. and Brown, D. J. (1973). Measurement of instantaneous left ventricular dimension and filling rate in man using echocardiography. *Brit. Heart J.*, **35,** 1141
4. Gibson, D. G. and Brown, D. J. (1974). Use of echocardiography in the evaluation of left ventricular function. *Proc. Roy. Soc. Med.*

52
Measurement of cardiac output in infants and young children using thermodilution
A. Rees

These studies in fact were made in the postoperative period. All the parameters which were used clinically in the intensive care ward were thought to be indirect indicators of the cardiac output. If the cardiac output could be measured directly, it could be a valuable guide to the management of the postoperative period, especially in infants and children. The Fick method although known to have a 20% error, is accepted as a standard but its performance is laborious and time consuming and requires complex apparatus, whereas the various dilution methods are simpler. But there are problems of discolouration, pyrogenic reactions and the problem of obtaining a free-flowing arterial cannula in infants. We chose a thermo-dilution method because of its simplicity and capacity for infinite repeatability, and because the fluid injectate which we use, dextrose 5% can be incorporated into the child's calculated fluid requirements. A two-part study was designed, in the first instance to establish the validity of thermo-dilution techniques as compared to the Fick in this situation, and the second part, which is a long-term project, to determine the clinical usefulness of serial cardiac output measurements in the postoperative period.

The Fick principle was used by taking arterial blood from the radial cannula, which was directly placed before operation. The mixed venous sample was taken from the pulmonary artery, via the cannula in which the thermistor probe was mounted. The oxygen content of both these samples was then estimated in a Lexicon oxygen cell. The expired gases were collected in a series of PVC Douglas bags, via a collect valve mounted on the endotracheal tube; this valve which was designed by Dr Fitzner of the Brompton anaesthetic department, is a low-resistance, low dead space, model. The volume of the expired gases is measured and the composition of inspired and expired gases analysed with a Beckban paramagnetic oxygen analyser and the oxygen consumption was then calculated from standard equations. This all took a considerable amount of time and by comparison the thermo-dilution method was simplicity itself. A known volume of dextrose 5% at room temperature was injected into the superior vena cava via the internal jugular line which was placed routinely prior to surgery. The pulmonary artery temperature, was measured by a Devices thermistor probe, which was inserted into the pulmonary artery at the end of the operation by an oblique stab incision in the right ventricular outflow tract. The probe was then brought out through the lower end of the skin incision, and directly connected to the Devices cardiac output monitor which gave an instantaneous read out on a meter.

In the last four patients, as a check, a thermo-dilution curve was recorded on a paper strip and the cardiac output calculated by manually integrating the area under the curve. We intend to repeat this measurement in subsequent patients but though it is marginally more accurate, it lacks the immediacy of the meter read out for clinical purposes.

In the first instance we compared the thermo-dilution cardiac output values with those obtained by the Fick method and they are comparable favourably in the majority of instances. In fact, the correlation coefficient turned out to be .93. However, the Fick values tended to be somewhat lower than that obtained than that obtained by the thermo-dilution method but we found that this was corrected in those patients in whom we manually integrated the area under the curve. These values for the thermistor were slightly higher and more closely approximating to the Fick value. We, therefore, feel confident that as further studies are performed, confirmation of the validity of thermo-dilution in this situation will be obtained. Most individual readings show a fairly close association to the mean even those which were taken over 12 to 26 hours postoperatively. The lowest mean cardiac index was 2.2 litres and the highest was just a little over 5, with an average, or overall mean cardiac index of 3.6 litres per minute per m^2. So far in this small series we have not found the mean cardiac index to be of any prognostic value, for instance, the child with the lowest cardiac index, that of 2.2, had no postoperative troubles, but the ones who died, had cardiac indices of 3.4, 3.1 and 5.

Similarly, the stroke indices showed a close grouping around the means. Again, these were taken over the first 26 hours postoperatively and corresponded closely to the cardiac indices in individual patients, but again appeared to be of no prognostic value. The mean stroke index was 25 mls per beat per m^2, which is perhaps a somewhat low value compared with suggested normals. It may be related to the postoperative tachycardia which is very common and certainly not physiological.

Published cardiac output studies in infants and small children are surprisingly scanty. Of the published studies, many are concerned with neonates, and much of the emphasis is placed on the problems of measuring left-to-right shunts through a patent duct. In the neonatal group, from published studies, the mean cardiac index shows a wide range from 2 to 4.1 and in the older children a smaller range of 3.5 to 4.9 litres is quoted. At present the study is continuing and there has been no morbidity, and certainly no mortality attributable to the method. Although at present the cardiac output does not seem to be the ultimate parameter for deciding postoperative treatment that I at least thought it might be, it certainly is of prognostic value where there is a very low cardiac index, that is below 1 to 1.5 litres. This has been indicated by a personal communication from Dr Kirkland in Alabama to Mr Lincoln.

In summary then, we have performed serial cardiac output studies in 16 children, with a mean age of 4, a mean weight of 14.3 kilos, and a mean surface area of .58 square metres. The cardiac index meaned at 3.6 litres per minute per m^2, with a mean stroke index of 25 mls per beat per m^2.

53
Cardiac output and its derivatives using an implantable electromagnetic flow probe and intra-cardiac manometers

A. F. Rickards, J. H. Chamberlain and B. T. Williams

Following cardiac surgery, the cardiac output probably provides the best basic estimate of cardiac performance and its response to various therapeutic interventions.

The use of indirect indices of cardiac output, such as arterial blood pressure and urinary output has been repeatedly shown to correlate poorly with measured cardiac output. However, the standard techniques for cardiac output determination are difficult to institute in the postoperative clinical situation and their well-recognised errors are compounded by small degrees of valvular regurgitation, shunts or low output states, all of which may be present in this group of patients.

Conversely, the electromagnetic flowmeter is entirely linear over a wide range of values for blood flow, this being expressed as a continuous, electrical signal with an excellent frequency response. Subsequent electronic manipulation of such a signal, especially when combined with a high fidelity blood pressure signal allows access to many more sophisticated indices of cardiovascular function, such as cardiac power, work and vascular impedance.

It was for these reasons that an electromagnetic flow probe for clinical use was developed.

THE WILLIAMS–BAREFOOT FLOW PROBE (MK. I) *

This device was originally described in 1969 and used clinically the following year.[1-3] Details of its transducer characteristics were presented to the Cardiac Surgical Course in 1971.[4]

The basic design concept involved rearrangement of the standard components of the electromagnetic flow probe so that they could be housed in a soft, pliable, silicone rubber moulding of uniform cross-section (Figure 53.1). This allowed the device to be positioned around the ascending aorta of a patient undergoing cardiac surgery and subsequently withdrawn by traction on the protruding cable. The probe head is fixed in position by a nylon snare which may be released externally; this

*See Chapter 60

maintains a good fit of the probe on the aortic wall and prevents changes in the size of the annulus with arterial pulsation, up to the time of withdrawal.

Preoperative, *in vitro* calibration yields a linear plot; after insertion, beat-by-beat zero flow reference is provided by the end-diastolic portion of the flow trace.

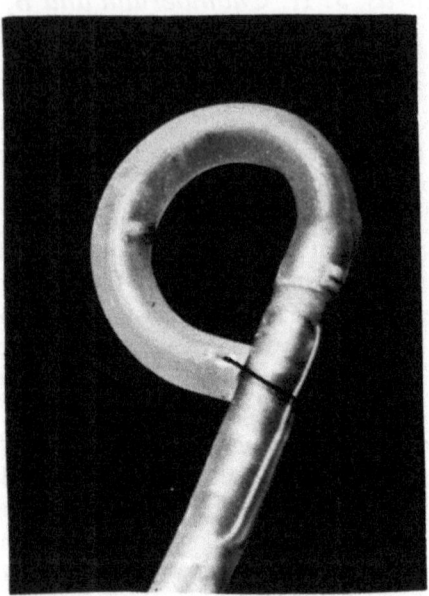

Figure 53.1 Williams–Barefoot probe in closed position

RECENT DEVELOPMENTS

Since 1971, improvements in the design of the probe and its associated flowmeter have been introduced. The sensitivity and signal: noise ratio of the probe itself have been enhanced by increasing the amount of soft iron within, and the number of turns of wire upon, the electromagnet.

A new model of flowmeter* has been introduced for clinical use with simplified controls and the incorporation of autoranging and electronic zero facilities.

CLINICAL USE

This device has now been used in more than sixty patients for monitoring the cardiac output after cardiac surgery.

*Carolina Medical Electronics Inc. King, North Carolina, U.S.A.

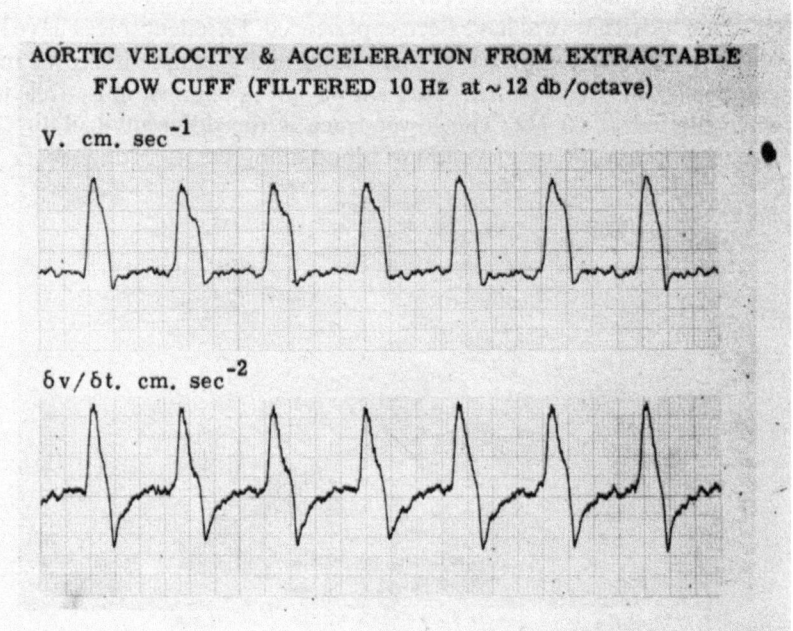

Figure 53.2 Upper: Ascending aortic flow trace in a patient following mitral valve replacement, Lower: Differential of flow signal

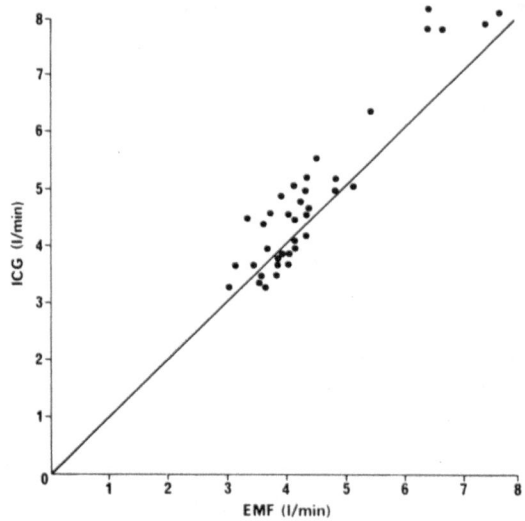

Figure 53.3 Comparison of mean cardiac output by extractable electromagnetic flow probe and indocyanine green dye

No complications have occurred due to its implantation and no difficulties in its withdrawal have been experienced. Excellent traces have been obtained from the majority of these cases and a sample is shown in the upper part of Figure 53.2. This shows an essentially noise-free trace when filtered at 10 Hz. The lower trace is the differential of the flow signal, representing acceleration of blood along the ascending aorta.

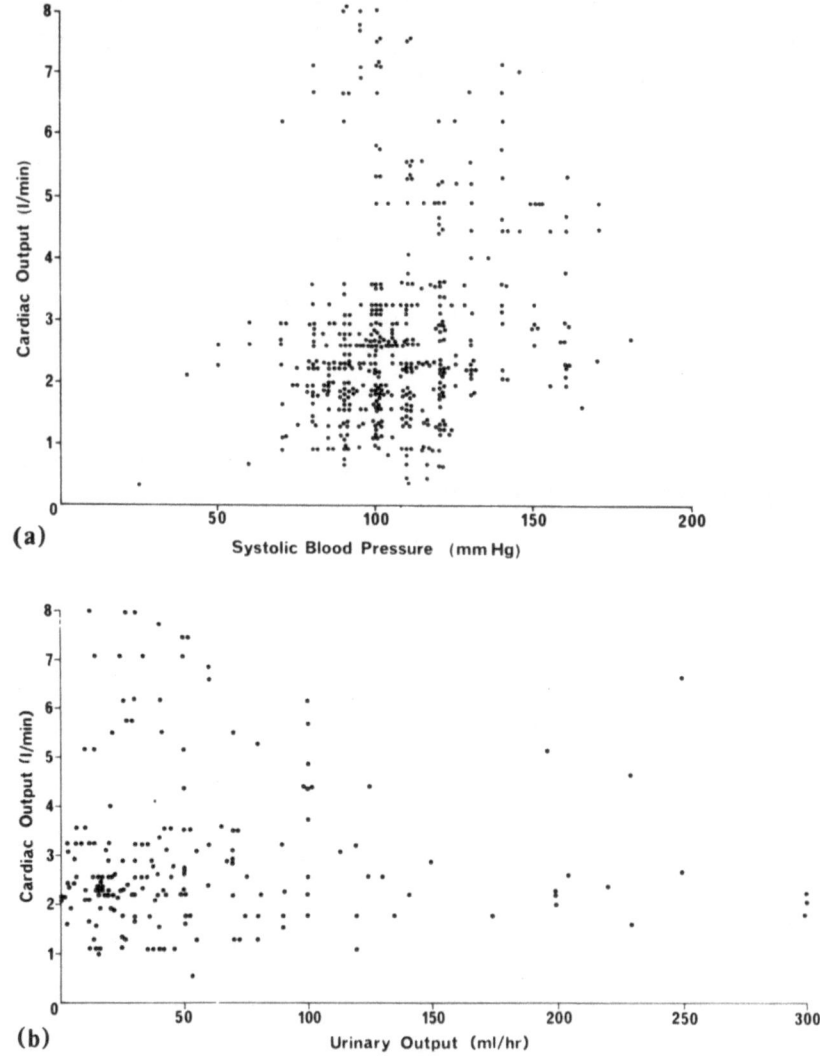

Figure 53.4 Comparison of mean cardiac output with, (a) Systolic arterial blood pressure (b) Urinary output (c) Pulse rate

Comparison of mean flow data with those obtained using indocyanine green dye and standard densitometer measurements has been carried out. Figure 53.3 shows the results of these studies in four patients and confirms the results of previous comparative studies in both models and experimental animals.[5, 6] There is good overall correlation $(R > 0.9)$, although as previously reported the electromagnetic flowmeter shows better reproducibility than indocyanine green dye, the latter also tending to overestimate the cardiac output.

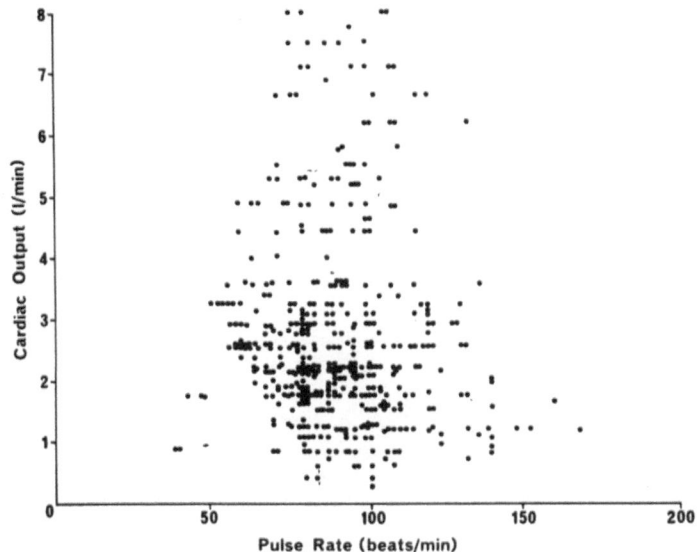

Figure 53.4 c

The results of comparison of the mean cardiac output with arterial blood pressure, pulse rate and urinary output are shown in **Figure 53.4**. They all confirm the poor correlation reported by other workers.

Manometric studies have been conducted simultaneously with flow studies. A Millar catheter tip pressure transducer has been passed retrogradely into the thoracic aorta from the femoral artery using the Seldinger technique. The same transducer may be introduced into the left ventricle through the vent site at the end of operation. The simultaneous pressure and flow signals have been recorded on a PI analogue tape recorder. This new data, together with any derivatives may be displayed off the tape in the clinical area or stored for subsequent analysis.

In deriving other indices of cardiovascular function from flow and pressure measurements, it is important to remember that the cardiovascular is a phasic or a.c. system, to which a.c. circuit theory should be applied.

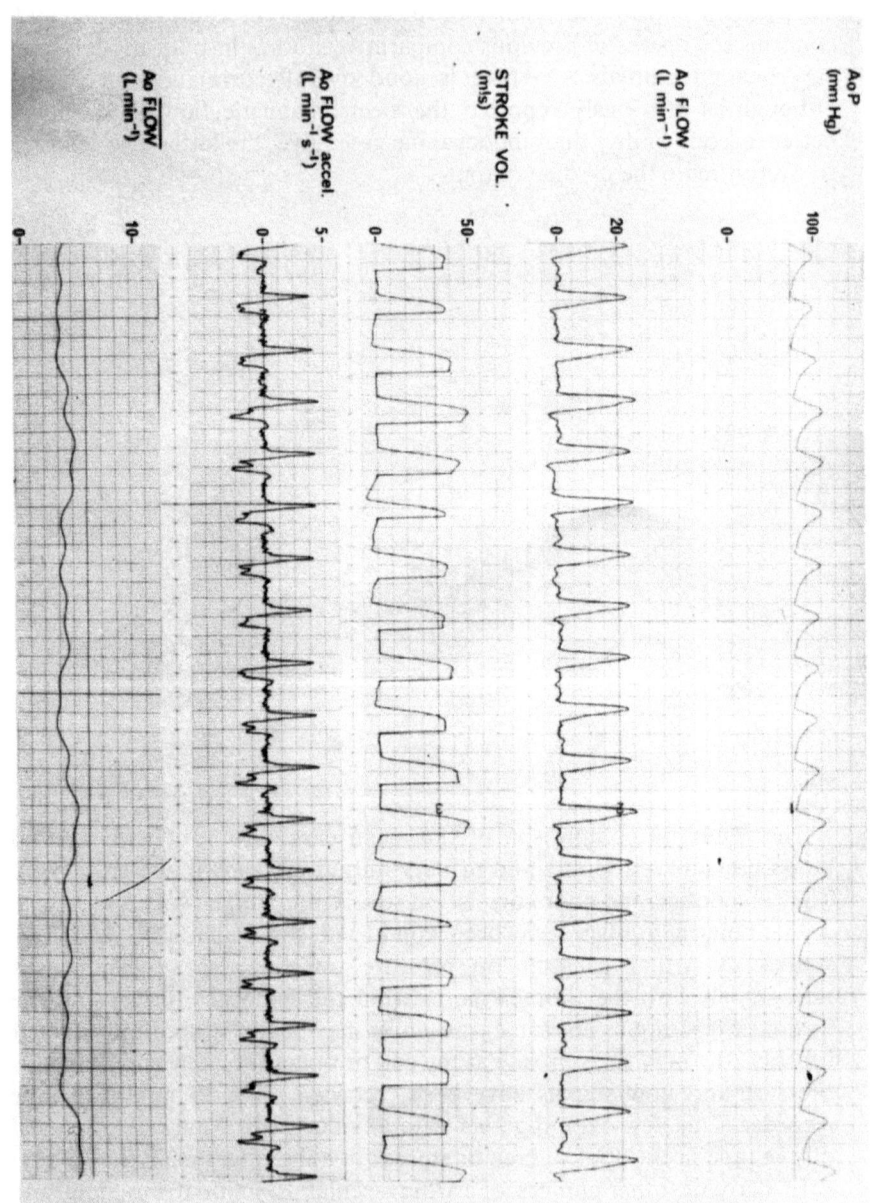

Figure 53.5 Data derived from the phasic ascending aortic blood flow signal

The use of mean flow and pressure data to derive other functions is highly inaccurate.[7] We have used simple analogue multiplying, integrating and differentiating amplifiers to obtain beat-by-beat stroke volume, cardiac power, stroke work and mean peripheral vascular impedance, from phasic pressure and flow signals.

Figure 53.5 shows some derivatives of the flow signal and Figure 53.6 the effect of 2 μg of isoprenaline on these measurements. Figure 53.7 shows some derivatives of simultaneous phasic ascending aortic blood flow recordings and Figure 53.8 the effect of 1 μg of isoprenaline on these.

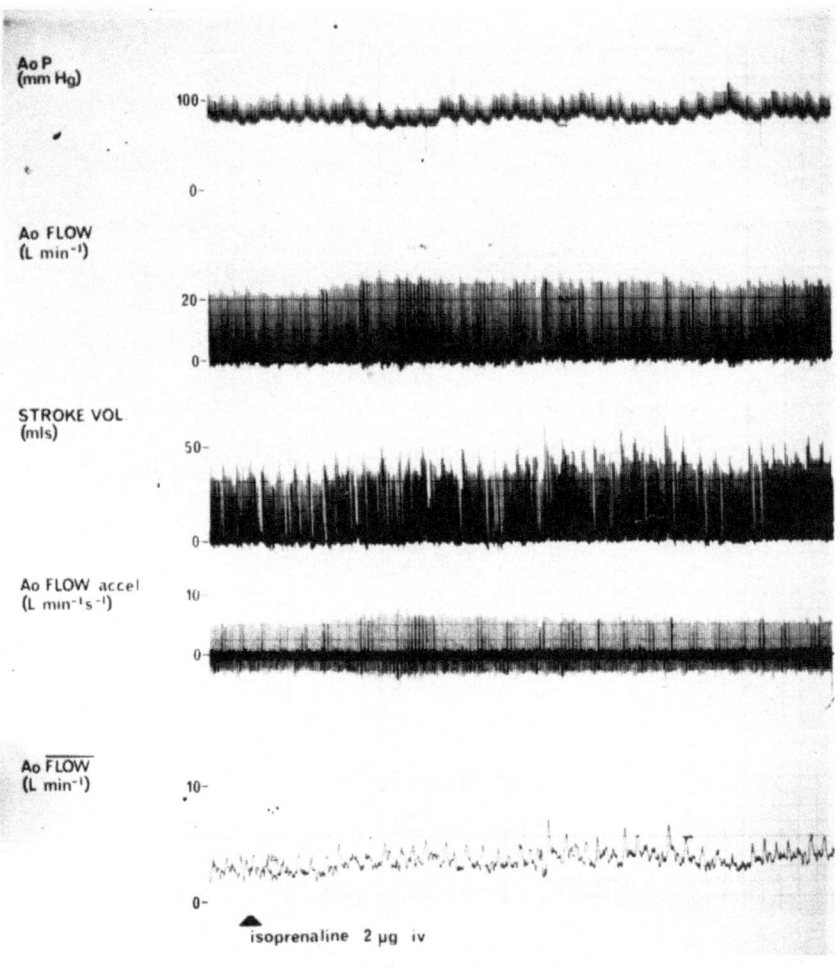

Figure 53.6 The effect of isoprenaline on aortic flow and its derivatives

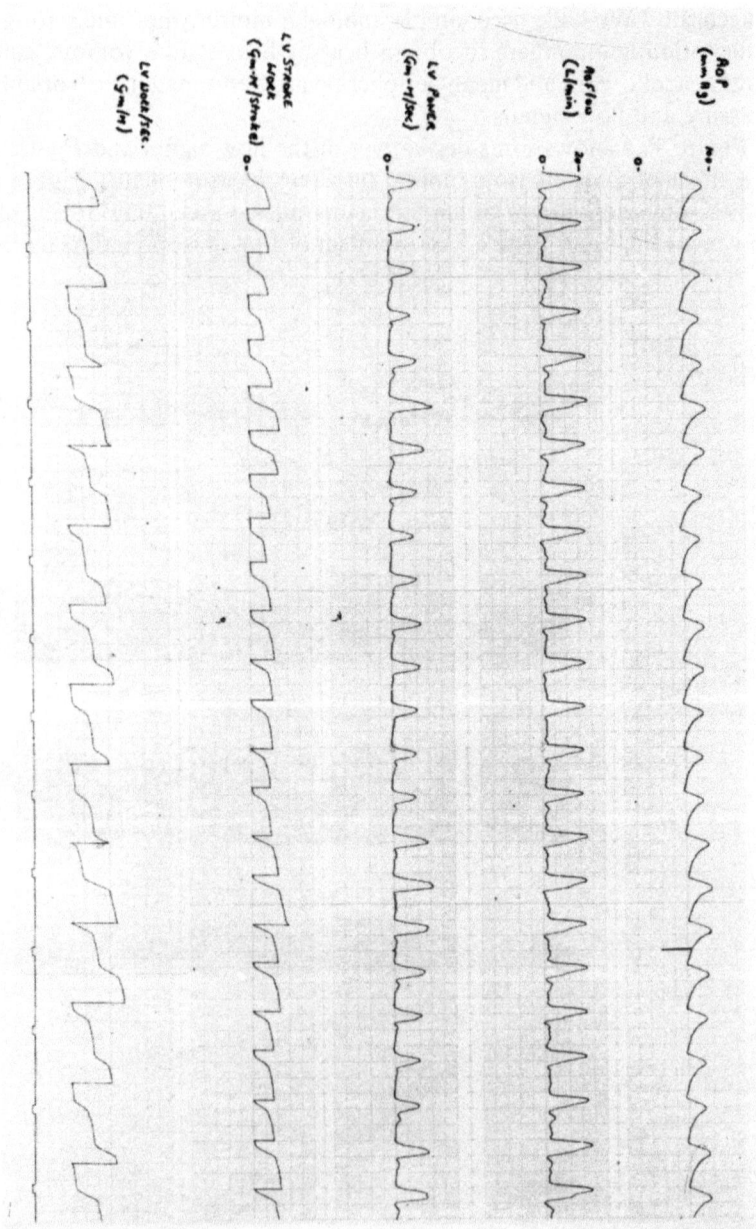

Figure 53.7 Data derived from the simultaneous recordings of phasic ascending aortic flow and pressure

The authors believe that the application of modern technology of this kind of cardiovascular surgical practice will not only upgrade current patient management, but also provide completely new information about cardiovascular disease.

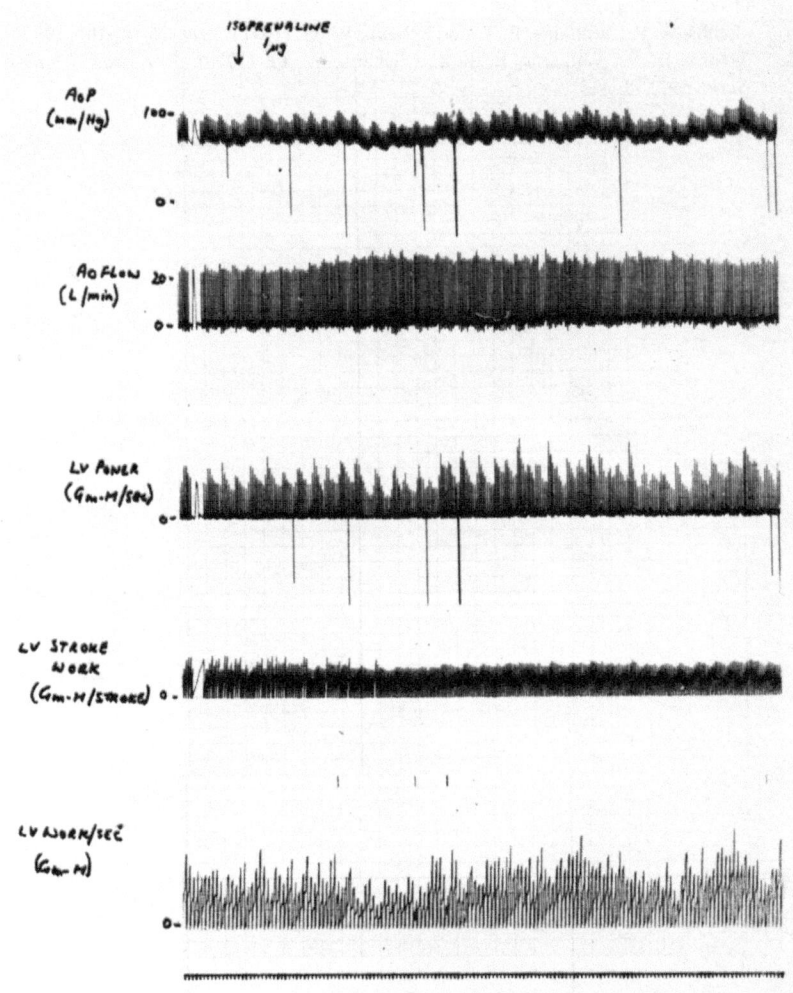

Figure 53.8 The effect of isoprenaline on pressure flow derivatives

References
1. Williams, B. T., Barefoot, C. and Schenk, W. G. (1969). *Res. Surg.*, **26,** 227
2. Williams, B. T., Sancho-Formos, S., Clarke, D. B., Abrams, L. D. and Schenk, W. G. (1971). *Ann. Surg.*, **174,** 357

3. Williams, B. T., Sancho-Fornos, S., Clarke, D. B., Abrams, L. D., Schenk, W. G. and Barefoot, C. (1972). *J. Thorac. Cardiovasc. Surg.*, **63,** 917
4. Williams, B. T., Sancho-Fornos, S., Clarke, D. B., Abrams, L. D. and Schenk, W. G. (Jan. 1972). In: *Blood Flow Measurement* (C. Roberts, editor)
5. Jacobs, R. R., Heyden, W. C., Williams, B. T., Schmitz, U. T. and Schenk, W. G. (1970). *J. Surg. Res.*, **10,** 25
6. Jacobs, R. R., Williams, B. T. and Schenk, W. G. (1971). *Arch. Surg.*, **102,** 199
7. Jacobs, R. R., Williams, B. T. and Schenk, W. G. (1970). *J. Thorac. Cardiovasc. Surg.*, **59,** 558

54
The place of the computer and automation in postoperative care
T. D. Preston

The growing application of physiological knowledge and measurement in postoperative care has led to a data explosion. Traditionally, nurses monitored a patient's vital signs and kept records on a fairly simple chart. The increasing pace of development in electronic monitoring equipment and the widening field of biochemical investigation, coupled with the fast-changing situations in modern intensive therapy, led to the supposition that use of automated data handling would be advantageous. However, at the present time almost all applications of computers in medical care are at an experimental stage. Uses of computing in administration, record keeping, diagnosis and research will not be discussed here, but applications of computers to patient care will be considered in three categories.

1. *Applied research.* The computer may indirectly assist in patient care by assisting in medical research. Grodins[1] used techniques of computer modelling to simulate and investigate the mechanisms controlling ventilation. The results of this work could lead to automatic control of a ventilator.[2]

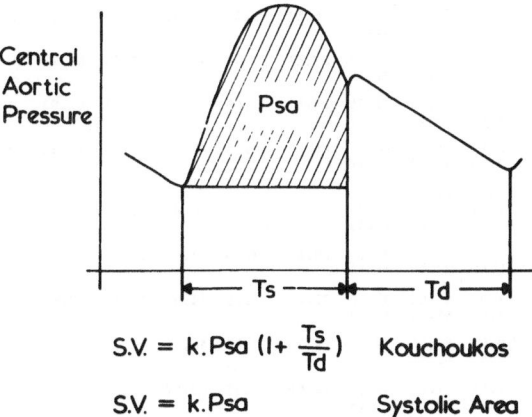

$$S.V. = k.Psa \left(1 + \frac{Ts}{Td}\right) \quad \text{Kouchoukos}$$

$$S.V. = k.Psa \quad \text{Systolic Area}$$

Figure 54.1 Derivation of stroke volume (SV) by integration of the area P_{sa} beneath the central aortic blood pressure. k is calibration constant

357

2. *Physiological monitoring.* Computers may assist in physiological investigation of patients as in the calculation of cardiac output from dye or thermal dilution measurements. Though this work has often been carried out by digital computation, it should be noted that a general purpose analogue computer is just as efficient at less cost. A special purpose calculator is even more efficient and still cheaper. It should not be supposed that programmable digital computers have no part to play. Where a method of measurement is under development, the flexibility of a digital computer allows effects of changes in technique to be evaluated by

KB 16 FILE 4 PT.325447. CODE 99-6

SAMPLE 16 ALREADY ON DISK
DATE   16/10/72
BAR. PRESSURE   760.0 MMHG
LOW CO2 CYL.   4.0 %
HIGH CO2 CYL.   8.0 %
WEIGHT   11.2 KG
ASTRUP TEMP.   37.9 C

LINE 2 IS TEMP. CORRECTED *

SAMPLE	TIME	TEMP.	PH	PO2	PCO2	STD.HCO3	BASE	HCRIT	HB.	SATN.	O2CONT	ETCO2	ETPCO2
1	1025	35.60	7.37	60.00	45.00	23.69	−0.19	40.00	13.16	89.63	16.55	5.64	40.18
			7.40	52.50	40.69								
2	1340	21.50	6.67	190.00	135.00	7.28	−22.69	19.00	6.25	96.74	8.66	9.53	67.96
			6.91	85.50	65.88								
3	1350	23.80	******	198.00	******	******	******	******	******	******	******	******	******
			*****	0.00	******								
4	1355	16.60	6.72	405.00	92.00	6.96	−22.88	15.00	4.93	99.39	7.59	5.48	39.06
			7.03	259.08	36.23								
5	1517	21.50	6.88	170.00	140.00	14.94	−11.19	21.00	6.91	97.31	9.59	9.22	65.75
			7.12	82.20	68.32								
6	1543	36.80	7.06	77.00	64.00	13.85	−12.71	23.00	7.56	87.89	9.46	6.90	63.48
			7.08	73.27	60.99								
7	1625	36.10	7.10	64.50	55.50	13.77	−12.98	30.50	10.03	82.65	11.70	7.10	50.63
			7.13	58.22	51.30								
8	1655	34.50	7.20	89.00	49.00	16.51	−9.19	29.00	9.54	94.51	12.75	6.38	45.50
			7.25	74.30	42.23								
9	1800	34.90	7.38	56.00	44.00	23.89	0.05	42.00	13.81	87.79	16.99	5.23	37.30
			7.42	46.46	38.59								
10	2045	37.00	7.44	35.00	37.00	24.42	0.65	29.00	9.54	67.52	9.05	5.23	37.28
			7.45	33.74	35.57								
11	2145	37.50	7.45	38.00	44.00	28.15	4.96	29.00	9.54	72.00	9.66	6.35	45.29
			7.45	38.00	43.24								
	DATE		17/10/72										
12	15	37.50	7.27	35.00	50.00	19.84	−4.90	40.00	13.16	57.01	10.53	6.59	47.02
			7.28	35.00	49.13								
13	200	37.50	7.41	33.00	32.00	20.89	−3.58	41.00	13.48	62.66	11.84	4.03	28.71
			7.42	33.00	31.44								
14	220	37.50	7.39	44.00	38.00	22.22	−1.95	41.00	13.48	77.96	14.74	5.09	36.32
			7.40	44.01	37.34								
15	845	37.50	7.42	41.00	39.00	24.24	0.47	46.00	15.13	75.54	16.01	5.63	40.15
			7.43	41.00	38.32								
16	1545	36.60	7.45	57.00	39.00	26.05	2.57	49.00	16.12	90.44	20.42	5.41	38.61
			7.47	53.59	36.84								

Figure 54.2 Computer output from program which calculates acid-base data; correcting for temperature

making changes to the program. Attempts have been made to measure cardiac output by a method not involving the injection of an indicator.[3, 4] These rely on analysis of the blood pressure contour at the foot of the aorta. The area $k.P_{sa}$ in Figure 54.1 is roughly proportional to stroke volume, but the correlation may be improved by the application of correction factors.[5]

Redesign of a special purpose device for each modification of the experiment is clearly not realistic, but if the measurement has passed from the stage of development to implementation, design of a special purpose computer should be considered.[6]

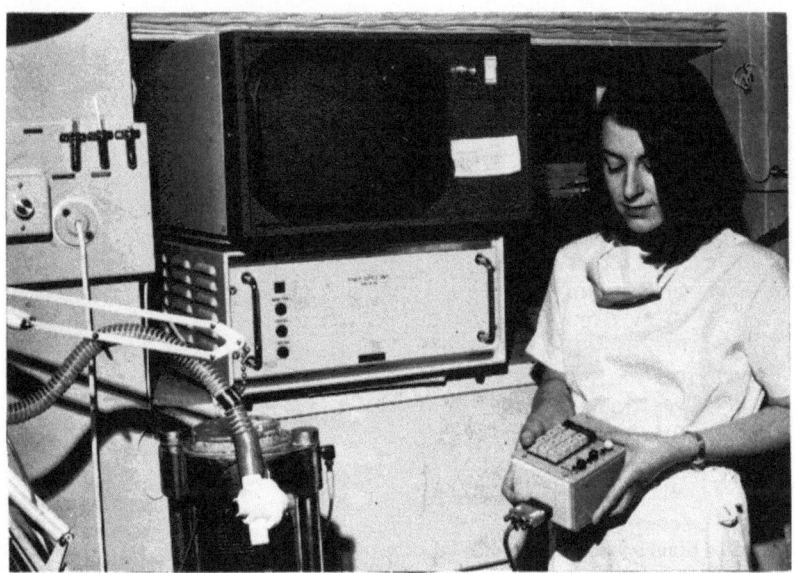

Figure 54.3 Keyboard and VDU in use in the recovery ward

3. *Computer-assisted patient care.* In a third approach, the ability of a computer to

(a) perform mathematical calculations and

(b) acquire, process, STORE and display data,

is used to assist and inform those people at the bedside directly concerned with the day-to-day care of the patients. This approach has been adopted at Westminster Hospital in the cardiothoracic operating theatre and recovery room.

BLOOD GAS ANALYSIS

Due to the technique of profound hypothermia used for cardiac surgery[7, 8] results of blood gas analysis must be corrected not only for a temperature gradient between the sample and the analyser but also for a large amount of haemodilution.[9] This is very conveniently done using an on-line terminal to the IBM 1800 computer in the hospital's Computer

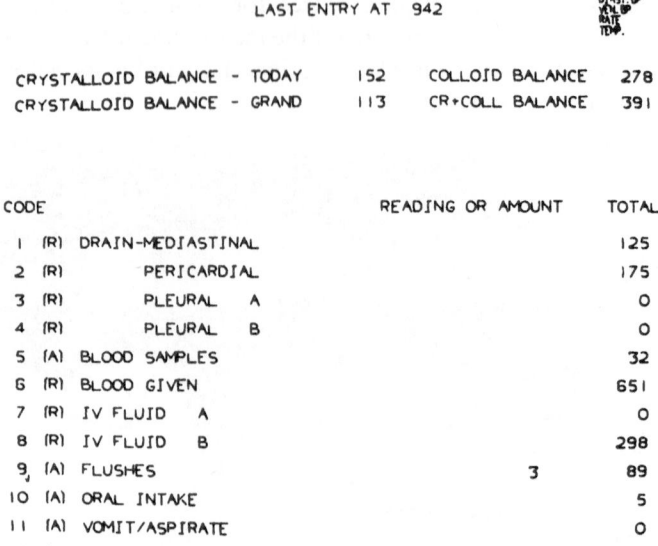

Figure 54.4 Fluid balance resumé on VDU. Current values of physiological variables appear at top right

Centre (Figure 54.2). New algorithms for the temperature correction factors appear daily and use of a digital computer allows any of unusual merit (e.g. Thomas[10]) to be easily and quickly incorporated.

POSTOPERATIVE CARE – FLUID BALANCE

Crystalloid prime is used for the extracorporeal circulation. The resultant haemodilution is corrected by transfusion of fresh blood and administration of a diuretic at completion of the operation. For this and the usual reasons careful fluid replacement in the postoperative period is a *sine qua non*.

Data for fluid balance calculations are entered by the nurses into the computer which keeps separate totals of crystalloid and colloid balance together with individual values for the several input and output routes and displays these on a Visual Display Unit (VDU) at the bedside (Figures 54.3 and 54.4). The format of the display and the methods and timings of the entries were arrived at by close collaboration between the medical and nursing staff and members of the Medical Computer Centre. Computers will make an impact on patient care only if such cooperation exists, so that the work done by the computer is clinically relevant and acceptable to the staff who actually use it.

PHYSIOLOGICAL MONITORING

As well as calculating the fluid balance, the computer samples the outputs from the standard ward monitors once each minute. The current values are displayed on the VDU and a five minute average value for each variable is stored permanently in the computer's files. Graphical displays of the recorded data may be requested by entering a suitable code through the keyboard (Figure 54.5). The display facility is mainly used

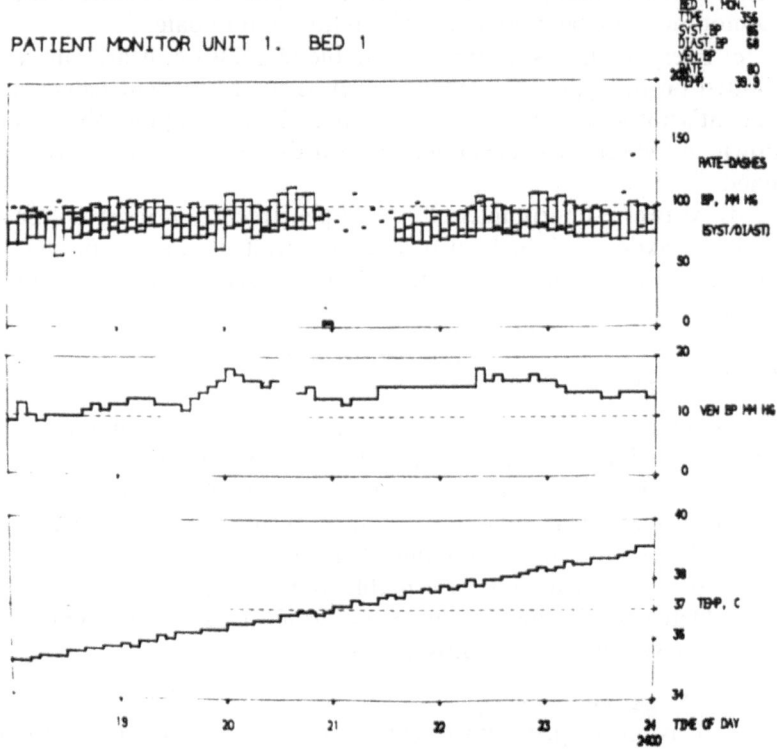

Figure 54.5 VDU graph of cardiovascular variables and rectal temperature

by the medical staff during their assessments of the patient, but the system helps the nurses by relieving them of the purely repetitive task of writing down the values from the monitors. It will continue to do this whilst the nurse is dealing with an emergency. Manual charts have not been kept in the Unit for over a year.

SECURITY OF DATA

The Unit is coming to depend on automation but it must not be forgotten that if a computer breaks down there is in general no way of retrieving the data until the computer is repaired. For this reason a number of fail-safe procedures should exist:

(a) The current physiological variables are ALWAYS available at the bedside. Systolic–diastolic blood pressure (for example) is derived by bedside monitors and not by the computer. The computer monitors these monitors and not the patient directly.

(b) Every half an hour sufficient data to allow a manual chart to be commenced is dumped on a typewriter. The fluid balance summary cannot therefore be more than half an hour out of date.

(c) Every six hours a graph of the blood pressure, heart rate, etc. is plotted on the typewriter. This is used as the permanent record in the patient's notes, replacing the nurse's chart. If the computer should break down, at the very worst six hours of records need to be reconstructed by hand.

(d) At twelve-hourly intervals a complete record of every transaction and a breakdown of the fluid balance are printed on a line-printer. This allows erroneous entries to be traced and is used as a master record for research purposes.

CONCLUSION

Computers may assist in routine patient care by facilitating applied research and physiological measurement. They may also be used to acquire and present data to the staff in a ward. In order to operate routinely in a clinical environment the following features are mandatory.

1. The exercise should be clinically relevant.
2. The system should be acceptable to doctors and nurses.
3. Data entry should be simple and display clear and unambiguous.
4. The system must be fail-safe.

Acknowledgments
The ideas developed above spring from close collaboration with C. E. Drew, Esq., FRCS, Cardiac Surgeon, Dr Percy Cliffe, Director of

the Department of Clinical Measurement and Mrs Gillian Tobin, Sister in charge of the Recovery Unit at Westminster Hospital. Systems Analysis and programming for the system described was carried out by Anna Mikolajczuk, D. J. Browń and P. J. Carrington of the Medical Computer Centre.

References
1. Grodins, F. S., Buell, J. and Bart, A. J. (1967). Mathematical analysis and digital simulation of the respiratory control system. *Scand. J. Clin. Lab. Invest.*, **19**, 29
2. Hilberman, M., Schill, J. P. and Peters, R. M. (1969). On line digital analysis of respiratory mechanics and the automation of respiratory control. *J. Thorac. Cardiovasc. Surg.*, **58**, 821
3. Warner, H. R. (1969). The role of the computer in medical research. *JAMA*, **196**, 944
4. Kouchoukos, N. T., Sheppard, L. C. and McDonald, D. A. (1969). Estimation of stroke volume from central arterial pressure contour in postoperative patients. *Surg. Form.*, **20**, 180
5. Seeley, H. F. (1973). Some methods of deriving cardiac output from central aortic pressure. *Proc. Roy. Soc. Med.*, **66**, 478
6. Stott, J. R. (1974). *A device to Extract Parameters from Blood Pressure Waveforms* (Thesis submitted for Diploma of Membership of Imperial College)
7. Drew, C. E. and Anderson, I. M. (1959). Profound hypothermia in cardiac surgery. *Lancet*, **1**, 748
8. Drew, C. E., Kreen, G. and Benazon, D. B. (1959). Profound hypothermia. *Lancet*, **1**, 745
9. Nunn, J. F., Bergman, N. A., Bunatyan, A. and Coleman, A. J. (1965). Temperature coefficients for P_{CO_2} and P_{O_2} of blood *in vitro*. *J. Appl. Physiol.*, **20**, 23
10. Thomas, L. J., Jr (1972). Algorithms for selected acid base and blood gas calculations. *J. Appl. Physiol.*, **33**, 154

Part 7

Ischaemic Heart Disease

55
Selection of patients for coronary artery surgery

J. L. Waddy

The introduction of saphenous vein graft surgery by Favaloro in 1967 has taken away from cardiologists one of their few remaining areas of peace. Patients with ischaemic heart disease who were previously treated to a monologue of rather hollow reassurance and given a few Anginine tablets, now pose difficult and critical problems of decision as to the desirability of investigation and later surgical intervention. It was easy, even up to and including the time of saphenous vein implants, to brush aside the surgeon's claim to take an active part in the treatment of this disease. However, these days are gone and medico-surgical co-operation in the selection of patients for the saphenous vein graft operation has become mandatory.

Much has been said about the long-term uncertainties of the operation and many crocodile tears have been shed about the absence of respectable clinical trials. In the event in this disease of such diversity, it seems unlikely that clinical trials would produce the necessary information because of the probability that differences would be confounded by variations of surgical skill and case selection. Rather than bemoaning what is not known about the operation it seems more productive in our decision making to consider the factors which are known.

Firstly there seems little doubt from numbers of series, including the author's, that complete or worthwhile relief from angina can be obtained in a large number – at least 75% – of the cases operated on and in a high proportion of those with pain relief, improvement in myocardial function and exercise tolerance can also be demonstrated.

Secondly, over a wide range of series, mortality figures varying between 1·5 and 20% have been claimed. Many of these series were done early in surgical experience and it now can be stated that mortality of less than 5% can be expected and that figures above this value imply either errors in case selection or deficiencies in surgical skill.

The operation, though technically demanding, is not a particularly dangerous one, provided that surgeons are not prepared to sacrifice myocardial protection in the interests of ease of operative procedure. It must be accepted at this stage that the operation is a palliative one.

Revascularisation is much too grand a term to use to describe our attempts to shore up a failing arterial system.

It is clear that the outcome to the patient will depend, whether or not he has surgery, on the rate of deterioration of the peripheral parts of the coronary vascular tree and if he has surgery, on the expected duration of life of the vein graft itself. It is usually stated that it is too early to evaluate the effect of the operation on longevity but we must be getting close to that time now. Indeed, a recent series from the admittedly heavily committed Cleveland Clinic suggests quite strongly that survival is better following vein graft operation. In a group of 1000 postoperative patients, the annual loss was just over 4·5% whereas the fall-off rate in a rather unsatisfactorily selected group of controls was of the order of 9% giving a substantial advantage to the operated group. Indeed there seems no valid reason why improving the supply of blood to an area of myocardium should decrease prospects of survival.

Although the number of pre-operative myocardial infarcts and the fate of the proximal coronary artery stumps following grafting are interesting topics for conversation, they really are not particularly relevant to the main issue when compared with such things as relief of symptoms, improvement of myocardial function and increase in longevity. The evidence in these important areas seems more than favourable.

The prime indication for investigation and perhaps subsequent operation is, of course, angina, which despite adequate medical treatment is disabling enough to disturb the life pattern of the patient. It goes without saying that angina acceptable to an elderly man who has retired would be intolerable to a 40-year-old labourer with a family to keep. The presence of significant angina is also important from another point of view. In this situation, to obtain adequate run-off through a saphenous vein graft, it is important to have a substantial pressure gradient across the graft. In other words, it is important to plug the graft into a low pressure coronary system and for this to occur, critical blocks of the coronary artery are needed. The presence of severe angina is good evidence that somewhere in the coronary tree, such critical blocks and low pressure areas exist.

Following investigation, adequate coronary arteriograms will provide the indication of whether or not to proceed with surgical operation. Cases can be divided roughly into three rather ill-defined groups. In the first group, severe proximal blocks can be seen with evidence often of adequately-sized peripheral vessels relatively free from disease. If then, normal left ventricular function can be found, it is probably not too strong a statement to say that it is bordering on malpractice not to offer the patient surgery. The author would also include in this category, those patients with single vessel disease. Much has been made of the fact that the mortality of these patients without surgery is very low, but in fact, with surgery, the mortality should be equally low and furthermore, the prospects of getting relief of symptoms is very high indeed. In many cases, it is the left anterior descending artery only which is involved. This is an artery which is easily reached surgically in which the technical problems involved are not great and the torsion and disturbances to the heart are minimal, so that subsequent myocardial embarrassment is almost always avoided. The whole group is an excellent one in which good results can be anticipated in the vast majority of cases and in which the risk of operation is absolutely minimal.

The second group shows much more widespread coronary artery disease and in many cases even in the presence of satisfactory angiograms, it will be difficult to decide whether adequate grafting points or run-offs can be obtained. We are looking here for vessels of 1 mm in diameter or more, and these critical facts are not always available from angiograms. More grafts will be required to attempt a satisfactory revascularisation and more myocardial disturbance can be expected as a result. From this graft will be drawn almost all of the fatalities and most of the unsatisfactory results. Surgical skill is all important in keeping these to a minimum.

The third group can show definite contraindications to surgery in two ways; firstly, by having a totally unsuitable coronary artery tree either with hypoplastic vessels, or with multiple peripheral obstructions and no areas which suggest the possibility of an adequate run-off; and secondly by showing on left ventricular angiography a poorly contracting left ventricle. A left ventricle which contracts badly in a diffuse manner is associated usually with large and diffuse areas of myocardial damage and on very few occasions has such a heart been improved by grafting. We are indebted to Frank Spencer for painfully demonstrating the futility of saphenous vein grafting for failing hearts and this after all is one of the radiological signs of left ventricular embarrassment. This diffuse myocardial contractile failure is not to be confused with that in which discreet areas of the myocardium are non-contractile. These are, of course, usually related to previous myocardial infarcts and in many cases grafting gives satisfactory results and the removal of the involved piece of myocardium may even result in improved myocardial function.

There are one or two other indications for surgery worth consideration. The Cleveland Clinic have shown conclusively the disastrous prognosis of those patients who have a block of their left main coronary artery or allied conditions in which the left anterior descending and circumflex are both blocked high up. It seems to be widely held that the presence of this lesion is an essential indication for early surgical interference. Should we be looking for this and other life threatening lesions without waiting for the tell-tale symptom of angina?

Coronary insufficiency, preinfarction angina or whatever term is used to describe the intermediate state, has been described by some as an immediate indication for investigation and operation but subsequent series from Michael Oliver and from Kraus in Boston among others, have demonstrated that perhaps this condition is not quite so serious as we have been led to believe. Kraus describes in his last series 1% mortality and 6% infarction. Perhaps we have over-reacted to this group and clearly with these sort of figures they are entitled to a period of observation. In the event, a certain number of these cases single themselves out by an unremitting pattern of pain over a period of three or four days and indicate their need for investigation and subsequent treatment, as opposed to the vast majority of the group who from the early stage begin to show signs of improvement.

The surgical approach to acute myocardial infarctions with excision plus or minus coronary artery grafting and with or without the assistance of balloon pumping is an interesting and disturbing field. Although notable cases have been quoted, the price in effort and manpower is extremely high and logistically there are few Units that can embark on this difficult and demanding field without materially prejudicing the outlook for the cases on their interval programme. Surgeon fatigue and intensive care fatigue, like pilot fatigue, can occasionally be dangerous.

In the author's Unit, just over half the patients investigated have been operated on. Not all of the rejects were inoperable; a significant proportion of those investigated showed lesions which were not serious enough to warrant surgery and some of them, of course, showed normal coronary artery trees.

Of the first 100 cases, 80 were operated on because of severe angina and 20 warranted the diagnosis of coronary insufficiency. 55 cases had a convincing story and confirmatory evidence of one or more previous myocardial infactions; 60 of the series, had a left ventricular end-diastolic pressure greater than 12 implying some degree of impaired left ventricular function. Four cases were complicated by the necessity to do an aortic valve replacement in addition and in four cases it was considered desirable to remove an area of left ventricular muscle either as an aneurysmectomy or an infarctectomy. 35 patients were given single grafts, 56 double grafts and nine had triple grafts. In the total series of 140 cases there was a hospital mortality of four cases (2·8%), a late mortality of five cases, 10 of the results have been described as bad and 121 (87%) of the series described as substantially improved. By far the majority of these 121 cases are actually angina free.

In summary then, the author's Unit are looking for patients with persistent and intractible angina, to submit to coronary angiography. From this group can be found a significant number of people to whom relief from a disabling and demoralising disease can be offered at the price of a very small mortality and there seems little evidence that this procedure reduces their subsequent expectation of life.

A further group of people defined by coronary angiogram can be offered the operation with some degree of uncertainty, with a higher rate of failure and a significantly higher mortality, but nevertheless with a very significant chance of substantial improvement.

A third group of people can be defined in whom no surgical procedure is likely to be successful. The more dramatic procedures on the acute coronary emergencies must be regarded, at the present time, as largely experimental.

However, the acceptedly low mortality rate of these supportive procedures must encourage us to look for specific and dangerous areas of ischaemic heart disease where prophylactic intervention can be contemplated without waiting for the premonitory anginal attack or for the so common unheralded fatal infarction.

56
Pre and postoperative investigation
R. Balcon

One of the problems with coronary artery disease is that it presents almost no physical signs and the symptomatology is intermittent. It is therefore very difficult to define the exact status of the patient. However, this has been attempted in order to follow the patients' course both with and without treatment. Routine investigations include chest X-ray, electrocardiogram and serum lipid analysis. Although the electrocardiogram is often abnormal and there is quite often evidence of previous infarction it rarely has any effect on the management of the patient. The chest X-ray is usually normal, but again of little diagnostic value. Finally, at this stage of the disease lipid analysis has little practical importance. Physical examination is also usually normal and so the routine Out-Patient investigations do not help when the patient is symptomatic.

The symptoms themselves are the most important factor in determining future management. It is therefore essential to use a stress test in evaluating patients. We have used bicycle ergometer exercise testing with the object of reproducing the symptom rather than looking for electrocardiographic changes. The electrocardiogram is however monitored and if there is severe ST segment depression (more than 2 mm) the test is terminated even though symptoms have not yet developed.

In the first 109 patients treated at the London Chest Hospital the preoperative exercise test was limited at an average of 488 kpm/min. It is of interest to note that in 12 patients the test was limited by dyspnoea and not angina, although the latter was the complained of symptom. A second stress test was routinely performed during the cardiac catheterisation when the heart was paced from the right atrium or ventricle at a progressively increasing rate. This often reproduces the symptom at which time there is a rise in left ventricular end-diastolic pressure, which is probably due to an abnormality of compliance that develops. This is another indicator of ischaemia. The pacing procedure has also been useful in following the course of patients with and without treatment. Ninety-two patients were paced, the others either had rest pain or there were technical difficulties in achieving capture. The limiting factor was angina in all but five patients, who either had dyspnoea or reached the maximum rate of 180 beats/min without symptoms.

This type of objective testing has proved extremely useful in following patients particularly after aorto-coronary bypass surgery. Angiography, however, is still the most important investigation. It includes selective injection into the coronary arteries and left ventriculography. Recent advances in angiographic equipment have made it possible to produce excellent pictures of these structures making anatomical diagnosis simple. About a third of the patients had a major lesion of one coronary artery, the rest having involvement of two or three vessels. Eight had a major lesion of the left main coronary artery. Approximately half the patients had an abnormal left ventricular angiogram. The left ventricular end-diastolic pressure at rest ranged from 5 to 46 mmHg with a mean of 14·6 mmHg.

Similar investigations as described above can be carried out post-operatively. Cardiac pacing and angiography involves recatheterisation, but exercise tests can be performed on all patients. The effects of major surgery persist for three or four months so evaluation after six months is more meaningful. At this time approximately 72% of patients were symptom free, 24% improved and 4% unchanged. These clinical findings were confirmed with the exercise test.

Thirty-three patients were recatheterised an average of eight months after surgery, 12 of them because of recurrent angina or an attack of chest pain at rest without evidence of infarction. Twenty of this group were also free of angina. Once again exercise testing showed a significant improvement which was confirmed by an improvement in the pacing test, the maximum rate rising from 134 preoperatively to 163 postoperatively. All of the patients had angina in the preoperative test and only ten in the postoperative. Left ventricular end-diastolic pressure did not change significantly nor did the state of the left ventriculer as judged angiographically. Coronary angiography was similar in both pre and post-operative studies, although there was a tendency for major stenotic lesions to become occlusions when the vessel was grafted distally. Forty-three (80%) of the 52 grafts were patent at the time of reinvestigation. 72% of the patients had all grafts patent, 18% had one graft patent and one occluded, three had no patent grafts.

In conclusion, stress testing has been used to follow the course of patients undergoing aorto-coronary bypass surgery. The results have given a factual evaluation of the effects of the procedure which has been of great value in helping to decide its future.

57
Problems of technique in aorto-coronary bypass operations

J. E. C. Wright

The first step in aorto-coronary bypass operation is to produce the vein graft that is going to be used. There are theoretical reasons for preferring the vein from the lower leg to the vein from the upper leg or thigh. The vein removed from the lower leg is of course of smaller calibre and is therefore more like the size of the coronary artery than is the large vein from the upper thigh. However, the vein in the lower leg has many more branches which can produce trouble. Conversely, the reported incidence of intimal hyperplasia might encourage use of a wide vein from the upper thigh in the hope that this will stay open longer. Initially the author used the vein from the upper thigh but later the vein from the lower leg was preferred. However, since many more multiple grafts are now being performed, it is often necessary to remove the whole length of vein which eliminates the need to make a choice.

Two methods can be used to obtain a long length of vein; one is to use a long incision. Alternatively multiple short incisions, the so-called 'step ladder' incision, can be used. The author prefers the long incision, because this method reduces the possibility of damaging the vein on removal. Having successfully removed the vein, it is necessary to test for leaks. However, recent reports have shown that the fluid which is injected into the vein to perform the test could possibly be responsible for intimal lesions, hyperplasia and medial degeneration. Initially the author used Hartman's solution, but having read the reports, now uses the patient's own blood to distend the vein. Distending the vein also reveals any twists or narrow segments where one of the side branches has been ligated too close to the main vessel.

During the waiting interval, the vein is stored in the patient's own blood. The next step is to isolate the coronary artery. To do this the author prefers to use two snares made of prolene, with a circumferential snare above and below the site of operation. This method has now been used for several months and has replaced the previous technique where no snares were used, but the technique was to cut straight down onto the coronary artery and then clamp the aorta. This latter technique can still be used when doing one or two grafts when the whole distal anastomosis can be performed under ischaemic conditions but in the case of multiple endarterectomies and triple vein grafts the duration of the operation does not allow for total ischaemia. For this reason the prolene snares are now used, when it is possible to leave the coronaries perfused while producing a dry field.

Having isolated the coronary artery, simple stay stitches are used to pull the fat aside in order to expose it. Once the coronary artery is

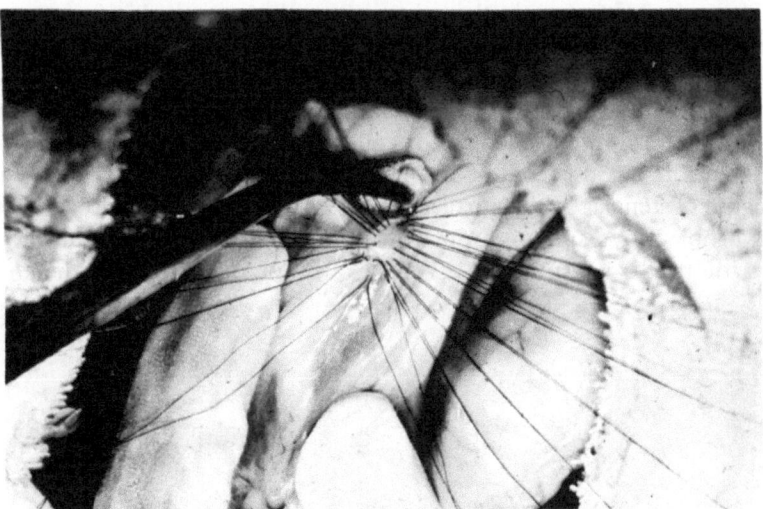

Figure 57.1 The use of multiple interrupted stitches in exposing the coronary artery

exposed a linear incision is made. The initial technique used to expose the coronary artery was to use multiple interrupted stitches (Figure 57.1). The edge of the vessel was stitched in this manner and then inserted through the obliquely cut distal vein by sliding it down rather like a prosthetic valve. This is a very reliable technique, produces excellent results, and avoids the problem which arises when using a continuous suturing technique where the ends of the incision may be narrowed by a purse-string effect. However, in multiple procedures the use of these multiple stitches is too time consuming so a continuous suture technique is now used. Initially the suture material was black silk but now monofilament prolene is used.

There are many techniques for inserting continuous stitches. Currently, the author places a single suture at one end of the incision, brings it half-way down one side, half-way down the other, puts another stitch in at the other end and brings them back to the middle. An alternative is to put a stitch in at one end, bring it all the way round and back again, and for the right coronary it is possible to put a stitch in at the distal end, go up half one side and then all the way round. Using prolene, this can be done with separation of the vein from the coronary and simply pulling up on the prolene slides the vein down. Just before the anastomosis is finally closed patency of the coronary at each end is checked. This is an obvious area for purse-stringing when using a continuous technique and may be responsible for some of the reported early incidences of block in the first few days following operation.

The next step is to join the vein graft to the aorta and it is necessary to decide whether to join the distal end or proximal end first. Theoretically it is desirable to put the proximal end on first and perfuse the coronary immediately the vein graft is completed, but this is not of great importance as it only saves five or eight minutes. Initially the simple slit in the aorta was used but again there were reports of vein graft closure because of stenosis at the aortic end. However, it is possible to overcome this problem by using an ordinary Cooley side clamp on the aorta and an orthopaedic instrument – a ronger – to bite out a piece of the aorta.

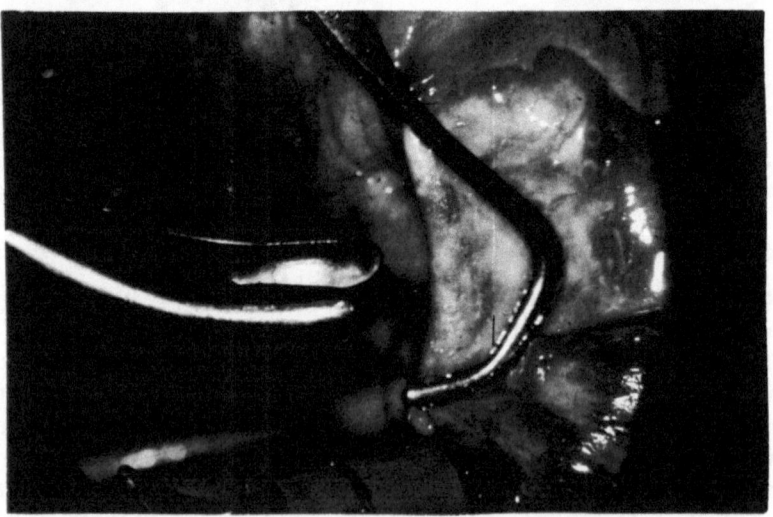

Figure 57.2 The use of a Cooley side clamp and a ronger in joining the vein graft to the aorta

This produces a disc of tissue or an elipse, leaving a clean-cut hole on which to sew the vein (Figure 57.2). It is also possible to put two veins into the same segment of aorta isolated by the clamp by taking a bite high up and low down getting two anastomoses from the one clamp – this technique solves the problem of finding room on the aorta when performing multiple vein grafts. Here again, a continuous technique would be used although the suture material is not as important and with a single

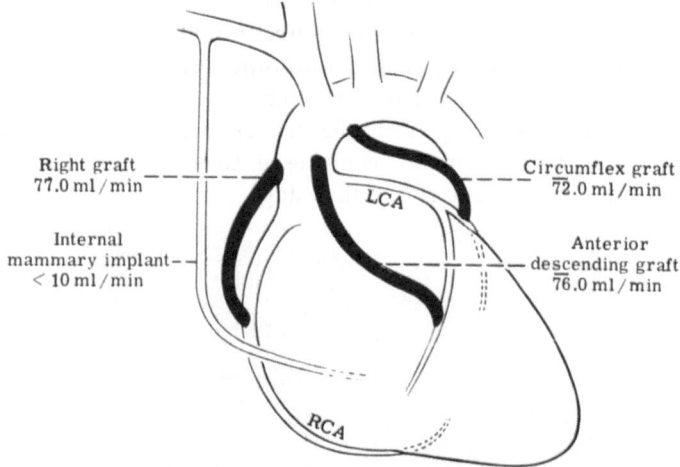

Right graft
77.0 ml/min

Circumflex graft
72.0 ml/min

LCA

Internal
mammary implant
< 10 ml/min

Anterior
descending graft
76.0 ml/min

RCA

Total coronary flow at rest ≈ 300 ml/min

Figure 57.3 Average flow rates in completed vein grafts

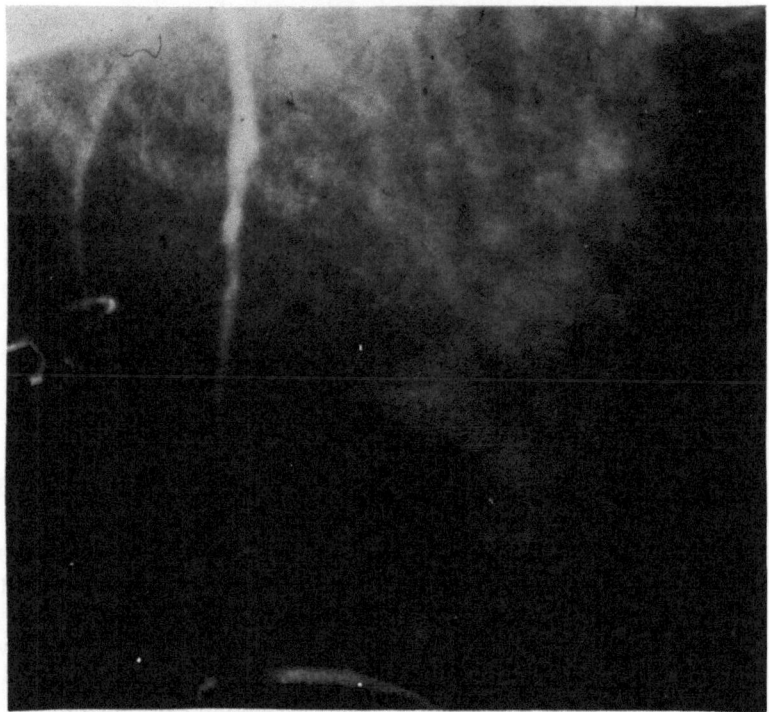

Figure 57.4 A vein graft in the process of occluding

377

stitch at the back and then straight round, the anastomosis can be
completed in a relatively few minutes. Sometimes this is done on bypass
and sometimes off, the author using normothermic bypass. If ischaemia
is used during the distal end of the anastomosis, then the top end is put
on while still on bypass to give the heart a chance to recover from the
ischaemic insult, but if ischaemia is not used, then it is possible to come
off bypass and do the aortic end at that stage.

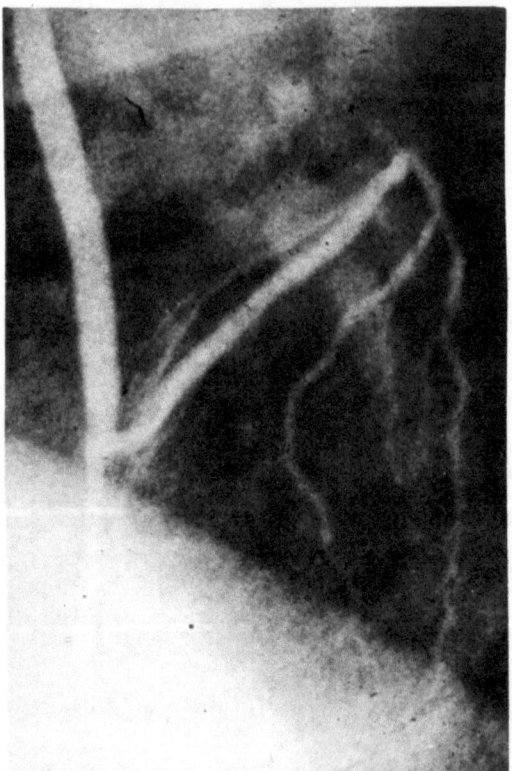

Figure 57.5 A vein graft in a distal right coronary with good run-off

Having completed the vein graft, it is now essential to measure the flow
in order to detect any defects. In the long-term, flow measurement has
been shown to be of prognostic value, both with regard to the patient's
relief of symptoms and to the long-term patency rate. World literature
seems to indicate that a flow of about 44 cc/min will ensure a patent graft.
Figure 57.3 shows some values for average flows. Figure 57.4 shows a vein
graft in the process of occluding. In this patient two vein grafts were
inserted, one into a distal right coronary with a good run-off (Figure 57.5)
and the other into an anterior descending with disease, a poor run-off and

a poor measured flow (Figure 57.4).

It is important to overcome the problem of a vessel with a poor run-off and one possible answer might be to use the internal mammary artery as the reported patency rates following this operation are significantly higher than those following vein grafting. At the London Chest Hospital vein graft patency rate is around 85% but world literature would indicate nearly 100% patency rate for the internal mammary artery. The technique for internal mammary implants is simply to dissect off the pedicle and take the vein with it if it happens to come. The side branches are managed with silver clips and the artery is left attached until needed, so that it is continually perfusing, the distal end only being detached when required. The most satisfactory mammary arteries are those which have a good stream of blood coming out of them when the bulldog clamp is taken off but often, when the artery is taken from other sources the amount of blood coming out of it is too poor for use. Another problem with internal mammary implants is that the arteries are not sufficiently long to reach the anterior descending if a very distal anastomosis is indicated, although occasionally the circumflex can be reached. Furthermore, the calibre of the artery is not large enough throughout its length and mammary graft flows are on average 30 or 40% less than rear vein graft flows. Therefore, although the patency rate is excellent, the actual amount of blood supplied by the mammary artery is probably not as good as a vein graft.

In cases with an isolated major stenosis in the coronary artery, but a good distal run-off, vein grafting or mammary artery implantation is the obvious procedure. However, what is the procedure when faced with diffuse disease in a dominant right coronary artery which has multiple distal branches going to the septum and the left ventricle all of which may narrow at their origin? A possibility would be to insert eight or nine small grafts into each small distal coronary ensuring a flow of 20 or 30 cc/min in each one. The alternative is to perform an endarterectomy.

In cases of endarterectomy, the distal right coronary artery is isolated between the marginal branch and the posterior descending and a simple Macdonald's dissector is hooked under the core, which then elevates. Gas endarterectomy is sometimes the method used, but the author prefers a manual approach using a simple blunt dissector, although gas probes are used for separating the core but are not connected to any gas supply. Having elevated the core, it is then pulled out from the aortic end, and usually breaks off. This does not present a problem since the alternative a divided flow situation, most of the blood going down the endarterectomised coronary and some going down the vein, in which situation they could both occlude. Therefore the proximal coronary is left with its disease and all the blood is diverted down the vein. The next

379

stage is to remove the cores of atheroma from the branches using probes and dissectors (Figure 57.6). To ensure that this procedure has been performed thoroughly the bits and pieces are always very carefully examined for good smooth cut-offs. Twenty-seven patients have been

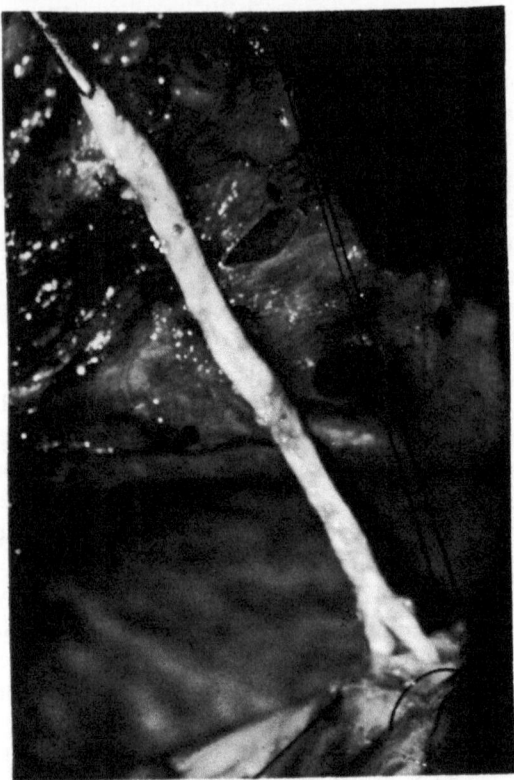

Figure 57.6 The use of probes and dissectors to remove cores of atheroma from branches of the proximal artery

operated on using this technique with no increase in mortality and no significant difference in ECG evidence of infarction following operation. In fact there was only one death in the series and this was the case of an unstable angina patient. The anterior descending can also be operated on in exactly the same way, elevating the core, pulling the core out from the proximal end and then pulling it out from the distal coronary and examining with the probe to make sure there has been complete clearance. If the core breaks, as it does occasionally, a fresh incision is made over the site of breakage and the rest of the core is removed. The incision is then closed with a vein patch. Flow measurements following endarterectomy give similar values to ordinary vein grafting.

58
The coronary bypass operation
A. Starr

For many years in Oregon, Dr Melvin Judkin pioneered the method of coronary arteriography, which was very reliable and very easy to teach to other cardiologists. Therefore, in Oregon there is a large group of cardiologists who are very skillful in performing coronary arteriography, having attained their skill relatively early in coronary artery surgery, and although the area is relatively small, there is a very large reservoir of patients from which to draw clinical material.

In evaluating the role of surgery in coronary artery disease, it is important to distinguish between different groups of patients who really have a different medical prognosis and also present different surgical problems. For example, there are patients with disabling chronic angina. This is a group that cardiologists in Oregon know a great deal about, and the results with this particular group will be discussed.There is also a group of patients with accelerated angina. The definition of this group of patients varies very much from one clinic to another, which makes it difficult to compare results. Therefore, when discussing these patients each clinic must be very specific about their definition of accelerated angina. In addition, there is a group of patients who really have chronic valvular heart disease but also in association with coronary artery disease. This poses some other problems in a completely separate group of patients that will be discussed later. Finally there are other groups of patients which need clarification, e.g. those patients with chronic angina and significant congestive failure. Cardiologists in Oregon do not have much experience with these patients and really do not know at this time the proper role of surgery in this situation. The situation is similar with patients who are in the immediate post-infarction period. Those patients with relatively small infarctions, do tolerate coronary arteriography and emergency surgery very well. Those patients with large infarctions studied late after their infarct with congestive failure, seem to do poorly, but this group has not yet been very clearly defined.

In this chapter the author will discuss the results with three groups of patients that have provided some very hard data, mainly in terms of the relief of symptoms, but also in terms of the effect of operation on longevity.

The overwhelming majority of these patients—532 with chronic disabling angina—were operated on between 1968 and July 1973. These operations were performed in the majority of cases using the saphenous vein, there were very few internal mammary anastomoses in this group. During the past two years, patients have been operated without a left ventricular vent or any venting of the left side of the heart. Reviewing this experience during the years beginning in 1968, a very marked increase in the number of operations per year can be seen. During the past few years the number of operations has almost doubled each year. Also, as is the case with most surgical procedures, the operative mortality diminishes with experience, beginning at about 12%, in early experience, and then rapidly falling so that in the first half of 1973 the operative risk of saphenous vein bypass graft for chronic disabling angina was only $1\frac{1}{2}$%. This is really a different form of intracardiac surgery from other more usual types. It is more like peripheral vascular surgery, operating on the surface of the heart and producing very little in the way of myocardial damage.

The total operative mortality is 3.4%. This includes deaths occurring in the first 30 days after operation. There was a late death rate of 3.2% The cause of death after surgery is of some interest. Most deaths are related to coronary artery disease and not the operation *per se*. For example, there were five patients who could not be weaned from bypass and there were 11 patients who had clear cut, myocardial infarction with low output syndrome and died in the first 24–48 h after operation. Therefore 16 of 18 patients died of a coronary artery disease and similarly late deaths have almost always been related to the presence of coronary artery disease.

An attempt was made to study graft patency in as many patients as possible after operation, but this was only successful in about 200 of the 500 cases. The time of study was a mean of six months after surgery and many patients were studied beyond the six month period. The patency rate for grafts was 76%, however 85% of the patients had at least one patent graft. This is possibly explained by the fact that in may cases an unsatisfactory vessel was grafted while at the same time placing the coronary graft on a vessel which is very suitable for grafting.

A study of the functional results in a series of more than 1000 cases reveals that most of the patients are in class 3 or 4 prior to operation. Post-operatively most patients are in class 1 or 2 but some gradually deteriorate into classes 3 or 4.

Is it the change in the nature of the operative procedure that accounts for this apparent deterioration in the late results after operation? In the beginning only 69% of the vessels that were diseased at the time of operation were being grafted. However, as experience increased, the percentage of diseased vessels which were grafted also increased. More multiple grafts were performed, so that in 1973 91% of the diseased vessels were being grafted. Therefore, if the patients are broken up into cohorts, depending upon the year of surgery, it can be seen that of those patients operated upon in 1973 in the first year after operation, a very small number were in functional class 3 or 4 after surgery, but of those patients operated upon in 1968, 1969 and 1970, relatively large numbers of patients were still in functional class 3 and 4 after operation. These are the patients who contribute to the curve which shows an apparent decline in the operative results. Therefore, although there must be some deterioration of results in terms of progressive coronary artery disease, this deterioration is slow and the apparent decrease in good results in this series is related to the nature of the operation as performed in the early days of coronary artery surgery.

The results in terms of an actuarial survival curve for patients with chronic disabling angina show that the chance for a patient surviving to the end of a four-year period after this operation is 89%. How does this survival rate compare with other recorded medical series of survival? In the present study, there was an 89% survival rate in a group of 532 patients. In the literature two interesting series of patients were found – the Cleveland Clinic series and the Johns Hopkin's series of 590 patients. The mean age of these patients compares very well with the age of the patients in the Oregon group, as does the distribution of single- and multiple-vessel disease. The Johns Hopkin's series showed a survival rate at the end of four years of 75% and the Cleveland Clinic group, a survival rate of 69% as compared with patients in the Oregon group who had the same disease – chronic disabling angina – and showed a survival rate of 89%. If these series are broken down into the presence of single-, double- and triple-vessel disease, the difference between surgical results and medical results becomes very significant. With the single-vessel disease there is a little operative and postoperative risk but by the end of four years, the survival following surgery is 96% and this includes operative, as well as late deaths. While the survival at five years in the medically-treated group with single-vessel disease is very good – 83% – there is still a significant difference. However, when the multiple-vessel disease is included, there is no question that surgery has something to offer the patient beyond the simple relief of angina pectoris, because the Oregon group has an 89% survival in patients with double-vessel disease at the end of four years, compared to 62% in patients with double-vessel disease treated without surgery. This is even further accentuated in patients with triple disease, where the Oregon group have an 84% four-year survival, compared to a 45% survival in patients treated without surgery. So patients with multiple-vessel disease discovered on coronary arteriography are very much at risk, and this risk is greatly alleviated by the performance of surgery.

There is a statistically significant difference in the long-term survival rates of patients who have single-, double- and triple- vessel disease. The survival rates for grafted patients are better than those for patients treated with medicine alone. The symptom of angina is simply an indicator that there is myocardial ischaemia. It is not possible to know from this indicator the extent of the coronary artery disease. Even the slightest symptom of angina is still a signal and this signal means that coronary arteriography must be performed – it is astonishing the extent of the disease that one will find even in patients with relatively mild angina. This doesn't apply to the group that has just been discussed, but is simply an aside remark concerning the author's own philosophy in dealing with patients who have angina.

In considering a smaller group of patients who have what is called unstable or accelerated angina, the problem has to be clearly and carefully defined. Firstly, these are patients who have been proven to have at least a 50% narrowing of a coronary artery. They are the patients described in the literature as having unstable angina. They have never had coronary arteriography and it is not even known if they have coronary artery disease. Some patients can exhibit typical symptoms and yet without coronary artery disease. Secondly, the patients in the author's series may have prior chronic angina or a previous myocardial infarction and finally, the angina increases in frequency and severity and culminates in recurrent chest pains at rest. The rest pain persists for more than 24 h after hospitalisation and there is the EKG evidence of ischaemia which almost invariably accompanies the pain. Fifty five such patients have been operated on – most of them men with a mean age of 53 years. 62% of them had previous chronic angina and 38% were of relatively recent onset – less than three months. Many had a previous infarction. These patients have been treated as rather urgent problems and the majority of operations were performed on the second day of hospitalisation. Some of the patients were operated on later in the week.

The clinical results obtained in this group of patients in terms of anginal free status are similar to those described by Dr Balcon and Dr Waddy. 42% of the patients were in functional class 1 following operation (this is a very difficult group to treat) and 35% were in functional class 2. 15% remained in functional class 3, 7% died either early or late after surgery and 2% in this group are lost to follow-up. The patency rate in this group is very similar to the patency rate for chronic angina – perhaps a little bit less. 90% of the patients had at least one patient graft and only three patients studied – 10% – had all grafts occluded. All the patients in functional class 3 were studied and 63% of the patients in functional class 2 were studied, while only 43% of the patients in functional class 1 were studied. Therefore these grafts patency rates lean very heavily towards the patient who is continuing to have symptoms following operation.

The author has tried to extract from the literature a group of patients that correspond to the group of patients being discussed and the report of Gazes – his worst group – corresponds. On an accurate actuarial display, the chance for a patient surviving four years after surgical management of accelerated angina is 93%. The chance for survival with this condition at the end of five years in a similar group of patients is 27%.

The survival rates in groups of patients are as follows in the chronic angina group – 89% at the end of 4 years; those patients in the Oregon series who have had isolated aortic valve replacement and those patients who have had aortic valve replacement with saphenous vein bypass grafts, superimposed on the aortic valve replacement alone. Therefore it can be said with some reasonable certainty, that the addition of coronary artery surgery to the saphenous vein bypass graft operation does not significantly increase the risk. In terms of mitral valve disease, there is a very significant difference. The important point here is that when saphenous vein bypass grafts are associated with rheumatic mitral valvitis, the mortality is quite low – 8% – but when mitral valve replacement is performed for non-rheumatic disease, usually ischaemic heart disease, then there is a very high mortality of combined mitral valve replacement and saphenous vein bypass grafting.

Finally, there are those patients with mild stable angina – there is no clear cut evidence of how these patients should be managed – and those patients that are asymptomatic following a myocardial infarction. These patients have demonstrated that they have had advanced coronary artery disease by having had an infarct and yet at the present time, neither of these two groups are considered as potential candidates for study and possible surgery if significant disease is found. The author believes that these patients need to be studied, perhaps even randomised and some determination made as to how to manage them.

59
Coronary endarterectomy
C. Hahn, N. Radovanovic and B. Faidutti

The results of aorto-coronary bypasses depend on good peripheral flow. Coronary artery disease is often the result of diffuse lesions of the distal segments of the coronary arteries. The possibility of revascularisation by venous graft is therefore limited due to the fact that this would cause obstruction of the distal part of the arteries.

To allow more patients to benefit from direct revascularisation of the myocardium, endarterectomy of the distal part of the coronary arteries has been recently brought back into use[1]. At the present time, endarterectomy of the coronary arteries has been advocated as an additional method in all those cases where the patency of the venous graft might be endangered by poor peripheral outflow.

A direct revascularisation of the myocardium has been performed on 513 patients since June 1968. The endarterectomy of one or more coronary arteries has been performed on 130 patients (25% of those operated on) (Table 59.1). The technique of endarterectomy consists of

Table 59.1 Coronary endarterectomies, June 1968–March 1974

Direct revascularisation:	513 Cases
Endarterectomies:	130 = 25·1%

Table 59.2 The frequency of endarterectomies performed on the different coronary artery branches. Mortality rate 13·8%

	No. of patients	Post-op mortality	Secondary mortality
Right coronary artery	102	10 = 10·2%	6 = 6%
Left coronary artery	19	2 = 10·5%	0
Right + ant. desc.	7	0	0
3 vessels	2	0	0
Total	130	12 = 9·3%	6 = 4·6%
	Mortality rate = 13·8%		

manual dissection with the aid of a dissector or a Crile forceps. Table 59.2 shows the frequency of endarterectomies performed on the different coronary artery branches. It demonstrates that 102 patients have had an endarterectomy of the right coronary artery with a postoperative mortality of 10·2%. Late mortality during a five year period is 6%. The endarterectomy of the left anterior descending and circumflex has been performed in 19 cases with a postoperative mortality of 10·5% and no late mortality. In nine patients a double and triple endarterectomy has been performed without mortality. In our experience, the risk involved in a left endarterectomy is no greater than for the right one.

RIGHT CORONARY ARTERY ENDARTERECTOMY

Table 59.3 shows the results of different lesions and surgical procedures involved in endarterectomy of the right coronary artery. It shows that the postoperative mortality in the treatment of the lesions of the right

Table 59.3 The results of different lesions and surgical procedures used in endarterectomy of the right coronary artery in 102 patients

Surgical procedure	No. of patients	Postop mortality	Secondary mortality
Single bypass	31	1	2
Vineberg	3	0	0
Lad bypass	40	2	1
Circ. bypass	3	1	0
Triple bypass	1	1	0
Aneurysmectomy			
Single bypass left side	14	4	2
Mitral replacement	1	0	0
Aortic or arterial procedures	9	1	1
Total	102	10	6

coronary artery without aneurysm of the left ventricle is about 6%. The surgical risk rises with the resection of the aneurysm of the left ventricle. The late mortality is also higher in this group. The postoperative mortality of patients with diffuse lesions and serious loss of myocardium is detailed in Table 59.4. Four patients had a large aneurysm of the left ventricle and one showed lesions of the abdominal aorta which were treated at the same time. Most frequently, the cause of death is postoperative infarcts, which was encountered in four patients. Cause of death in two cases was intractable ventricular fibrillation while in another case cerebral embolism was responsible. In one case, haemorrhagic diathesis, anaesthesia with Ketalar and bad extracorporeal circulation were responsible for severe renal and respiratory insufficiencies. In one patient where an endarterectomy of the right coronary artery had been performed together with a resection of a left ventricular aneurysm, the reason for death was a postero-lateral infarct, due to an absence of collaterals in the region of the left ventricle, while the venous graft remained patent. Causes of death in the late postoperative period are summarised in Table 59.5. Five out of six patients died of coronary

Table 59.4 The postoperative mortality of 102 patients with diffuse lesions and serious loss of myocardium. Postoperative mortality: 10 patients = 10·2%

Name	Surgical procedure	Time of death	Cause of death
P.W.	Right bypass aneurysmectomy	7 weeks	Ant.-sept. MI
P.D.	Right and lad bypasses	1st day	MI (thrombosis of right graft)
CH.CH	Bypass of 3 V.	1 hour	Irreductible ventricular fibrillation
F.R.	Right and circ. bypasses	8 days	Unknown
N.A.	Right bypass aneurysmectomy	1 hour	Irreductible fibrillation
F.L.	Right bypass aneurysmectomy	3 days	Post.-lat. MI open bypass
R.L.	Right and lad bypasses Aorto-bifemoral bypass	4 days	Left hemiplegia Cardiac arrest
M.W.	Right and lad bypasses	18 days	Renal + respiratory insufficiency
B.G.	Right bypass aneurysmectomy	2 hours	Bleeding
L.G.	Right bypass circ. explor.	30 min	Post.-lat. MI

artery conditions and one patient died of intestinal perforation. One patient died suddenly after 15 months of normal activity following a right coronary bypass with distal endarterectomy. The autopsy showed that the left anterior descending branch had been affected by important lesions,

Table 59.5 Causes of death in the late postoperative period of 102 cases of endarterectomy of the right coronary artery. Secondary mortality: 6 patients = 6%

Name	Surgical procedure	Time of death	Cause of death
M.J.J.	Right bypass	29 months excell. health	Septal MI Thrombosis of the graft
L.R.	Right bypass aneurysmectomy	36 months excell. health	Sudden death
B.W.	Right bypass aneurysmectomy Aneurysmectomy of abdom. aorta	42 months excell. health	Sudden death
R.G.	Right bypass Endart. of innom. art. and right vertebr. artery	4 months	Posterior MI Thrombosis of the graft
N.L.	Right bypass	15 months excell. health	Sudden death Open graft but lad. stenosis
C.R.	Right bypass	14 months	Intest. perfor.

while the venous bypass remained open. Five previously completely invalid patients survived from 14–42 months; in this kind of malignant disease, this is a good palliation. 81 patients were given check-ups after an endarterectomy of the right coronary artery.

The late results are shown on Table 59.6. Out of 25 patients with a survival of four to five years, the operative results in 18 are good, in three moderate and in two bad. Among the patients with a successful operation, we found 10 who were working at 100% of their normal capacity and two who were working at 50% of their normal capacity. These patients reached 100–150 watts in effort tests. Mitral insufficiency because of dysfunction of the mitral pillar has been responsible for a poor postoperative result in one case. In two other cases, unsuccessful results were shown to be caused by postoperative myocardial infarction due to obstruction of the venous graft. In the group of patients with a survival rate of three to four years, 21 patients have been checked and three have not been followed-up. Out of these 21 patients, 17 were in a healthy condition, while four were in a moderate condition. The condition of one of these patients, although

Table 59.6 Late results of 86 cases of endarterectomy of the right coronary artery. 1 month to five years

Follow-up	No. of patients	No. of controls	Good	Fair	Poor
4–5 years	25	2	18	3	2
3–4 years	24	3	17	4	0
2–3 years	12	0	10	2	0
1–2 years	12	0	11	0	1 (Post MI)
1 month–1 year	13	0	13	0	0

Table 59.7 Results relating to the lesions and surgical technique used in 19 endarterectomies of the left coronary artery

Surgical procedure	No. of patients	Postop mortality	Secondary mortality
Lad bypass	(2)	1	'0
Right and lad bypass	(7)	0	0
Lad and circ. bypass	(2)	0	0
Circ. bypass	(2)	0	0
Circ. bypass Fem.-popl. bypass	(1)	0	0
Lad and circ. bypass	1	0	0
Lad and right bypass Fem.-popl. bypass	1	0	0
Lad bypass Aneurysmectomy	2	1	0
Lad bypass Y bypass between aorta and subclav. and carotid art.	1	0	0

good during a two year period following the operation, has now declined due to dyspnoea on effort and angina.

ENDARTERECTOMY OF THE LEFT CORONARY ARTERY

Nineteen patients were given endarterectomies of the branch of the left coronary artery followed by a left aortocoronary bypass. The results relating to the lesions and the surgical technique are shown in Table 59.7. The postoperative mortality rises to 10·5%. Detailed analysis of the causes of death of the two patients is shown in Table 59.8. In one case, death was due to an insufficiency of the left ventricle after resection of an aneurysm, in the other case to heart tamponade with cardiac arrest and decerebration of the patient. In this later case, obstruction of venous graft four months after the operation necessitated a reintervention, during which an arteriotomy of the anterior descending branch at the level of the implantation of the graft showed a narrowing atheromatous plaque, which had not been removed at the first operation. This time an endarterectomy was performed, which allowed for a good back-flow. A new aortocoronary bypass was installed. It appeared to us that the omission of the

Table 59.8 Causes of death in two cases of endarterectomy of the left coronary artery. Postoperative mortality: 2 patients = 10·5%

Name	Surgical procedure	Time of death	Cause of death
W.P.	Lad bypass Aneurysmectomy	3 days	Cardiac insuff.
H.R.	Lad bypass (4 months after occl. of a lad graft without endarterect.)	31 days	Cardiac tampon. and arrest irreversible cerebr. damage

Table 59.9 Late results of 19 cases of endarterectomy of the left coronary artery. 1 month to five years

Follow-up	No. of patients	No. of controls	Good	Fair	Poor
3–5 years	5	1	4	0	0
1–3 years	6	1	5	0	0
1 month–1 year	5	0	5	0	0

endarterectomy during the first operation had been responsible for the early obstruction of the graft.

Long-term results for up to five years are shown in Table 59.9. We have examined four patients out of five with a survival of three to five years. The patients are asymptomatic and have effort tests of over 100 watts and are reintegrated in social and professional life. In the group with a survival of one to three years, five patients out of six showed good results. Finally, in the third group, with a survival of one month to one year, there were five good results.

Table 59.10 Results of bilateral endarterectomy. Double endarterectomy + double bypass. Right coronary artery 3 + 3 lad: 7 patients

Postoperative and secondary mortality	:	0
Follow-up	:	9 months–4 years
Good results	:	6 patients (3 patients with full working capacity)
No. of controls	:	1 patient

BILATERAL ENDARTERECTOMY (Table 59.10)

There are seven patients in this group which was followed-up from nine months to four years. There were six good results in the controlled patients, of whom three work up to 100% of normal capacity.

Table 59.11 Results of triple endarterectomy. Triple endarterectomy + triple bypass. 2 patients

Name	Surgical procedure	Follow-up	Result
B.A.	Lad bypass Right bypass Circ. bypass	30 months	Good I (nyha)
V.E.	Lad bypass Right bypass Circ. bypass	38 months	Fair (full work capacity)

TRIPLE ENDARTERECTOMY (Table 59.11)

A triple endarterectomy with threefold bypass was performed on two patients. In one patient the result was good (he is asymptomatic), while the result for the second case can be considered as rather favourable, the patient being capable of an effort of 100 watts and a daily work capacity of 100%. However, he occasionally suffers from angina. In the last two groups of patients with multiple endarterectomies are cases of severe diffuse coronary artery disease of the three vessels. In this condition endarterectomy was the only possibility and led to a direct revascularisation of the myocardium by venous bypasses.

Table 59.12 The surgical risk for patients receiving endarterectomy

	No. of patients	Postop mortal.	Second. mortal.	Mortal. rate
Direct re-vascularisation of the myocardium (June 1968– 15th March 1974)	513	32 = 6·2%	19 = 3·8%	51 = 10%
Direct re-vascularisation of the myocardium without endarterectomy	383	20 = 5·2%	12 = 3·1%	32 = 8·3%
Direct re-vascularisation of the myocardium with endarterectomy	130 = 25·1%	12 = 9·3%	6 = 4·6%	18 = 13·8%

CONCLUSIONS

1. The surgical risk for patients receiving endarterectomy is not significantly greater than for those who did not undergo such a procedure since all the patients in the endarterectomised group had

a severe coronary artery disease with already one or more infarcts and in most cases heavy damage of the left ventricle (Table 59.12). These patients would not have benefited from a revascularisation without an endarterectomy. There was no alternative in this kind of situation except that of leaving young patients as invalids. The author's experience and attitude is similar to that of Groves et al[4].

2. Experience has shown that there is no significant difference in the surgical risk of a right or left coronary endarterectomy.

3. In conclusion, an endarterectomy in coronary artery surgery is an additional method of permitting good outflow of an aorto-coronary bypass and can be performed on the left coronary-tree as well as on the right one. The surgical decision will depend on the pathological findings of arteriotomy. If the atheromatous plaque is ulcerated, endarterectomy is unavoidable. This conclusion enables the operative indications to be extended so that a greater number of patients can profit by the direct revascularisation of the myocardium.

SUMMARY

From June 1968 to March 1974, 513 patients have been operated on for a revascularisation of the myocardium. In 130 cases, it was necessary to add an endarterectomy of one or more coronary arteries. Endarterectomy is never performed as an isolated procedure but has always been associated with a venous bypass.

This procedure has been performed on the right coronary artery of 102 patients with an operative mortality of 10.2% and a late mortality of 6% over a five year period. When this procedure was performed on the left coronary artery of 19 patients, the operative mortality was 10.5% without late mortality during a five year period. Double and triple endarterectomies have been performed on nine patients without operative mortality. Total mortality was 13.8%.

References

1. Bailey, C. P., May, A. and Lemmon, W. M. (1957). Survival after coronary endarterectomy in man. *JAMA*, **164**, 641

2. Dumanian, A. V. *et al.* (1972). Endarterectomy of the branches of the left coronary artery in combination with an aorta-to-coronary artery reversed saphenous vein graft. *Ann. Thorac. Surgery*, **Vol. 14**, No. 6

3. Dilley, R. B., Cannon, J. A., Kattus, A. A., MacAlpin, R. N. and Longmire, W. P., Jr (1965). The treatment of coronary occlusive disease by endarterectomy. *J. Thorac. Cardiovasc. Surg.*, **50**, 511

4. Groves, L. K., Loop, F. D. and Silver, G. M. (1972). Endarterectomy as a

supplement to coronary artery-saphenous vein by-pass surgery. *J. Thorac. Cardiovasc. Surg.*, **64**, 514

5. Sawyer, P. N., Kaplitt, M., Sobel, S., Karison, K. E. *et al.* (1967). Experimental and clinical experience with coronary gas endarterectomy. *Arch. Surg.*, **95**, 736
6. Cooley, D. A., Hallman, G. L. and Wukasch, D. C. (1971). Myocardial revascularisation using combined endarterectomy and vein by-pass autograft: Technique and results. *Int. Surg.*, **56**, 373
7. Urschel, H. C., Jr, Razzuk, M. A., Nathan, M. J., Miller, E. R., Nicholson, D. M. and Paulson, D. L. (1970). Combined gas (CO_2) endarterectomy and vein by-pass graft for patients with coronary artery disease. *Ann. Thorac. Surg.*, **10**, 119

60
Postoperative blood flow in auto-coronary saphenous vein bypass grafts

A. F. Rickards, J. E. C. Wright, C. A. Barefoot and B. T. Williams

Bypass grafting of occluded coronary arteries using autologous saphenous vein is now an established surgical procedure for certain groups of patients. It has been estimated that in 1972, 55 000 operations of this type were carried out in the USA alone. In Britain, numbers are much smaller but increasing as the operation gains wider acceptance.

Although on-table measurement of blood flow along the vein graft is now regarded as mandatory, data on long-term blood flow in these grafts is sparse. For this reason an electromagnetic flow probe has been designed which could be left around the graft for postoperative measurement of blood flow and subsequently withdrawn from the patients without reoperation.

THE WILLIAMS–BAREFOOT PROBE (MK. II)*

The design criteria of this probe follows those of the extractable aortic probe, which is now in routine clinical use, in that the electronic components of the device are modified so that they may be housed in a soft silicone rubber moulding of uniform cross-section. The geometry of the electromagnet and collecting electrodes is rather more conventional than that of the aortic probe (Figure 60.1); this is made possible by the smaller size of vessel to be accommodated.

The annulus is at the tip of the silicone rubber moulding and encircles only two-thirds of the cirumference of the vessel, so that removal by traction on the protruding cable is easily achieved without risk of damage to the graft.

The position of the probe is maintained by two soft, pliable silicone rubber wings attached to either side of the probe head. When sutured to the epicardium these wings not only maintain the longitudinal position of the probe, but also prevent its twisting and consequent occlusion of the vein graft.

Calibration. This is carried out *in vitro* before operation, by passing blood along an excised length of saphenous vein immersed in a bath of warm saline. Correlation of the signal from the attached probe with the volume

* See Chapter 53

of blood collected over a timed interval provides a calibration factor which is used to adjust the flowmeter gain. A calibration plot for a wide range of blood flows yields a straight line graph.

Clinical use. The prototype model of this device has now been implanted into four patients, yielding good signals in three of these for up to five

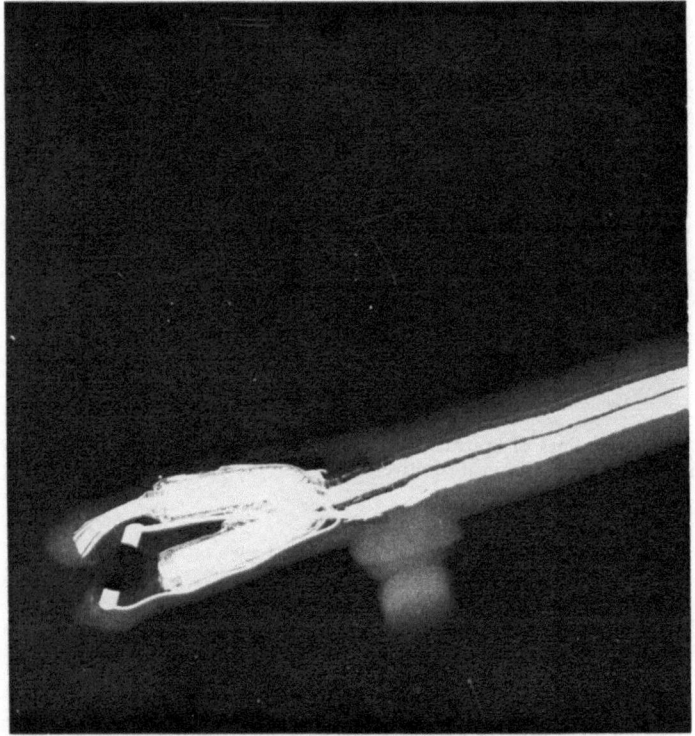

Figure 60.1 Lateral X-ray of the Williams–Barefoot (Mk. II) probe showing the geometry of the electronic components

days postoperatively. In the fourth patient the probe slipped off the graft in the immediate postoperative period.

The probe is attached to the epicardium using the rubber wings as previously described and the probe cable routed to the exterior immediately below the right costal margin.

Prior to closure of the chest temporary occlusion of the vein graft distal to the probe provides a reliable zero flow reference; subsequent drift in the zero point has been found to be negligible; zero flow in the graft has occurred between systole and diastole in some recordings and provided confirmation of the accuracy of the occlusive zero.

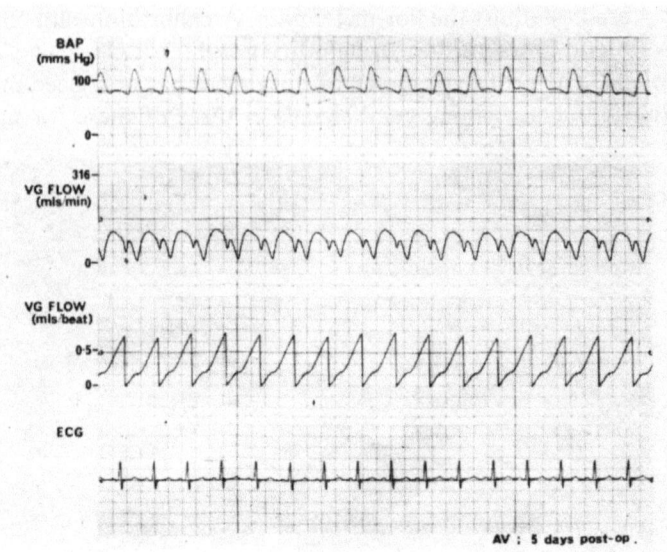

Figure 60.2 Recordings of brachial artery pressure, mean vein graft flow, flow/beat and ECG in a patient five days postoperatively

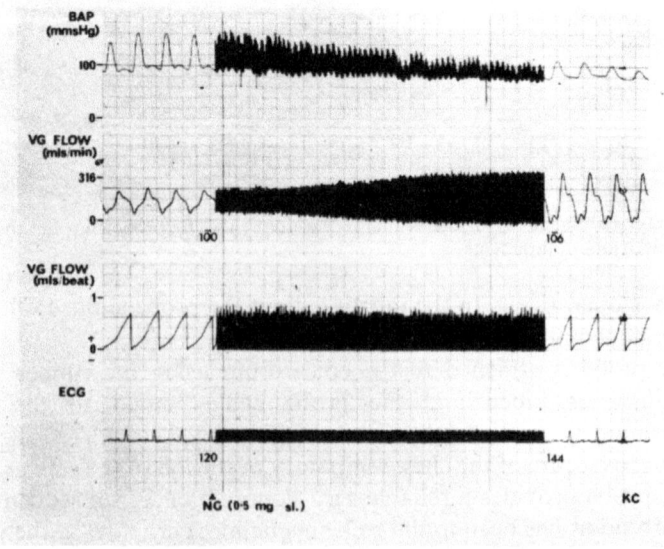

Figure 60.3 The effect of Trinitrin on vein graft flow and arterial pressure

Results. Graft flow has been continually studied in three patients for the first twenty-four hours after operation. Two of these have been further studied on the fifth postoperative day, by which time the patients were ambulant. Figure 60.2 shows the recordings obtained in an ambulant patient five days postoperatively. Vein graft flow, brachial artery pressure

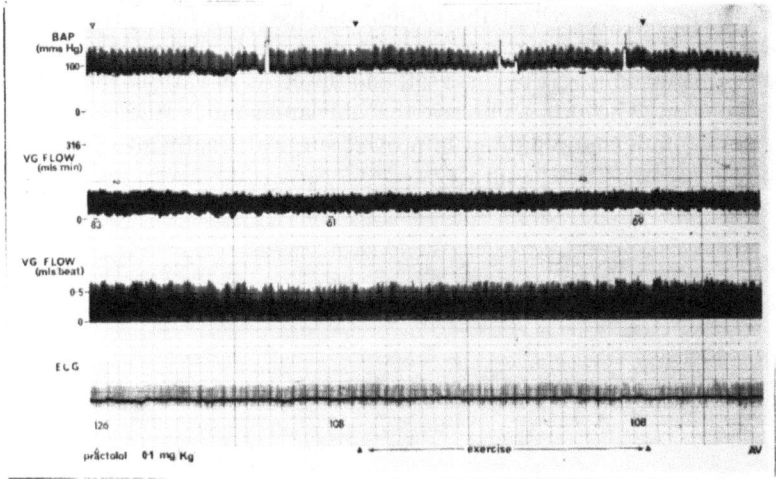

Figure 60.4 The effect of practolol on the response to Trinitrin

and ECG are shown. An integrating amplifier triggered 40 msec after the ECG QRS complex provided a display of flow/beat passing down the graft. As expected maximum flow occurs during diastole, although some flow also occurs during systole, possibly due to the passive conduit properties of the graft; this may also explain changes in the pattern of the flow trace with respiration.

Figure 60.3 demonstrates the effect of a Trinitrin tablet on these parameters, the ambulant patient chewing on the tablet in this case. The systolic arterial blood pressure fell from 160 mmHg to 105 mmHg. There was a striking increase in peak diastolic flow but a decrease in the flow/beat, in part due to the negative flow occurring during systole but also to reduction in the duration of flow for each beat. However an increase in the heart rate was contributory in maintaining the mean flow which was not significantly altered by the Trinitrin.

The effects of beta-blockade (in this case practolol) on the response to Trinitrin is shown in Figure 60.4. Isometric exercise produced an increased arterial diastolic pressure which resulted in increased vein graft flow and flow/beat. The administration of practolol before isometric exercise abolished the anticipated increase in graft flow, there being only a slight increase in the diastolic pressure.

SUMMARY

This chapter has described the design and use of a flow probe which allows long-term post-operative measurement of blood flow in an aorto-coronary saphenous vein bypass graft and the effect of various therapeutic agents on this. The authors believe that this and similar studies will lead to a better understanding and improved surgical treatment of patients requiring coronary artery surgery.

61
Pathological aspects of ischaemic heart disease
E. G. J. Olsen

The changes which occur in the heart following ischaemia have been extensively studied in the experimental animal and man.

Ordinarily, muscle damage becomes apparent to the naked eye approximately 15 h after cell death. Thereafter, the dead area becomes opaque and a well-defined haemorrhagic border appears three to four days later. After approximately one week, the centre becomes rubbery and after three weeks, if the damage is extensive, thinning of the myocardium appears. After six to eight weeks, scarring becomes clearly evident.

At light microscopic level changes become manifest five to six hours after cell injury, after which time myocardial damage proceeds along uniform lines. These events were tabulated by Lodge-Patch[1] in 1951 and have permitted dating of myocardial infarction with a fair degree of accuracy for the first three weeks.

In an effort to visualise myocardial damage at earlier periods, histochemical investigation must be undertaken. Macroscopically, this can be performed by perfusing the heart by Nitro-BT according to the method of Glagov *et al*[2]. It is a general dehydrogenase reaction and the procedure takes advantage of substrate and enzyme loss, which occurs as a result of cell damage. If muscle is intact, endogenous substrate, co-enzymes and dehydrogenases are present and reduce the Nitro-BT to a dark blue formazan. Damaged tissue fails to reduce Nitro-BT, the result of which is that the muscle remains pale in colour. The reaction becomes positive approximately eight hours after cell death has occurred.[3, 4]

At microscopic level histochemical changes have been extensively studied[5-8] and are summarised below.

Glycogen disappears from the damaged cells within minutes and is completely absent from the dead myocardial cells approximately six to eight hours after damage has occurred.

Succinic dehydrogenase apparently increases sharply after approximately two hours in the damaged area, which continues up to approximately six hours. The enzyme is particularly prominent in the A bands of the myocardial fibrils. Thereafter a gradual increase follows for the succeeding 18 h before a decrease occurs.

Cytochrome oxidase behaves similarly to succinic dehydrogenase.

Fat globules increase in size and number, two to four hours after ischaemic death of the cell. Globules become progressively larger up to seven hours, after which time they gradually disappear from the centre of the damaged area during the following 24 h.

Histochemical analysis at macroscopic, as well as light microscopic level, is dependent on autolysis.

A stain, the haematoxylin-basic-fuchsin-picric acid stain, (HBFP), recently evolved at the Mayo Clinic[9], is independent of autolysis and

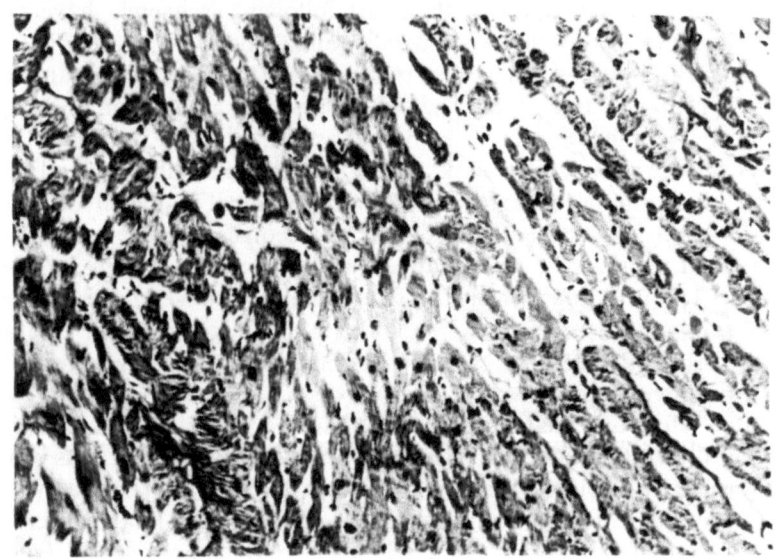

Figure 61.1 Photomicrograph from the junction of infarcted and normal area of a patient who died three hours after myocardial infarction. The darker myocardial fibres have retained the basic fuchsin. The paler myocardial cells are negative. Note the patchy distribution of positive and negative myocardial cells. HBFP × 200

shows ischaemic damage of myocardial cells 30 min after experimental ligation of a coronary artery. Damaged cells retain basic fuchsin (Figure 61.1). This stain can be applied to paraffin embedded material and has been used by Nayar and Olsen[10] in 1974, who retrospectively investigated myocardial infarction in patients who died within five hours after the episode. Clinical diagnosis of myocardial damage has been established in every case, but histological evidence at necropsy was lacking with conventional stains. The results of HBFP staining showed that if total occlusion in a coronary artery was present, every previously selected area of myocardium showed a positive reaction in the region supplied by that vessel (Group I, 28 patients). If there was moderately severe narrowing of the coronary arteries (Group II, 17 patients), 82% of the available material showed a positive reaction and in the absence of significant coronary arterial narrowing (Group III, 15 patients), 60% of cases showed retention of basic fuchsin in the area localised by electrocardiographic changes. This has been summarised in the Figure 61.2.

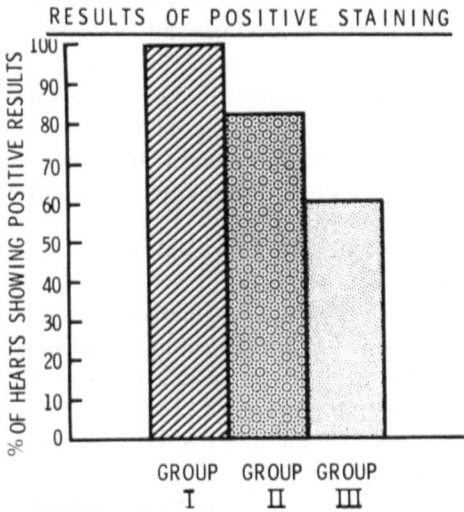

Figure 61.2 Results of HBFP staining

The best results offering understanding of the morphological sequential events that may be observed following myocardial cell damage are seen at electron-microscopic level. These changes, however, can be mimicked by autolysis and it is therefore essential that material must be examined in the fresh state. It is unrealistic to hope to achieve this in human material and most of the work has been carried out in experimental animals. In those patients where myocardial tissue removed at surgical operation had been studied, it has been confirmed that animal experiments closely mimic the findings which occur in humans.

Cellular necrosis may be produced by a number of different methods, but the resulting cell damage proceeds along recognisable and fairly uniform lines. Depending on the method employed to produce cell damage, either by anoxia, acute or chronic hypoxia, or by intermittent or permanent ischaemia, slight quantitative and qualitative differences occur, as well as changes in the chronological order. The findings are briefly summarised below.

Glycogen depletion begins at one to five minutes after acute hypoxic injury and after 40 min of ischaemia cellular depletion is virtually complete.[11]

Mitochondria. Mitochondrial swelling may begin after 10–20 min[11, 12] following cell damage, and vacuolation and decreased matrix density as well as disintegration of cristae may be seen. These changes become well-established after 30 min. Further vacuolation and calcium deposition become evident two hours after damage has occurred and rupture of mitochondrial membranes occurs approximately five hours after injury. Rupture may, however, be seen in some mitochondrial membranes as early as one to two hours.[13]

Nuclei. Nuclear change in cardiocytes is usually well-established 15 min after permanent ischaemia[11, 14]. Clumping of chromatin becomes evident, accompanied by drifting towards the nuclear membrane. This clumping subsequently becomes progressively more marked and rupture of the nuclear membrane occurs.

Sarcotubular system becomes swollen and shows vacuolation after approximately 30 min.

Myofibrils. The contractile elements are relatively resistant to ischaemia. Separation between myocardial fibrils becomes evident after 10–15 min and increase in the I-disc is clearly established at one hour and at four hours transverse tears of myofibrils can be seen.[12]

Sarcolemma. Following ischaemic heart injury, focal rupture has been observed four hours later.[13]

Intercalated disc. Separation, probably due to oedema[15] can be seen in rats after 10–30 min of hypoxia, but is usually not observed in the early stages of ischaemia.

Small lipid droplets make their appearance within the first hour of ischaemia.[16]

Chronic human ischaemia of cardiac muscles shows similar features to those described above and also resembles the changes observed in chronic hypoxia in the rat.[17] The subject has been reviewed by Heggtveit[18] and Olsen.[19]

These changes offer some understanding of the processes involved which lead to cardiac damage as a result of ischaemia and are similar to those observed in myocardial infarction. It may be concluded that irreversible damage to cells occurs approximately 20 min after total ischaemia, but may be somewhat longer, depending on the experimental methods employed. Hypothermia may also lengthen the survival of cells.

References
1. Lodge-Patch. I. (1951). *Brit. Heart J.,* **13,** 37
2. Glagov, S., Eckner, F. A. O. and Lev, M., (1963). *Arch. Pathol.,* **76,** 640
3. Nachlas, M. M. and Shnitka, T. K. (1963). *Amer. J. Pathol.,* **42,** 379
4. Ramkissoon. R. A. (1966). *J. Clin. Pathol.,* **19,** 479

5. Wartman, W. B., Jennings, R. B., Yokoyama, H. O. and Clabaugh, G. F., (1956). *Arch Pathol.*, **62**, 318
6. Shnitka, T. K. and Nachlas, M. M. (1963). *Amer. J. Pathol.*, **42**, 507
7. Fine, G., Morales, A. and Scerpella, J. A. (1966). *Arch. Pathol.*, **82**, 4
8. Morales, A. R. and Fine, A. G. (1966). *Arch. Pathol.*, **82**, 9
9. Lie, J. T., Holley, K. E., Kampa, W. R. and Titus, J. L. (1971). *Mayo Clinic Proc.*, **46**, 319
10. Nayar, A. and Olsen, E. G. J. (1974). *Cardiovasc. Res.* **8**, 391
11. Jennings, R. B., Baum, J. H. and Herdson, P. B. (1965). *Arch. Pathol.*, **79**, 135
12. Caulfield, J. and Klionsky, B. (1959). *Amer. J. Pathol.*, **35**, 489
13. Grosgogeat, Y., Scebat, L., Renais, J. and Lenègre, J. (1966). *Arch. Mal Coeur*, **59**, 203
14. Miller, D. R., Rasmussen, P., Klionsky, B., Cossman, F. P. and Allbritten, F. F. Jr (1961). *Ann. Surg.*, **154**, 751
15. Büchner, F. and Onishi, S. (1967). *Beitr. Pathol. Anat.*, **135**, 153
16. Korb, G. and Totovic, V. (1967). *Virch. Arch. Pathol. Anat.*, **342**, 85
17. Sulkin, N. M. and Sulkin, D. F. (1965). *Lab. Invest.*, **14**, 1523
18. Heggtveit, H. A. (1969). *Bull. WHO*, **41**, 865
19. Olsen, E. G. J. (1973). In: *The Pathology of the Heart*, 52, 56 (New York: Intercontinental Medical Book Corporation)

62
The intra-aortic balloon pump
R. J. Donnelly

Temporary mechanical support of the myocardium was first successfully achieved in 1953 with the development of cardiopulmonary bypass.[1] However, since the use of this new technique was limited to a time period of only a few hours, a variety of longer-term assist devices were subsequently developed, including methods of left heart bypass[2-4], of direct mechanical compression of the heart[5] and systems based upon the principles of counterpulsation[6-11].

These principles were initially described by Clauss et al.[6] in 1961. Using bilateral femoral cannulation, arterial blood was withdrawn from the circulation during systole and reinfused in diastole. The effect of the withdrawal was to reduce left ventricular afterload and thereby peak left ventricular pressure and myocardial oxygen consumption. Reinfusion raised the systemic arterial diastolic pressure. Mean coronary perfusion pressure and, in theory, coronary blood flow to stenosed and pressure-dependent areas would thereby be increased. Perfusion of other vital organs would also be enhanced.

It soon became apparent that the same haemodynamic effects could be achieved using an inflatable balloon in the aorta, timed to deflate during systole and to inflate during diastole and this was reported by Moupopoulos et al.[7] in 1962. Subsequently, balloon-assist units were devised by several other groups of workers. However, this chapter will not describe the relative merits of the different balloon-pump systems commercially available. The experience of the author has been with the MGH-Avco balloon pump, developed by Dr Buckley and his colleagues at the Harvard Medical School, the Massachusetts General Hospital, Boston and the Avco Research Laboratories in Everett, Massachusetts and it is this system which is referred to in this chapter.

INSERTION AND OPERATION

The MGH-Avco balloon is made from Avcothane, a proprietary product which has been shown to be compatible with blood over prolonged periods of time[12] and to be non-destructive of blood elements.[13] It is comprised of three segments. The holes admitting gas to the middle segment are larger than those admitting gas to the two end segments. This ensures that the middle segment inflates first and improves the efficiency of pumping.

The balloon is inserted under local anaesthetic. The largest balloon which can be inserted into the femoral artery is selected and an estimate made of the length to be inserted by comparison with the distance between the groin and the angle of Lewis. Before commencing, an X-ray plate is placed behind the patient's chest. The femoral artery is exposed and tourniquets positioned above and below. The balloon is passed through a short segment of 12 mm Dacron tubing and inserted into the femoral artery through a vertical arteriotomy. It is advanced to the estimated length, when some resistance is usually felt at the aortic arch. The balloon should lie just distal to the left subclavian artery. A chest X-ray is then taken and, while the film is being developed, the piece of Dacron tubing is sutured to the arteriotomy. When the correct position of the balloon has been verified on the X-ray, one or more stout ligatures are secured around the tubing to prevent blood leaking back past the catheter. The snares are removed and the wound closed. It is important to tape the catheter securely to the leg to prevent excessive movement which could lead to infection of the wound or displacement of the balloon. Later, when the balloon is removed, the Dacron is cut short and closed in the form of a patch.

Complications from the use of the balloon are minimal.[14] It is probably contraindicated in severe peripheral atherosclerosis because of the danger of lifting athermatous plaques or of dissection. On rare occasions it is impossible to pass the balloon because of tortuosity of the iliac vessels. Rupture of the balloon is a theoretical risk but no instance of this has yet been reported. The gas used in the MGH-Avco system is helium, the low density of which facilitates inflation and deflation at rapid heart rates. An isolation chamber is incorporated into the system so that the helium is constantly recycled. The unit is fitted with a sensitive leak-detection mechanism which immediately exhausts the balloon and stops pumping in the event of even a very small balloon leak. Clot formation and arterial embolisation have not been seen. However, it is recommended that the balloon should not be left uninflated in the circulation for more than a short period but that it should be inflated at least once in every eight heart beats. Low molecular weight dextran (20 ml h $^{-1}$) is given intravenously and heparin is given to all but postoperative patients.

The control mechanism is regulated from a standard surface electrocardiogram and the timing of inflation and deflation is adjusted so that deflation occurs immediately prior to the onset of systole and inflation at the end of systole. At the optimal point there will be maximum reduction of arterial systolic pressure and maximum increase of diastolic pressure. A regular ventricular rhythm (and it may be necessary to use pacing to achieve this) is necessary for efficient working of the machine. A competent aortic valve is also clearly a necessity.

CLINICAL APPLICATION

The principal protagonists of balloon pumping over the last few years have been Dr Buckley and Dr Mundth and their colleagues at the Massachusetts General Hospital in Boston. This group have made the major contribution to the understanding of the principles of balloon pumping in relation to its clinical application and reference will be made to several of their publications.

Cardiogenic shock

Initially the balloon pump was used exclusively in the management of patients in cardiogenic shock following myocardial infarction. The persistence of shock in such patients, in spite of full medical treatment, carries a very high mortality with medical treatment alone. Dunkman *et al.*[15] reported the haemodynamic changes observed with balloon pumping in 40 patients in cardiogenic shock unresponsive to medical treatment. They defined cardiogenic shock as:

1. Arterial systolic pressure less than 90 mmHg.
2. Urine output less than 20 ml h[1].
3. Signs of poor peripheral perfusion.

The mean haemodynamic changes observed in their group of patients were:

1. Cardiac index increased by 44%.
2. Mean arterial pressure increased by 10%.
3. Pulmonary capillary wedge pressure reduced by 23%.

The addition of balloon pumping reversed cardiogenic shock in 80% of patients but improved only marginally the ultimate prognosis.

It is clear that balloon pumping in this situation is only a temporary measure which affords time for full investigation and, if feasible, corrective surgical action. A trial without balloon support should be attempted after 24 h. A small proportion of patients can be weaned from the balloon and revascularisation surgery in appropriate cases carried out later as an elective procedure.[14] The majority of patients will remain balloon-dependent and may be suitable for urgent surgery. Balloon-dependence can be defined as:

1. Mean arterial pressure less than 60 mmHg.

2. Pulmonary capillary wedge pressure greater than 20 mmHg.
3. Cardiac index less than 2 l min $^{-1}$ m $^{-2}$.
4. Recurrent pain, with temporary cessation of balloon support.

Of 68 patients who were balloon-dependent in a series reported by Mundth *et al.*,[14] 14 patients (24%) died because the shock state could not be reversed. A further 17 (25%) were not considered suitable for surgery on the basis of coronary and left ventricular angiography. These patients also died. 35 patients (51%) underwent surgery and 13 of these (37% of those operated on) survived. This is small return for a great deal of effort but it is likely that the results of this form of treatment would be much improved by accepting only those patients who have been in shock for a short time. This time has not yet been clearly-defined but the shorter the better and 12 h is probably the maximum. It is the duration of the shock and not the severity which should limit the choice of patients for balloon assistance. It is, of course, true that others have successfully investigated and operated on these patients without balloon assistance but a strong case can be made for its use. It is safe, effective, simply controlled and minimally invasive. It provides a greater margin of safety during the investigation and pre and postoperative care of these seriously-ill patients.

Post bypass

Buckley *et al.*[16] have reported 26 patients who failed to come off cardiopulmonary bypass following elective surgery. None of these patients underwent surgery for the complications of acute myocardial infarction or had required balloon support for preoperative cardiogenic shock. Eleven of the 26 patients survived and were discharged from hospital. Balloon pumping was most effective when applied early to patients with acute ischaemic injury to the myocardium at the time of operation and in patients with left ventricular hypertrophy and a small chamber volume. 15 patients had double or triple saphenous vein grafts and 55% of these survived.

Ventricular septal defect and mitral incompetence

Buckley *et al.*[17] have reported seven cases of ventricular septal defect and nine cases of mitral incompetence following myocardial infarction in whom balloon-pump support was instituted because of deteriorating cardiac function. Shunting through the VSD and mitral regurgitation were both reduced during balloon assistance. All patients were submitted to coronary and left ventricular angiography and all but one then underwent surgery. Two out of six patients with VSD survived and both these had defects in the anterior part of the septum. Six out of nine patients with mitral regurgitation survived. It was concluded that postinfarction VSD and mitral incompetence were amenable to surgical treatment if a sufficient amount of residual functional muscle could be preserved in the left ventricle and that intra-aortic balloon pumping allowed time to stabilise the condition of the patients. reduced myocardial ischaemia. allowed coronary and left ventricular angiography to be carried out with safety and afforded continued support in the postoperative period.

Ventricular arrhythmias
Mundth *et al.*[18] reported seven patients operated on for intractable arrhythmia problems within six weeks of infarction. Balloon support was used preoperatively in four of these for haemodynamic instability. The cardiovascular status was improved. ventricular irritability reduced but not abolished and angiography carried out with safety. Balloon support was used postoperatively in all seven patients. Four of these survived and it was considered that balloon pumping had helped substantially in supporting the heart and in reducing postoperative arrhythmia problems.

Impending myocardial infarction
Mundth *et al.*[14] have described 12 cases of impending myocardial infarction treated surgically in eleven of whom intra-aortic balloon pumping was instituted preoperatively. Impending infarction was defined as:
1. Pain lasting longer than 30 min.
2. ECG changes of ischaemia associated with pain.
3. No evidence of evolution of infarction by serial ECGs or enzymes.

Balloon pumping effectively abolished pain and improved altered haemodynamics in nine patients. Two others also received significant benefit. Full angiographic study was completed safely in all patients and revascularisation surgery carried out. All twelve patients survived.

Acute myocardial infarction with impending extension
Six patients with recurrent pain and impending extension during the recovery period of acute myocardial infarction have been reported by Mundth and his colleagues.[19] All six patients received balloon-pump assistance prior to angiography and revascularisation surgery. Five of the six patients survived. the only death occurring in one patient in whom balloon support was not instituted until after angiography had precipitated deterioration.

CONCLUSION

In conclusion. it can be stated that intra-aortic balloon-pump assistance is a useful and established addition to the armamentarium of the cardiac physician and surgeon. It is effective in reversing cardiogenic shock in the majority of patients following myocardial infarction but the duration of the shock is of major importance in determining the eventual survival of these patients.

Balloon support will salvage some patients who would not otherwise come off cardiopulmonary bypass, particularly those with either left ventricular hypertrophy and a small chamber volume or an acute intra-operative ischaemic injury.

In the management of the complications of acute myocardial infarction, balloon-pump assistance allows time for haemodynamics to be improved and stabilised, permits safe coronary and left ventricular angiography, increases the safety of anaesthetic induction and provides continued support in the postoperative period.

References

1. Gibbon, J. H. Jr (1954). Application of a mechanical heart and lung apparatus to cardiac surgery. *Minn. Med.*, **37**, 171
2. Dennis, C., Hall, D. P., Moreno, J. R. and Senning, A. (1962). Left atrial cannulation without thoracotomy for total left heart bypass. *Acta Chir. Scand.*, **123**, 267
3. Zwart, H. H. J., Kralios, A. and Kwan-Gett, C. S. (1970). First clinical application of transarterial closed-chest left ventricular (TaCLV) bypass. *Trans. Amer. Soc. Artif. Int. Organs*, **16**, 386
4. DeBakery, M. E. (1971). Left ventricular bypass pump for cardiac assistance. *Amer. J. Cardiol.*, **27**, 3
5. Anstadt, G. L., Schiff, P. and Baue, A. E. (1966). Prolonged circulatory support by direct mechanical ventricular assistance. *Trans. Amer. Soc. Artif. Int. Organs*, **12**, 72
6. Clauss, R. H., Birtwell, W. C., Albertal, G., Lunzer, S., Taylor, W. J., Fosberg, A. M. and Harken, D. E. (1961). Assisted circulation. I. Arterial counterpulsator. *J. Thorac. Cardiovasc. Surg.*, **41**, 447
7. Moulopoulos, S. D., Topaz, S. and Kolff, W. J. (1962). Diastolic balloon pumping (with carbon dioxide) in the aorta. Mechanical assistance to the failing circulation. *Amer. Heart J.*, **63**, 669
8. Brown, B. G., Goldfarb, D., Topaz, S. and Gott, V. L. (1967). Diastolic augmentation by intra-aortic balloon. *J. Thorac. Cardiovasc. Surg.*, **53**, 789
9. Kantrowitz, A., Tjonneland, S., Freed, P. S., Phillips, S. J., Butner, A. N. and Sherman, J. L. (1968). Initial clinical experience with intra-aortic balloon pumping in cardiogenic shock. *JAMA*, **203**, 113
10. Buckley, M. J., Leinbach, R. C., Kastor, J. A., Laird, J. D., Kantrowitz, A. R., Madras, P. N., Sanders, C. A. and Austen, W. G. (1970). Haemodynamic evaluation of intra-aortic balloon pumping in man. *Circulation*, **41 (Suppl. II)**, II-130
11. Soroff, H. S., Giron, F., Ruiz, U., Birtwell, W. G., Hirsch, L. J. and Deterling, R. A. (1969). Physiologic support of heart action. *New Eng. J. Med.*, **280**, 693
12. Schoen, F. J., DeLaria, G. A. and Bernstein, E. F. (1973). Morphology of blood surface interaction on intra-aortic balloons. *J. Thorac. Cardiovasc. Surg.*, **65**, 304

13. Leinbach. R. C., Nyilas. E.. Caulfield. J. B.. Buckley. M. J. and Austen. W. G. (1972). Evaluation of haematologic effects of intra-aortic balloon assistance in man. *Trans. Amer. Soc. Artif. Int. Organs.* **18,** 493

14. Mundth. E. D.. Buckley. M. J.. Leinbach. R. C.. Gold. H. K.. Daggett. W. M. and Austen. W. G. (1973). Surgical intervention for the complications of acute myocardial infarction. *Ann. Surg..* **178,** 379

15. Dunkman. W. B.. Leinbach. R. C.. Buckley. M. J.. Mundth. E. D.. Kantrowitz. A. R.. Austen. W. G. and Sanders. C. A. (1972). Clinical and haemodynamic results of intra-aortic balloon pumping and surgery for cardiogenic shock. *Circulation.* **46,** 465

16. Buckley. M. J.. Craver. J. M.. Gold. H. K.. Mundth. E. D.. Daggett. W. M. and Austen. W. G. (1973). Intra-aortic balloon pump assist for cardiogenic shock after cardiopulmonary bypass. *Circulation.* **47** and **48 (Suppl. III),** III-90

17. Buckley. M. J.. Mundth. E. D.. Daggett. W. M.. Gold. H. K.. Leinbach. R. C. and Austen. W. G. (1973). Surgical management of ventricular septal defects and mitral regurgitation complicating acute myocardial infarction. *Ann. Thorac. Surg.,* **16,** 598

18. Mundth. E. D.. Buckley. M. J.. DeSanctis. R. W.. Daggett. W. M. and Austen W. G. (1973). Surgical treatment of ventricular irritability. *J. Thorac. Cardiovasc. Surg.,* **66,** 943

19. Mundth. E. D.. Buckley. M. J.. Gold. H. K.. Daggett. W. M.. Leinbach. R. C. and Austen. W. G. (1973). Intra-aortic balloon pumping and emergency coronary arterial revascularisation for acute myocardial infarction with impending extension. *Ann. Thorac. Surg..* **16,** 435

63
Infarctectomy

C. Hahn, E. Hauf and B. Faidutti

The term infarctectomy is defined as a resection of the myocardium in the first two weeks after infarction. After this time, the operation is not an infarctectomy; it may be an aneurysmectomy or a resection of scar tissue but the technical problem in the first two weeks after infarction is completely different.

The indications for infarctectomy in the eight patients operated on, were six cases of low cardiac output, one case of severe arrhythmia, with repeated intractable ventricular fibrillations and one case of acute mitral insufficiency. In five of these eight cases, VSD also occurred one and one half to two days after infarction.

The results were good in three cases aged 63, 60 and 73, all with low cardiac output, and these patients are all well after more than four years. However, there were also five failures. Two of these failures were due to the fact that these patients had tight stenosis of the first part of the right coronary artery, but because they were referred in a very bad condition, there was no time for preoperative investigation which would have revealed

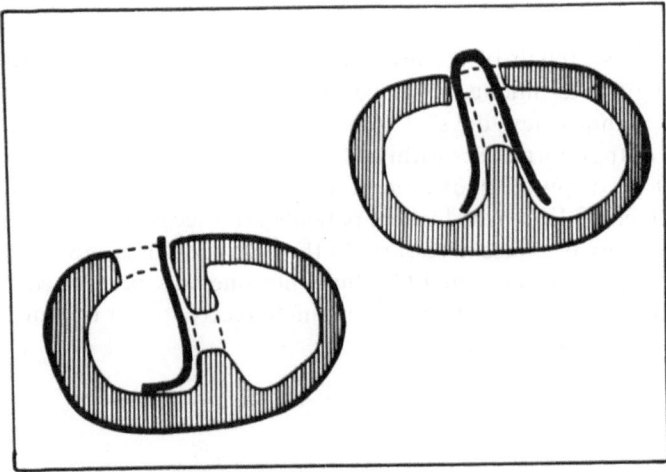

Figure 63.1 The use of a large folded patch to repair the septum

413

this condition.

The technique involves resecting a part of the left ventricle, part of the septum and part of the right ventricle in several instances. When this operation was first performed it was found very difficult to repair the septum and this led to the use of a large folded patch (Figure 63.1). The right and left ventricles are then sutured with a continuous stitch on a piece of Teflon felt (Figure 63.2). This technique therefore allows effective repair of the septum with no residual VSD.

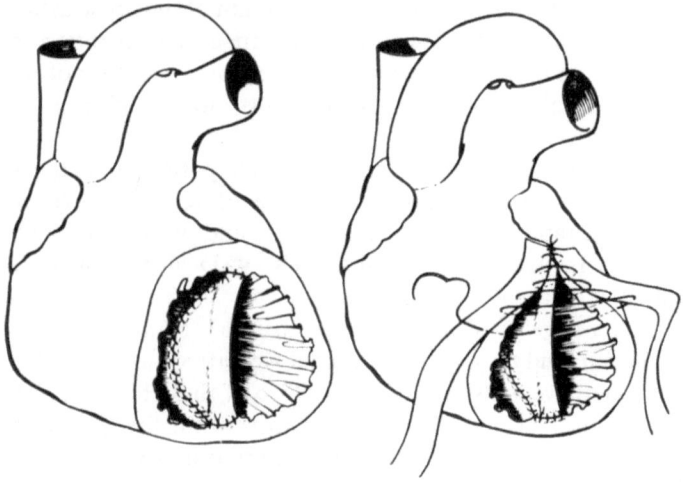

Figure 63.2 The right and left ventricles are sutured with a continuous stitch on a piece of Teflon felt

In the past, repair of the myocardium was thought to be impossible, but using the technique described above an infarctectomy can be performed within a few days of infarction. As a result of the operation cardiac output normalises within a few hours. The value of this technique can not be disputed. However, it would obviously be preferable if a situation could be reached where patients are successfully treated before infarctectomy becomes necessary. In the author's series, seven infarctectomies were performed in 1972, but only one was performed in 1973. This indicates that patients are beginning to receive better treatment in the early stages of their condition.

64

Surgical treatment of left ventricular aneurysm

H. H. Bentall

Ventricular aneurysm is defined as a full thickness gross dilatation of the ventricle (usually anterior) which occurs late. In most cases the aneurysm follows many weeks after occlusion of the artery. This Chapter excludes discussion of patients who have had infarctectomy and those who have only akinetic areas or a slight bulge of the ventricular wall.

The indications for operation are embolic and cardiac. Many patients not operated on have disastrous major cerebral emboli or repeated small embolic episodes. The cardiac hazards of unoperated ventricular aneurysm are:

1. The danger of rupture; there are often 'paper thin' areas of scar.
2. The reduction of cardiac output due to paradoxical movement of the wall of the ventricle.

Patients are operated on using conventional cardiopulmonary bypass. The temperature is reduced to 33 °C and electrical fibrillation and ankle cross-clamps are applied before opening the ventricle, to minimise the risk of coronary and cerebral embolism. Care is taken to avoid manipulation of the aneurysm before the aortic cross-clamp is applied. The importance of this was learnt from an early case in whom a major cerebral embolism was caused.

Figure 64.1a & b shows that the aneurysm is often full of soft clot which is loosely adherent to the ventricular wall. Once the clot is removed it is usually easy to see where the good ventricular muscle gives way to scar tissue. It is usually also possible to see on both the cavity and outside surfaces of the ventricle where to place the mattress sutures.

OPERATIVE TECHNIQUE

Heavy silk or Dacron is used for the repair and the technique is similar to the 'Mayo' repair of a ventral hernia. Almost all of the wall of the aneurysm is excised and the first row of mattress sutures is placed through the fibrous tissue at the edge of the normal muscle so as to leave as much contractile tissue as possible (Figure 64.2). A second layer of continuous mattress sutures ensures that the suture line is watertight (Figure 64.3). The usual procedure is to vent the left ventricle through the apical portion of the incision. The aortic clamp is released as soon as all clot has been removed and established in the ventricle.

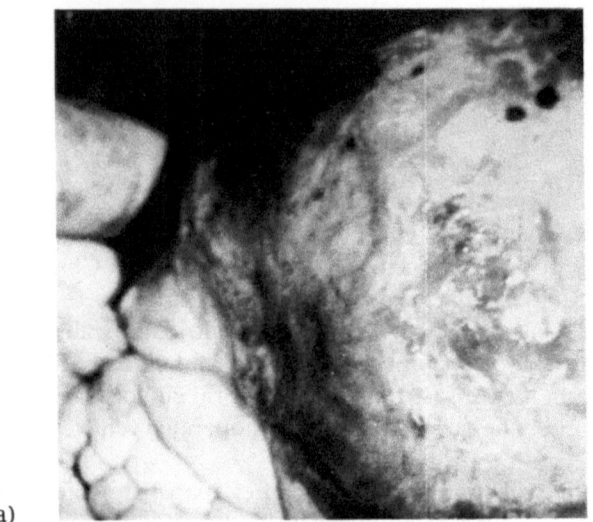

(a)

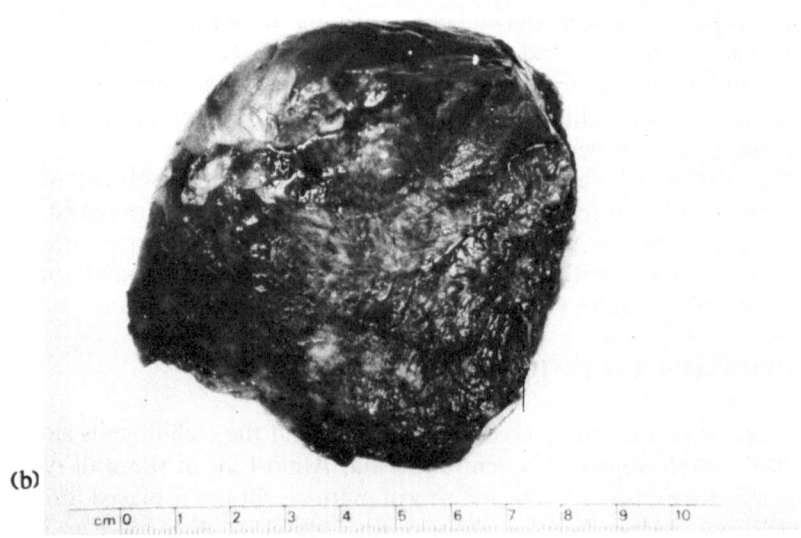

(b)

cm 0   1   2   3   4   5   6   7   8   9   10

Figures 64.1 a and b The aneurysm is full of soft clot which is loosely adherent to the wall of the ventricle

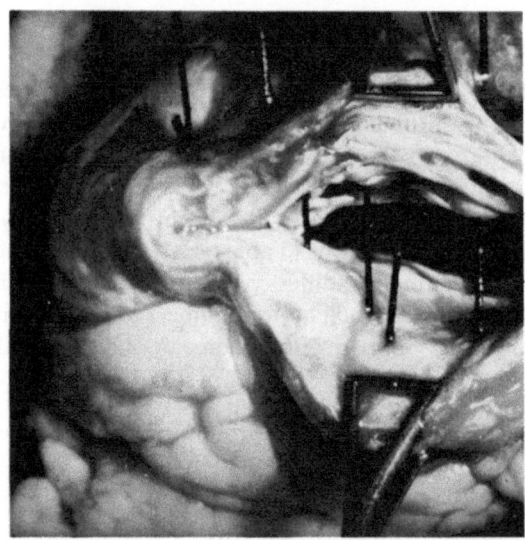

Figure 64.2 Shows the first row of mattress sutures placed through the fibrous tissue at the edge of normal muscle

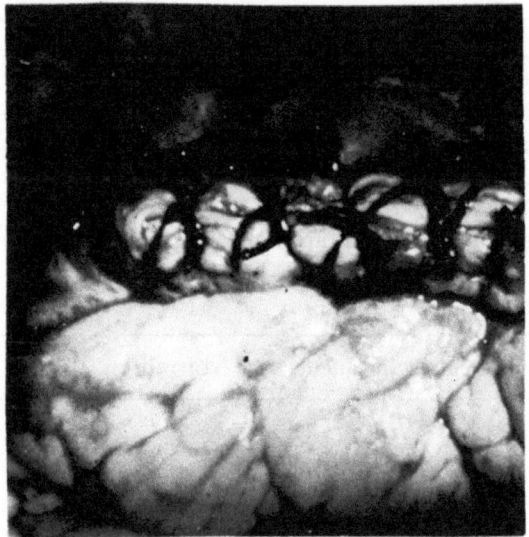

Figure 64.3 A second layer of sutures ensures a blood-tight ventricle

RESULTS

The total number of patients operated on at Hammersmith Hospital between 1961 and 1973 is 45. The age range of these ischaemic aneurysms varied from 21 years to 67 years, with a mean age of 53. The sex ratio was 39 males : 6 females, the proportion of females being slightly higher than is usually quoted (Table 64.1) Ten patients died in hospital (Table 64.2). One of the patients had, in fact, gone to convalescence and had another infarct in the convalescent home, but he is included in the hospital mortality (Table 64.3). The late mortality, so far, has been six patients, 13%, in a period between seven months and seven years, the mean being two years and 10 months (Table 64.4). These late mortality figures are completely meaningless, unless one considers either actuarial curves, such as one can show for much larger numbers of patients in valve disease, or one can show every patient; only then can one get a really satisfactory

Table 64.1 Resections of left ventricular aneurysms between 1961 and 1973

Total number	45 patients
Age range	21–67 years
Mean age	53 years
Sex ratio	39 males : 6 females or 6·5 : 1

Table 64.2 Left ventricular aneurysms. Causes of hospital deaths (10)

3 patients had arrested before operation; one having ruptured aneurysm.
3 patients died from respiratory infection (2 also had cerebral embolism).
3 patients had a further infarction (one had also CABG).
1 patient died on table (also CABG).

Table 64.2 Left ventricular aneurysms. Mortality

Hospital mortality
10 patients 22%
(1 day–2 months)
(Mean 19 days)

Late mortality
6 patients 13%
(7 months–7 years)
(Mean 2 years 10 months)

idea of the true expectation in the bulk of the patients (Table 64.5).

The question which remains open is whether multiple coronary artery grafting should always be done in association with the aneurysmectomy. Obviously it would be preferable to do coronary artery radiology prior to aneurysmectomy, although there were no coronary artery studies in this

Table 64.4 Left ventricular aneurysms. Causes of late deaths (6)

Further infarctions	5
Complications of gastric surgery	1

Table 64.5 Left ventricular aneurysms. The fate of the 29 survivors

Alive and well	29 (65%)
Dyspnoea on effort	3
Residual hemiplegia	2
Severe angina needing graft	1

series of patients for the bulk of them were operated on long before selective coronary artery angiography became commonplace.

Heretofore, any combination of coronary artery surgery with left ventricular aneurysmography has not been shown to produce good results and care must be taken when attempting to improve the blood supply of the right coronary artery on which the patient is almost certainly living. Any coronary artery surgery which would place this vessel in jeopardy might prove to be disastrously harmful. It is because of this that a study has been started on patients who have had coronary artery angiography and have then been operated on, possibly influenced by the results of the angiography.

65
Management of postinfarction mitral regurgitation

M. H. Yacoub

Mitral regurgitation secondary to ischaemic heart disease overloads an already damaged ventricle and if uncorrected might lead to death in the acute stage or produce chronic disability. A rational approach to the management of these patients can only be achieved if the following conditions can be fulfilled:

1. Accurate diagnosis of the presence and severity of regurgitation. This might be difficult in the acute stage as· massive mitral regurgitation produces a blowing early and midsystolic murmur which can easily be ignored if one is not aware of this possibility.
2. Clinicopathological classification into definite clinicopathological syndromes.
3. Defining the natural history and prognosis of each type.

In this chapter each of these points will be discussed and experience with surgical treatment of this condition will be described. Before doing so some anatomical and physiological factors which may have a bearing on the development, degree and type of postinfarction mitral regurgitation will be discussed. Each papillary muscle controls about half the anterior and posterior cusps (Figure 65.1). Total rupture of one of these muscles leads to massive mitral regurgitation. This, fortunately, is rare as each papillary muscle is formed of several heads (Figure 65.1), each controlling a limited area of one or both cusps. Rupture of one of these heads (partial rupture) results in less severe mitral regurgitation. The blood supply of papillary muscle has an important bearing on the development and type of mitral regurgitation (Figure 65.2). The papillary muscles are vulnerable to ischaemic injury because of the particular arrangement of their blood supply. The major coronary vessels run in the atrioventricular groove and give rise to fairly large branches which run on the epicardial surface of the ventricles generally towards the apex. From these branches the left ventricular myocardium is supplied by two types of vessels, Type A vessels which divide almost immediately into many ramifications to supply the outer part of the left ventricular wall and Type B vessels which pass perpendicularly through the thickness of the left ventricular wall to the subcudocardium

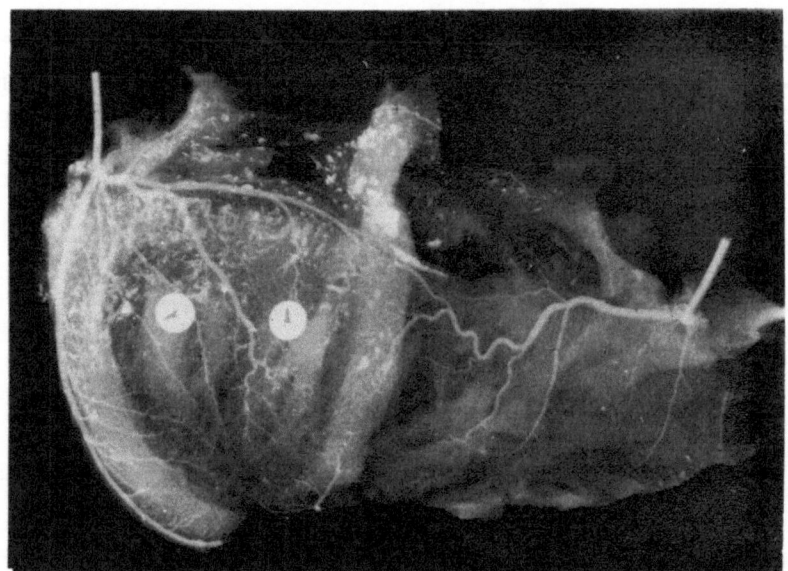

Figure 65.1 The papillary muscles, formed of several heads. Each muscle controls about half the anterior and posterior cusp

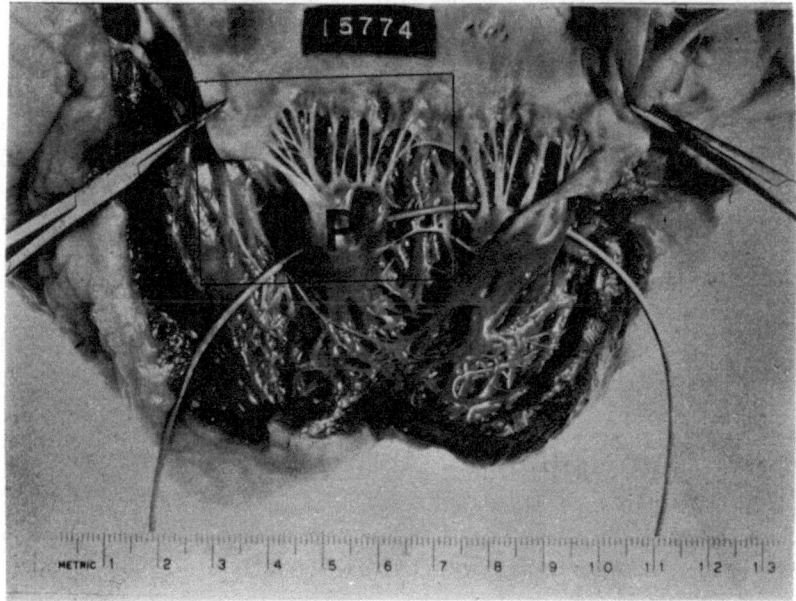

Figure 65.2 The blood supply of the papillary muscle. Type B vessels pass perpendicularly through the thickness of the left ventricular wall to the subcudocardium and papillary muscles

and papillary muscles (Figure 65.3).

The blood supply from each papillary muscle is derived from at least two main vessels (Figure 65.2). The posterior papillary muscle is supplied by branches from the anterior descending and circumflex. As is apparent from Figure 65.2, the blood supply to the anterior papillary muscle is usually better than that to the posterior papillary muscle, as the former is

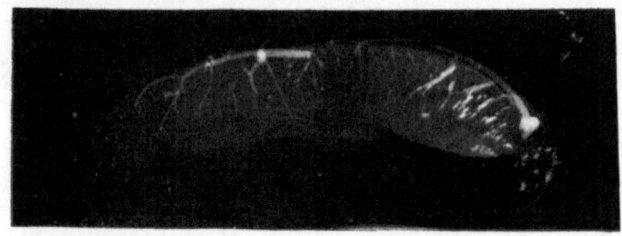

Figure 65.3 The blood supply from each papillary muscle is derived from at least two main vessels

surrounded by several large vessels and is nearer the main left coronary ostium than the posterior papillary muscle, which is further removed from both the right and left coronary ostia. This might explain the predominance of posterior papillary muscle affection observed in this, and other, series.

In addition the papillary muscles are more vulnerable to ischaemia because of the fact that their oxygen requirement is higher than the rest of the myocardium. This is because wall tension in papillary muscles is high throughout systolic, whereas in the remaining left ventricular myocardium, wall tension progressively falls during systole with the diminishing diameter of the left ventricular cavity (Laplace Law). As wall tension is one of the major determinants of myocardial oxygen consumption, it follows that papillary muscles have a higher oxygen requirement and are more vulnerable to ischaemia.

In the author's experience mitral regurgitation secondary to myocardial infarction could be classified into three separate clinicopathological syndromes.

1. Acute rupture of the whole or major part of one papillary muscle.
2. Subacute mitral regurgitation due to stretching of one papillary muscle by an evolving left ventricular aneurysm.
3. Chronic mitral regurgitation due to partial rupture, or stretching of one or both papillary muscle.

Acute rupture of one papillary muscle
This condition is rapidly fatal if uncorrected within 24–48 h of its onset.

The rupture usually occurs five to seven days after the onset of myocardial infarction. The rupture results in the sudden development of cardiogenic shock which is associated with pulmonary oedema (Figure 65.4). Clinical examination shows typical blowing early and midsystolic

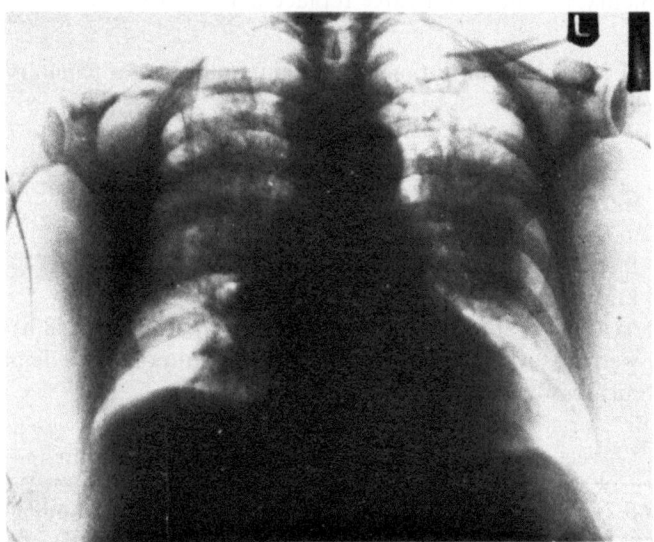

Figure 65.4 Acute rupture of one papillary muscle is usually associated with pulmonary oedema

murmurs which fade during late systole due to equalisation of pressures in the left atrium and left ventricle. This, plus the low cardiac output, results in the murmur being 'unimpressive'. The localisation of the murmur is apical and, in the author's experience, was not confused with the typical parasternal murmur associated with rupture of the interventricular septum. During the last four and a half years four patients with this syndrome were treated surgically at the Harefield Hospital. The clinical details are summarised in Table 65.1. In all four patients the posterior papillary muscle was affected. Emergency mitral valve replacement using a prosthetic valve resulted in immediate improvement in the haemodynamic state in all four patients. Two patients died one and two weeks respectively after operation, from acute infection of the previously oedematous lung in one and renal failure in the other. Two patients are long-term survivors.

Subacute mitral regurgitation due to evolving left ventricular aneurysm
This syndrome results from progressive stretching of one papillary muscle by a developing mitral regurgitation. It has an insidious onset

and a steadily progressive course. It presents approximately six weeks after myocardial infarction with signs of mitral regurgitation and an enlarging heart with progressive severe cardiac failure. We have encountered two patients with this syndrome who were treated by emergency resection of the aneurysm and mitral valve replacement. Both patients died in the

Table 65.1 Mitral regurgitation due to acute rupture of a papillary muscle. (Harefield Hospital)

4 patients

—all were males
—all in seventh decade (64, 64, 65)
—no history of previous infarcts in 2
—no known history of hypertension
—interval between onset of infarction and operation (< 48 h)
—all were in severe cardiogenic shock and pulmonary oedema (clinical and radiological)
— characteristic early systolic murmur
—ECG: recent posterior (inferior) myocardial infarction

Table 65.2 Mitral regurgitation due to stretching of papillary muscle secondary to acute ventricular aneurysm (Harefield Hospital)

Name	Age Sex	Interval between infarct. & operation	Site	Clinical pres.	Murmur	Operation	Outcome
J.G.	M 61	4 weeks	Post.	Shock & pulmonary oedema	Pan. SM	MVR & excision of aneurysm	Died 3 days (renal failure)
A.J.	F 71	6 weeks	Ant.	Low output & pulmonary oedema	pan. SM	MVR & excision of aneurysm	Died 7 days (recurrence of low output)

postoperative period three and seven days after operation from recurrence of the low output state (Table 65.2).

Chronic mitral regurgitation secondary to papillary muscle dysfunction or partial rupture

This syndrome presents months or years after infarction, with classical signs of mitral regurgitation of varying severity, and is due to partial rupture of one papillary muscle (rupture of one of the heads) or progressive stretching of infarcted and fibrosed papillary muscles. Sixteen patients suffering from this syndrome have been treated (Table 65.3). Coronary artery bypass graft was performed at the same time in eight patients and excision of posterior left ventricular aneurysm in two. The mitral valve was replaced in 14 and repaired in two. There were no operative deaths

Table 65.3 Chronic mitral regurgitation due to ischaemic heart disease

Procedure	No. of patients	Deaths	
		E.	L.
MV repair & CABG	2	0	1
MVR alone	8	0	1
MVR & CABG	4	0	0
MVR, CABG & ex. of LV aneurysm	2	0	1
	16	0	3

(within the first four weeks after operation) and three late deaths (Table 65.3). The degree of clinical improvement was dependent on left ventricular function prior to operation.

It is concluded that surgical treatment of mitral regurgitation secondary to ischaemic heart disease can be life saving in patients with acute rupture of a papillary muscle. Limited experience with the subacute syndrome secondary to evolving left ventricular aneurysm has been disappointing. In the chronic stage surgical correction can be achieved with a very low operative mortality and encouraging late results.

66
The treatment of postinfarction VSD
B. N. Pickering

Rupture of the ventricular septum is a relatively uncommon complication of myocardial infarction; in most autopsy series the incidence is 1–2%[1,2]. The defect is almost always associated with ECG evidence of either anterior or inferior infarction and most commonly occurs in the inferior part of the septum towards the apex[3].

Table 66.1 VSD after myocardial infarction. Mortality

	Non-surgical patients[4]	*Surgical patients*
	24% in 1st day	—
	65% in 2 weeks	—
	82% in 2 months	42% in 2 months
	—	50% in 6 months
	93% in < 1 year	68% in 1 year

The prognosis is very poor (Table 66.1). Sixty-five per cent of patients die within two weeks, 82% within two months and only 7% survive for more than one year[4,5]. *Approximately one quarter of the patients die within 24 h.* Ideally therefore, operation should be undertaken as soon as possible. From the surgeon's point of view, however, the easiest time for operation is some two or three months after the infarction – when the margins of the defect are fibrosed and capable of holding sutures. By this time, however, most of the patients are dead. Operation at an early stage carries a high mortality (Table 66.2); the longer one can wait the better the prospect of a good result, but unfortunately in many patients haemodynamic deterioration will compel the surgeon to intervene within two weeks of the infarct.

These patients fall, therefore, into two groups:
1. A subacute group who can just be controlled on maximal medical treatment to await elective and definitive surgery.
2. An acute group, who present as emergencies, uncontrollable by

supportive therapy, in cardiogenic shock and with a prognosis (untreated) measurable in hours.

This will be illustrated by quoting patients treated at Hammersmith Hospital under the consultant care of Mr W. P. Cleland and Professor

Table 66.2 VSD after myocardial infarction. Operation within 14 days of rupture

Days from infarct	Result
1	D.O.T.
2	D.O.T.
4	D. 6 days
5	D.O.T.
6	D.O.T.
10	D. 1 day
11	D. 22 days
11	A. 15 Mo. (Res. shunt)
13	D.O.T.
13	D. 30 days
15	D.O.T.
16	D.O.T.
16	A. 12 Mo. (Res. shunt)
19	A. 18 Mo.
30	A. 9 Mo.

Table 66.3 Treatment of postinfarction ventricular septal defect in a group of subacute cases

Case	1	2	3	4	5	6
Sex	M	F	M	M	M	M
Age	64	61	63	56	54	65
Infarct site	Inferior	Anterior	Inferior	Inferior	Anterior	Inferior
Rhythm	SR	SR	SR	SR	SR	SR
Rupture site	Apical	Apical	Apical	Apical	Apical + LVA	Apical
Rupture to op.	1/12	3/12	2/12	3/12	3/12	6/52
Ventriculotomy	Right	Right	Right	Right	Lt. via LVA	Right
Repair	Suture	Patch	Suture	Suture	Suture · plication	Suture
Deaths	1 month	—	1½ years	—	—	—
Survivors	—	6 years	—	2 years	1½ years	3 days
	1965	1968	1969	1972	1973	1974

H. H. Bentall. In the first, less urgent, or subacute group there are six patients as shown (Table 66.3).

The patients are mainly male, in the 50–60 age group and suffered inferior infarctions; interestingly, all were in sinus rhythm. All had sustained a rupture of the apical region of the septum. All managed to survive a period of from one to three months before operative repair of the defect. In all except one case (vide infra) the defect was repaired via a right ventriculotomy. There was one 'hospital death' at 30 days as a result of anuria coupled with lung infection in 1965. One patient subsequently died a year and a half later from further infarction. Four patients out of six have survived for more than one year – 66%, compared with the 7%[4] in the unoperated group. One patient is alive and well six years after operation.

Turning now to the more acute – and even more surgically challenging – group, there are four patients (Table 66.4). Again these patients are in the sixth decade (49–64 years), again all with inferior infarctions. All patients had the typical apical rupture, but one of these had in addition a so-called 'subacute rupture of the heart'[6], and one had so large a rupture that it extended to the midseptal region and involved the moderator band and papillary muscles of the tricuspid valve, resulting in additional free tricuspid regurgitation. In all cases there was the development of a pansystolic murmur at the left sternal edge, followed by a rapid and

Table 66.4 Treatment of postinfarction ventricular septal defect in a group of acute cases

Case	*1*	*2*	*3*	*4*
Sex	M	M	F	M
Age	62	49	64	51
Infarct site	Inferior	Inferior	Infero-Lateral	Inferior
Rhythm	SR	SR	2 : 1 block	SR
Rupture site	Apical	Apical	Apical + ruptured LV	Midseptal + T.I.
Infarct to op.	13 days	8 days	2 days	14 days
Rupture to op.	7 days	7 days	2 days	9 days
Ventriculotomy	Right	Right	Right	Right
Repair	Suture	Suture	Suture	Patch + TVR
Deaths	—	10th day	2nd day	3 weeks
Survival	3 years 1971	— 1971	— 1971	— 1972

continuing deterioration in the patient's condition, with hypotension, oliguria, peripheral vasoconstriction, cyanosis and cerebral confusion.

The differential diagnosis from subvalvar mitral regurgitation was assisted by the disproportionately severe and rapid rise of right atrial pressure. The diagnosis was confirmed in each of these four cases by bedside catheterisation using a Swan-Ganz catheter, which showed a step-up in O_2 saturation at right ventricular level. All the patients operated upon were suffering from cardiogenic shock and were thought to have a prognosis of less than 24 h. Case one has survived for three years and has resumed his normal occupation. Case two died on the tenth postoperative day from a combination of acute myocardial infarction and hepato-renal failure associated with pre-existing diabetes and alcoholism, the severity of which was not known at the time of his presentation. Case three became asystolic as the chest was being opened and was found to have ruptured the left ventricle as well as the septum. The defects were successfully repaired but both inotropic stimulation and external pacing were required to maintain a circulation. The cardiac output did not improve and the patient died the next day. Case four survived for three weeks but on the day before he was due to be discharged from hospital he developed a dysrhythmia from which he could not be resuscitated. In the patients who died, the defects were found to have been successfully closed at autopsy.

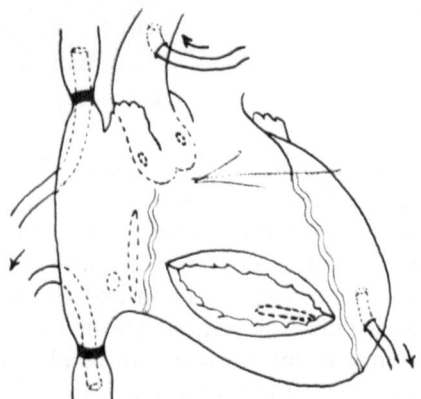

Figure 66.1 Bypass set-up and right ventriculotomy

OPERATIVE TECHNIQUE

The approach in all four cases was via a median sternotomy. Normothermic total cardiopulmonary bypass was employed with caval and aortic cannulation and a suction vent in the left ventricle. The aorta was left unclamped in order to maintain coronary perfusion throughout and the heart was not fibrillated. A right ventriculotomy was used, which gave excellent exposure of the septum without the need to manipulate the heart (Figure 66.1). The infarcted area of the septum was immediately apparent and the rupture was easily identifiable (Figure 66.2).

In the first three cases the defect was closed by direct suture with 2/0 silk on large needles passed through Teflon felt buttresses (Figure 66.3).

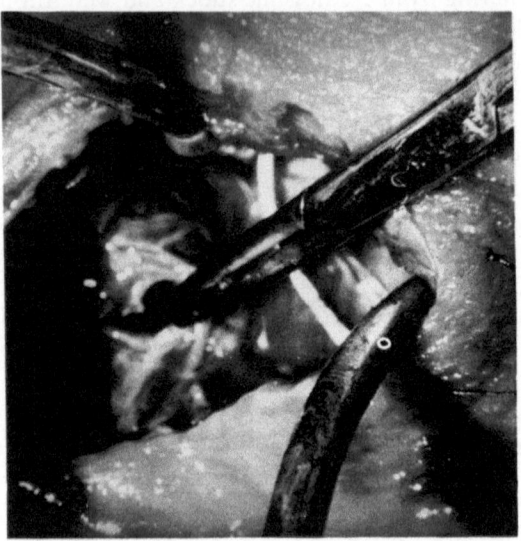

Figure 66.2 Suckers retract while scissors, in centre, indicate VSD, showing excellent exposure

The sutures were placed wide of the more obviously necrotic tissue, mindful also that these defects are often larger on the left side of the septum, and all the sutures were inserted before any were tied. In the fourth case the rupture had occurred in the centre of the septum and the infarct also involved the moderator band and the tricuspid apparatus, producing severe tricuspid regurgitation. The defect was repaired using a Teflon patch sewn in with interrupted sutures placed well clear of the margins of the hole. The tricuspid valve was replaced with a Bjork prosthesis.

SUMMARY

Cases of ventricular septal defect due to myocardial infarction show a predictable similarity in presentation with regard to age, sex and to site of infarction. Coronary ischaemic disease is still largely the perogative of the male and it seems likely that it is only those in their fifth or sixth decades whose physiology can survive the haemodynamic insult long enough to reach a hospital intensive care unit alive.

Thereafter they fall into two groups: (a) A (self-selected) subacute group who can just survive on maximal medical therapy to await elective

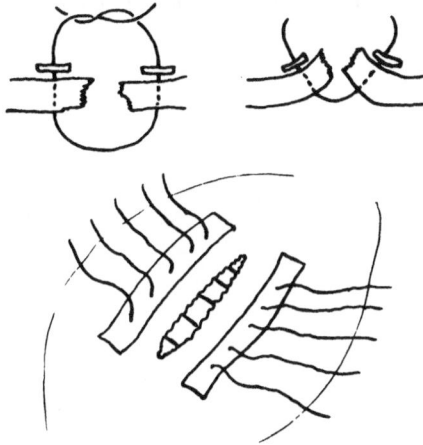

Figure 66.3 Simple direct ties over Teflon buttresses

operation after two or three months with a correspondingly increased chance of survival. (b) An acute group with a prognosis measurable in hours whose only hope lies in emergency operation and who may have additional and equally lethal complications such as mitral and/or tricuspid regurgitation or rupture of a ventricle. There will clearly be individual cases who become relegated from the subacute group by reason of the delayed development of such further complications.

Whilst all cases of VSD due to myocardial infarction should be repaired, early operation – if necessary within days of the infarct – should be undertaken in any patient who shows progressive deterioration in spite of maximal medical therapy.

References

1. Lee, W. Y., Cardon, L. and Slodki, S. J. (1962). Perforation of the infarcted interventricular septum. *Arch. Int. Med.*, **109**, 731
2. Lundberg, S. and Soderstrom, J. (1962). Perforation of the interventricular septum in myocardial infarction: a study based on autopsy material. *Acta Med. Scand.*, **172**, 413
3. Swithinbank, J. M. (1959). Perforation of the interventricular septum in myocardial infarction. *Brit. Heart J.*, **21**, 562
4. Oyamada, A. and Queen, F. B. (1961). Spontaneous rupture of the interventricular

septum following acute myocardial infarction with some clinico-pathological observations on survival in five cases. *Presented at the Pan Pacific Pathology Congress,
Tripler U.S. Army Hospital*

5.   Sanders, R. J., Kern, W. H. and Blount, S. G. Jr (1956). Perforation of the
     interventricular septum complicating myocardial infarction: a report of eight cases, one
     with cardiac catheterisation. *Amer. Heart J.*, **51**, 736

6.   O'Rourke, M. F. (1973). Subacute heart rupture following myocardial infarction.
     Lancet, **00**, 124

Part 8

Results of Surgery in Rare
Congenital Heart Disease

Part 5

67

Results of surgery in rare congenital heart disease*

Ch. Dubost

CONGENITAL AORTIC STENOSIS

Most patients presenting with this condition have supravalvular aortic stenosis either in a localised form or associated with hypoplasia of the aortic arch. This localised form is not difficult to correct since the narrowing can easily be opened up from above the constriction to below and then a diamond patch can be sutured in at the level of the stenosis in order to enlarge the constricted area. Those cases in which there co-exists hypoplasia of the ascending aorta or of the aortic arch are more difficult to treat and it has only been during the past few years that these special forms have met with surgical success.

Figure 67.1 shows hypoplasia of the ascending aorta including narrowing at the first centimetre of the innominate artery. On the right is the aortic arch and on the left is the origin of the left carotid artery which was normal. The narrowing of the ascending aorta involved the entire ascending aorta and the innominate artery but not the aortic arch nor the aortic vessels on the left. Therefore, in this case – a girl of 16 years – it was possible to enlarge the ascending aorta and the origin of the innominate artery with a patch and to restore both the aorta and the artery to normal size. The calibre of the ascending aorta is the same as that of the descending aorta.

COARCTATION OF THE AORTA

In coarctation of the aorta the interesting point to remember is that it is possible to operate without complications on patients over 50 or 60 years of age. Six patients of over 50 years of age and three patients of over 60 years of age have been operated on. In all nine patients a substantial reduction in the blood pressure level was obtained, and none of them required the insertion of any prosthetic materials. Therefore, age makes no difference in the surgical treatment of coarctation of the aorta and the

*Only patients in childhood, adolescence or adulthood will be discussed in this Chapter as the author has had no experience with infants or newborn babies.

435

same rate of success can be achieved in the older age group as has been found in younger patients.

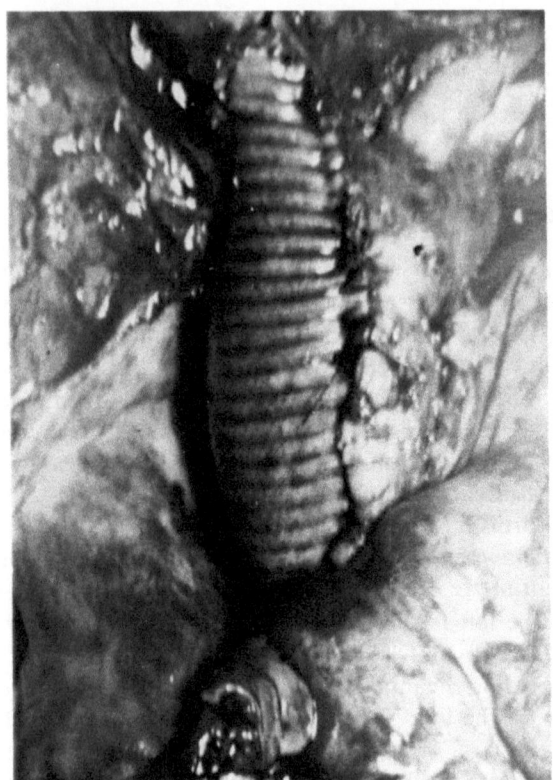

Figure 67.1 Hypoplasia of the ascending aorta including narrowing of the innominate artery.

CONGENITAL CORONARY ARTERY DISEASE
Two main types of disease of the coronary artery exist. The first group consists of the anomalous origin of left coronary artery from left pulmonary artery and the second group of fistulae between the coronary artery and a cardiac chamber.

The anomalous origin of left coronary artery from pulmonary artery
There are two types of anomalous origins of the left pulmonary artery; the first one, designated the infant type, is the one in which there is no anastomosis between the two coronary systems. This type carries a very bad prognosis. On the other hand, the other type in which there are several anastomoses between the two coronary systems has a better outlook, as it can be surgically corrected.

Figure 67.2 shows a case of this type where it was not particularly difficult nor dangerous to connect the left subclavian artery to the left coronary artery with a saphenous vein graft. However, ligation of the left coronary artery would probably have had the same result in this case, because of the existing anastomosis between the two coronary systems.

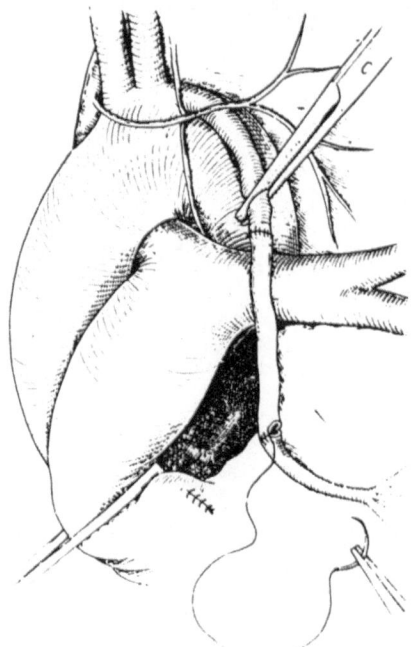

Figure 67.2 Correction for anomalous origin of the left coronary artery from the left pulmonary artery by connection of the left subclavian artery to the left coronary artery with a saphenous vein graft.

Fistulae between the coronary artery and a cardiac chamber
This is an interesting and quite rare affliction. At the present time less than 100 cases of this anomaly have been recorded and 16 of these cases have been operated on at Broussais in Paris.

Table 67.1 shows that in the majority of cases, the right coronary artery and either the right atrium or right ventricle or the pulmonary artery or the coronary sinus are involved. Fistulae on the left side are less frequent. Figures 67.3 and 67.4 show the various openings of the fistulae into the cardiac chambers. In some instances, these fistulae may be complicated by aneurysmal dilations (Figure 67.5). The diagnosis of this disease is not difficult. The symptomatology is clear and catheterisation of the heart alone, or in association with angiography, gives an indication of the abnormal communication of the vessels with the relevant

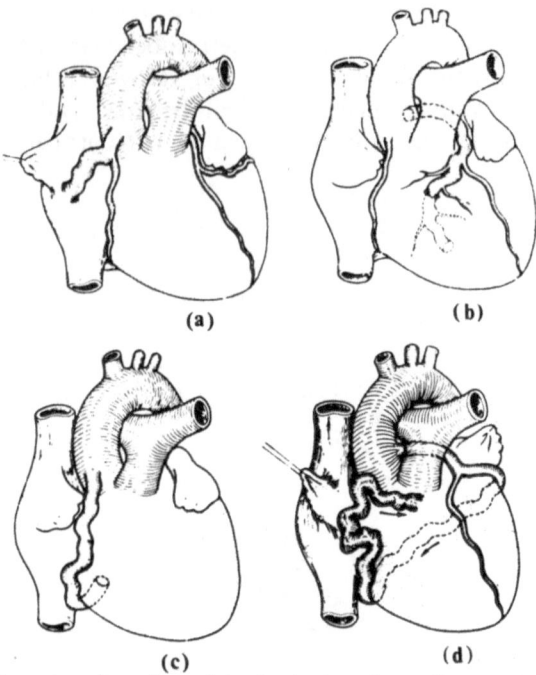

(a)   (b)

(c)   (d)

Figure 67.3 Examples of openings of the fistulae into the cardiac chambers.†

Table 67.1 Distribution of cases with a fistula between the coronary artery and cardiac chamber.†

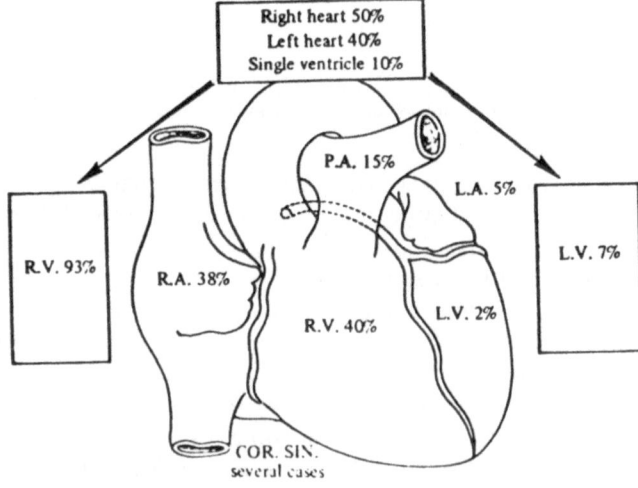

† From "Nouveau Traite de Technique Chirurgicale: coeur-gros vaisseaux T. IV" by P. Blondeau and E. Henry, Masson and Cie, Paris 1972.

438

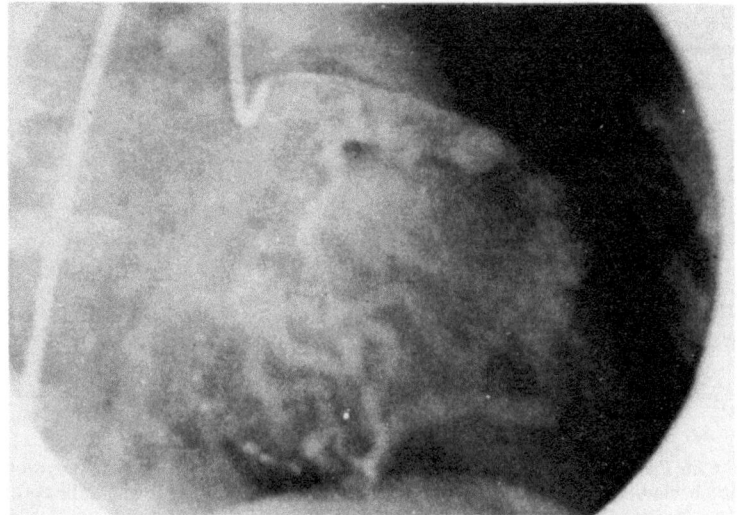

Figure 67.4

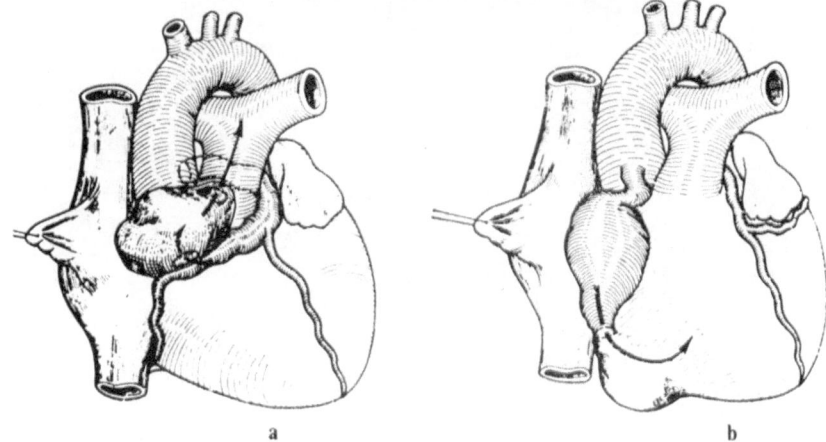

a   b

Figure 67.5 Fistulae with aneurysmal dilations.†

cardiac chamber. Figure 67.6 shows an anomalous communication of the left coronary artery to the coronary sinus, the exposure behind the heart and the sectioning of the artery just before it enters the coronary sinus. Figure 67.7 shows an enormous dilation of the left coronary artery opening into a common chamber with the coronary sinus on the posterior aspect of the heart. In this case it was easy to dissect the coronary

†From "Nouveau Traité de Technique Chirurgicale: coeur-gros vaisseaux T. IV" by P. Blondeau and E. Henry, Masson and Cie, Paris 1972.

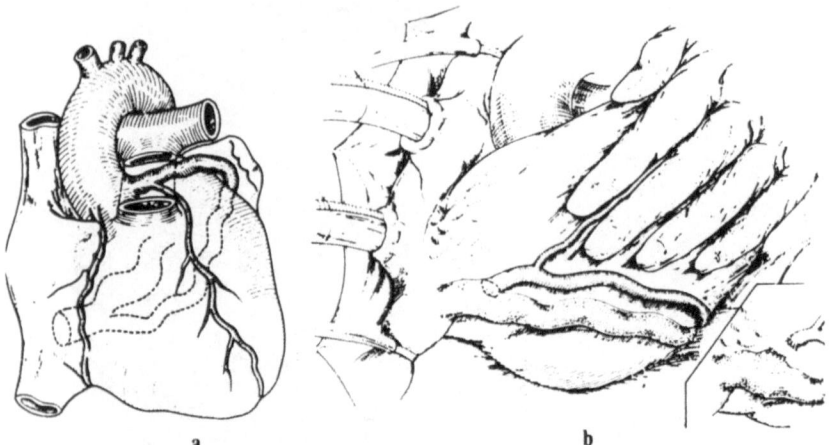

a   b

Figure 67.6 Fistula between the left coronary artery and the coronary sinus showing the exposure behind the heart and the sectioning of the artery just before it enters the coronary sinus.†

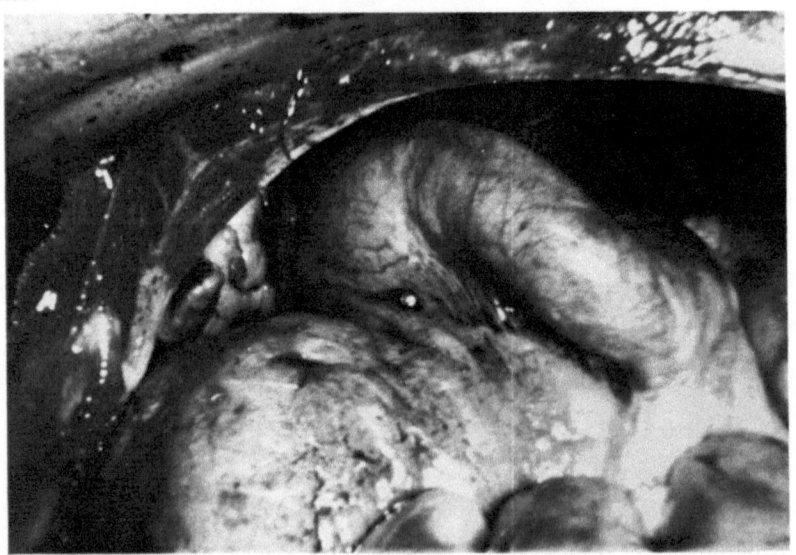

Figure 67.7 Showing an enormous dilation of the left coronary artery opening into a common chamber with the coronary sinus on the posterior aspect of the heart.

artery free before the point of entry into the common chamber and to suture both ends in order to suppress the shunt. Figure 67.8 shows a single left coronary artery with multiple fistulae opening into the outflow tract of the right ventricle. This case was more difficult to treat in that

†From "Nouveau Traité de Technique Chirurgicale: coeur-gros vaisseaux T. IV," by P. Blondeau and E. Henry, Masson and Cie, Paris 1972.

every abnormal communication had to be located so as not to leave any remaining shunt.

VENTRICULAR SEPTAL DEFECTS AND AORTIC INSUFFICIENCY

Another point of interest in congenital heart diseases involving the aortic area is the association of two lesions – ventricular septal defect and aortic insufficiency. Associations of these lesions were first described

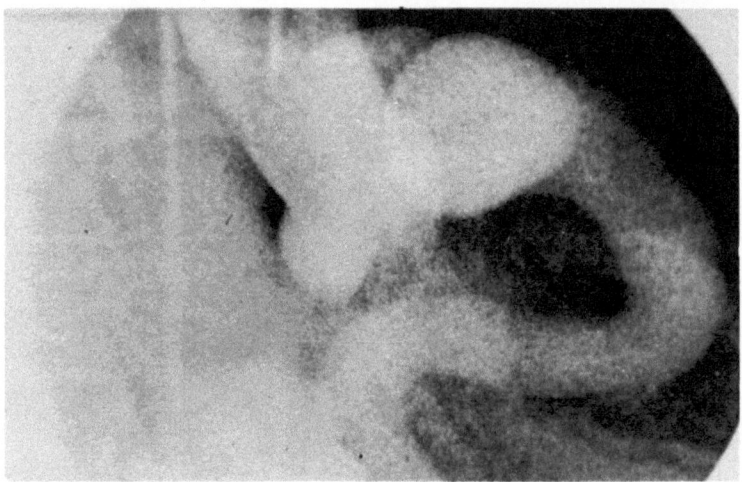

Figure 67.8 Showing a simple left coronary artery with multiple fistulae opening into the outflow tract of the right ventricle.

by Laubry and Pezzi many years ago. They are characterised by a high anterior septal defect located below the right valve - very often the defect is small – and the right valve is prolapsed with an excessively long free margin. This association raises a difficult surgical problem; that of closing the ventricular septal defect and also correcting the aortic insufficiency. The surgeon's problem is greatest when this occurs in young patients in whom one does not want to replace the valve with a prosthetic valve. Therefore, many conservative techniques have been developed to try and render these valves competent.

Some of these techniques consist of the plication of the free border of the right aortic valve or plication of the area of the commissures. These methods leave much to be desired. Some surgeons have suggested enlarging the right cusp using a piece of pericardium, but then the free margin of leaflet remains elongated and therefore this operation does not solve the main problem. Other surgeons have proposed replacing the diseased cusp using a homograft cusp but this is technically a very difficult operation.

The author, therefore, tried another technique in addition to the many already suggested. The method is to suture the free border of the right aortic valve cusp in order to reduce its length and give it the depth which is lacking (Figure 67.9). This is a short operation which is simple to perform. Four young patients have been operated on using this

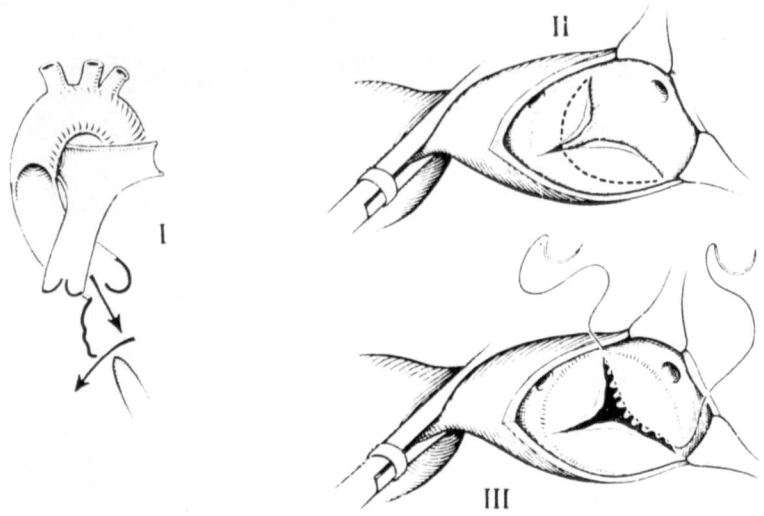

Figure 67.9 Showing the method of suturing the free border of the right aortic valve cusp in order to reduce its length.

technique, either by plicating the free border of only one valve cusp, or of two cusps, the right and the non-coronary cusp. All these patients have retained a slight diastolic murmur but the diastolic blood pressure is only slightly lower than normal and remains adequate. However, it must be emphasised that all these patients were young – in the five to eight year age bracket. Therefore this operation provides a good palliative technique for young patients who can probably then wait until a valve replacement is possible in adult life, but it is not claimed to be a definitive technique for correction of aortic insufficiency in association with VSD.

AORTA TO LEFT VENTRICULAR TUNNEL

The aorta to left ventricle tunnel is a very curious disease and only a few cases have been published in the literature. These cases are often associated with aortic insufficiency and with aneurysm of sinus of valvsalva. In the four cases operated on at Broussais both ends of the tunnel have been closed and an aortic prosthetic valve inserted. This was because the patients were young adults. When at operation an enormous dilation of the anterior root of the aorta is seen, the surgeon knows he is dealing with an aorto-ventricular tunnel, which represents a challenge as the operation is not always straightforward. The aim is to obtain complete closure of the tunnel. To ensure that the closure will not leak, two patches are used, one to close the distal end and the other the proximal end of the tunnel. In these cases it was necessary to replace the aortic valve with a prosthetic valve because the valves of these patients are very often damaged.

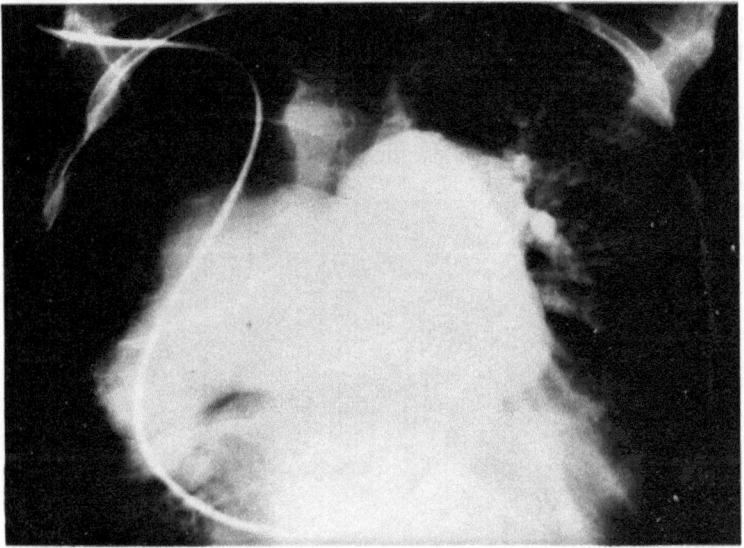

Figure 67.10 Angiogram of the first patient operated on for agenesis of the pulmonary valve five years ago.

SINGLE VENTRICLE

Single ventricle is also an interesting lesion and may prove difficult to correct, firstly because it is not easy to recognise at operation and secondly because once the diagnosis has been made it remains difficult to localise the bundle of His. A third difficulty arises in how to create a new septum and how to manage the valves. This explains why out of five patients operated on at Broussais, three have died. It is now believed that with the precise localisation of the bundle of His as developed by Dr. Malm it may be possible to avoid heart block and obtain better results in the future. Of the two patients who survived, one patient had a tricuspid valve replacement and in the other it was possible to preserve the tricuspid valve.

AGENESIS OF THE PULMONARY VALVE

The agenesis of the pulmonary valve is a fascinating problem in congenital surgery. It is associated with VSD and very often with an aneurysmal dilation of pulmonary arteries and infundibular stenosis. The surgical treatment consists of closure of the VSD, resection of the infundibular stenosis and inserting a frame-mounted aortic heterograft to complete the repair. Figure 67.10 shows the angiogram of the first patient operated on at Broussais five years ago. The calibre of the right pulmonary artery and of the left pulmonary artery can be seen; the trunk of the pulmonary artery is also widely dilated. However, the right branch was so enormous and the pressure inside was so high that there was compression of the

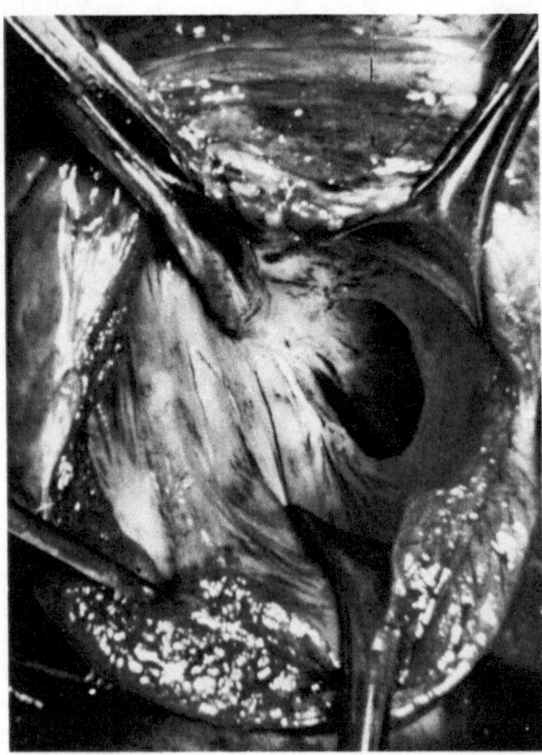

Figure 67.11 Infundibular chamber of a 13-year-old boy with pulmonary valve absent.

right main stem bronchus, sufficient to cause complete destruction of the right lung. The boy was 13 years old at the time of the operation. He was slightly cyanotic and had loud systolic and diastolic murmurs at the left sternal border, which was thought at first to be due to aortic insufficiency. It was only at catheterisation that the diastolic murmur was shown to be due to pulmonary insufficiency. This poor respiratory condition naturally caused concern at operation. Figure 67.11 shows what was found after opening the infundibular chamber of the right ventricle. In the area where the pulmonary valve should be there was nothing that indicated that there had ever been a pulmonary valve at this level as there was a ring without anything which could play the role of the pulmonary valve. It was possible to place a frame-mounted heterograft without enlargement of the right outflow tract. This boy has done well and continues to do well, showing no alteration of this porcine heterograft after five years.

Figure 67.12 shows another example of a 14 year old girl in whom a fibrous ring is located in the area of the pulmonary valve. There are no pulmonary valve cusps and nothing at all that resembles a pulmonary valve. In this case the ring was too small to permit the insertion of a heterograft and it was necessary to open the pulmonary artery in order to place the heterograft. It was also necessary to enlarge the outflow tract of the right ventricle after having resected the hypertrophic infundibular area and after having closed a large VSD. This girl did well and seven out of the eight patients operated on are doing well. Six of them had a patch reconstruction of the outflow tract of the right ventricle and seven had a closure of the VSD. Only one in the series had no VSD but had the same lesions at the level of the pulmonary valve, at the level of the trunk of the pulmonary artery and at the level of the branches of the pulmonary artery. Two had severe infundibular stenosis and the others had no infundibular stenosis at all. These interesting lesions are correctable using surgical techniques which are not too difficult nor too dangerous for the patient.

TETRALOGY OF FALLOT

A few special problems associated with tetralogy of Fallot will be discussed, particularly those having had previous palliative shunts. The most widely performed shunts at the present time are the Waterston and Blalock, left or right, whilst on the other hand the Potts operation and the Glenn operation have been largely abandoned. However, it is still necessary to treat patients who have been operated on in the past and are referred with end-to-end Blalock anastomosis or a Potts shunt or a Glenn shunt.

The Waterston shunt is easy to close but Waterston shunts are not performed at Broussais because, as mentioned at the beginning of the chapter, the author has no experience with infants or new born babies.

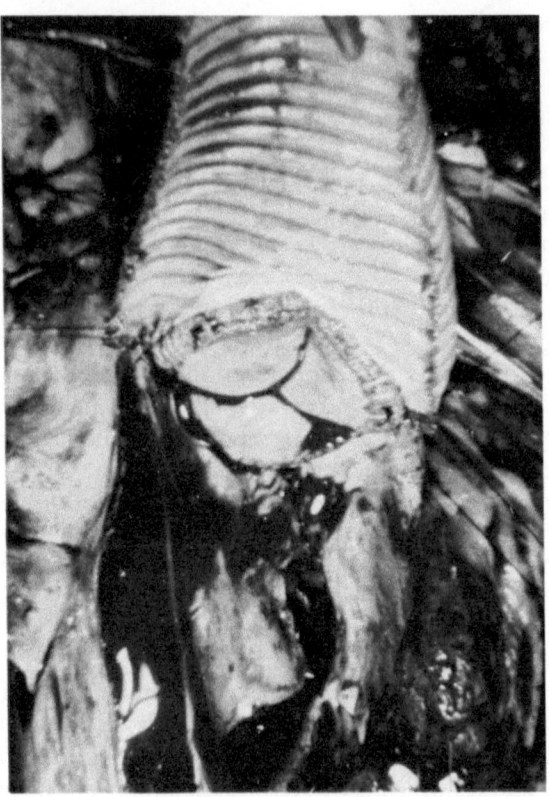

Figure 67.12 Another example in a 14-year-old girl where a fibrous ring was present in place of the pulmonary valve.

However, one patient was referred from another institution in a very poor condition, in intractable heart failure. This was due to the shunt being too large and the boy – 3 years old – was moribund on admission and had to be operated on as an emergency. The closure of the shunt was easily performed through the aorta after which it was possible to perform a total correction of the tetralogy of Fallot. The boy is now doing perfectly well and since there was no kinking at the level of the anastomosis the flow through both lungs is equal at present, four years after operation.

In the past 500 Blalock shunts have been performed at Broussais and of course most of these 500 patients are now returning for total correction. Most have had a left end-to-side Blalock operation which can be readily ligated. A few patients having had one end-to-side Blalock operation on the left side 25 or 26 years ago are now so well (some have married and have raised a family) that they refuse total correction. Their general condition is perfect, their exercise tolerance is almost normal and they understandably refuse operation. At Broussais there are about 12 of these patients in the series. However, the majority of these patients don't do as well and in many the shunt has closed because they have grown and the artery has been stretched, or if the shunt remains patent it is too small for the size of the patient. In this latter group the end-to-side Blalock must be closed in order to achieve complete correction of the lesion. The difficulty lies in the closure of the end-to-end subclavian to pulmonary artery anastomosis and in the total correction at the same time. Some teams have proposed total correction of the tetralogy of Fallot for the right side after having ligated the left subclavian artery. However, the author prefers in the majority of cases to attempt a reconstruction of the left pulmonary artery. This is a difficult and time-consuming procedure which adds to the risk of the total correction. Figure 67.13a shows a narrowing at the level of the anastomosis between the left subclavian and the left pulmonary artery. It was possible in this case, as in many other cases that have been published in the literature, to perform reimplantation of the left pulmonary artery using a Dacron tube to the right pulmonary artery thus obtaining a complete anatomical repair (Figure 67.13b).

The Potts operation presents a great challenge to the surgeon because in many instances the anastomosis is kinked and it is difficult to assess the degree of kinking of the Potts anastomosis prior to operation. Frequently trouble develops during the operation which may be difficult to understand. When under profound hypothermia, the left pulmonary artery is opened in order to find the shunt and close it through the pulmonary artery (according to the technique described by Kirklin) and no abnormal communication is found between the left pulmonary artery and the aorta, the surgeon is puzzled because he knows that the Potts operation was done and therefore a shunt must exist at that level. He therefore goes ahead and opens the left pulmonary artery further and deeper until after an hour's effort he understands. However, by this time it is too late because, by dissection, a part of the wall of the left pulmonary artery has been destroyed. This is difficult to reconstruct and the opening in the aorta is difficult to close in the depth of the chest. This then is the real problem with closing a Potts' shunt when it is not known how the shunt was performed.

Dr Soyer has developed an ingenious technique for closure of the Potts' anastomosis. It consists of perfusing both the ascending and descending aorta. The femoral cannula may be clamped and unclamped in order to determine with precision where the blood flow out from the

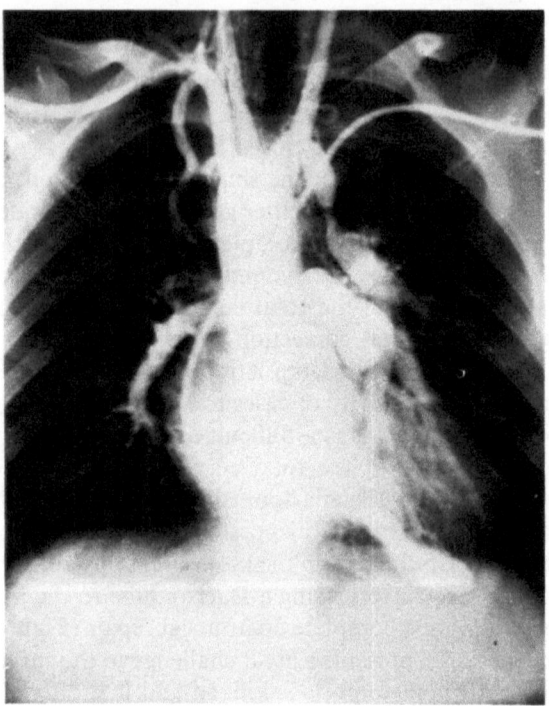

Figure 67.13a Narrowing at the level of the anastomosis between the left subclavian and the left pulmonary arteries.

aortic side with the pulmonary artery opened. This can be of great help in finding the site of the shunt, but it is not always enough. For example, in one case it was necessary to repair the aortic wall. This was done with great difficulty because when using the mid-sternotomy incision the descending aorta is very far away. It was then necessary to reconstruct the left pulmonary artery using a Dacron tube and to anastomose the tube to the right pulmonary artery. There was considerable bleeding and the patient died after two days from low cardiac output. Therefore the major risk is a left pulmonary stenosis following the Potts operation.

The case of teralogy of Fallot which had had three previous operations – two Blalocks, one left and one right, plus a Glenn procedure – was also quite a challenge to repair, because the right pulmonary artery must be

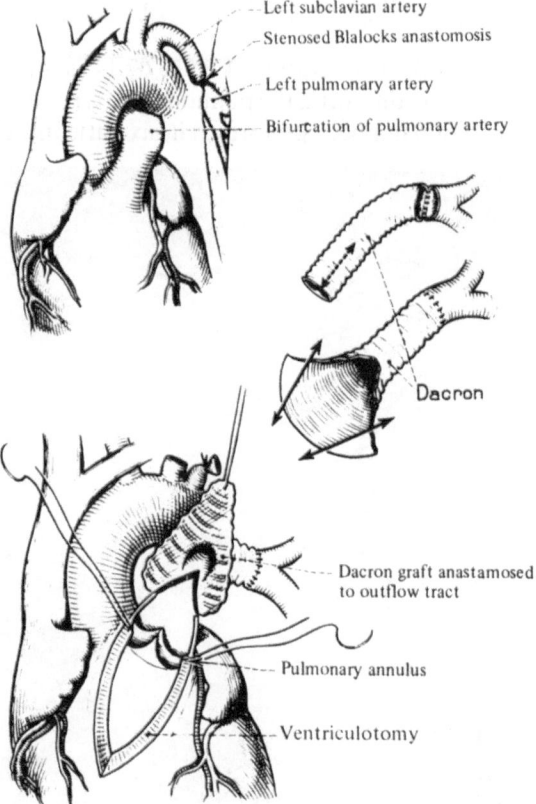

Left subclavian artery

Stenosed Blalocks anastomosis

Left pulmonary artery

Bifurcation of pulmonary artery

Dacron

Dacron graft anastamosed to outflow tract

Pulmonary annulus

Ventriculotomy

Figure 67.13b Reimplantation of the left pulmonary artery using a Dacron tube to the right pulmonary artery.

reconstructed at the same time as the total correction of the tetralogy of Fallot is undertaken. The Glenn procedure is performed between two venous structures and after its completion many adhesions develop in the area. The dissection of the vena cava and the right pulmonary artery may be controlled by placing an inflated Foley catheter in its lumen. This makes it possible to obtain a dry field in order to find the blind end of the proximal right pulmonary artery which is hidden in connective tissue behind the aorta. When it has been found, it is clear that there is only a short segment of proximal right pulmonary artery to use to sew a tube at this level, and it is necessary to try and complete the anastomosis by suturing it to the distal pulmonary artery. All of these corrective operations following Potts and Glenn operations are time-consuming, bloody and represent a very high risk to the patient.

TRANSPOSITION OF THE GREAT ARTERIES WITH VSD

This is a very dangerous operation. Figure 67.14 is a photograph taken at operation, showing the aorta, the pulmonary artery and the venae cavae. The Wheat operation has been performed in six patients at Broussais, with

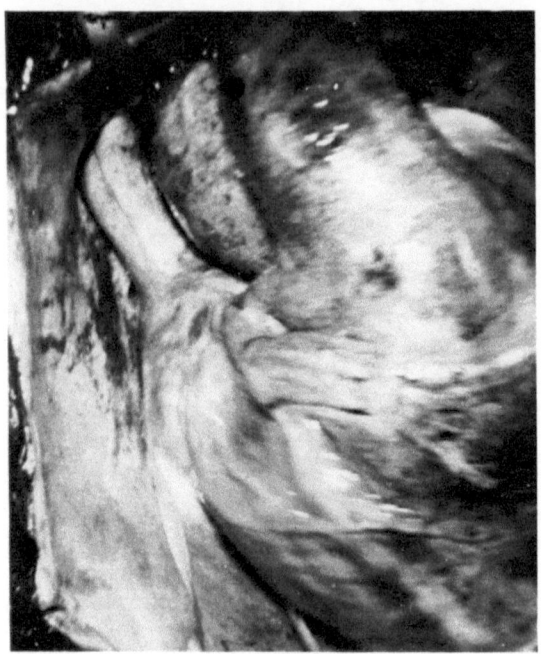

Figure 67.14 Transposition of the great arteries.

good results in three of these patients. A good result was obtained in a 20 year old medical student (Figure 67.15). The right ventriculogram shows that there is no communication with the other cavities. In the three failures there were complications – mainly complete heart block. The device used by Malm should prove to be of great interest in these cases, but at the present time it is not known what is the best operation to use.

EBSTEIN'S DISEASE

This disease may be alleviated either by a Lillehei Hunter plication or by the implantation of a prosthetic valve at the tricuspid level. There are two types of Ebstein's disease, the good case and the bad case. The good case is the one in which the anterior leaflet of the tricuspid valve has conserved enough length and enough tissue to be preserved in order to make possible a Lillehei Hunter operation. In the bad case, in which there is a very large atrialisation of the right ventricle, it is not possible to preserve this valve and it is necessary to resect what there is of the tricuspid valve and replace it using a Björk–Shiley, Starr or heterograft or homograft valve.

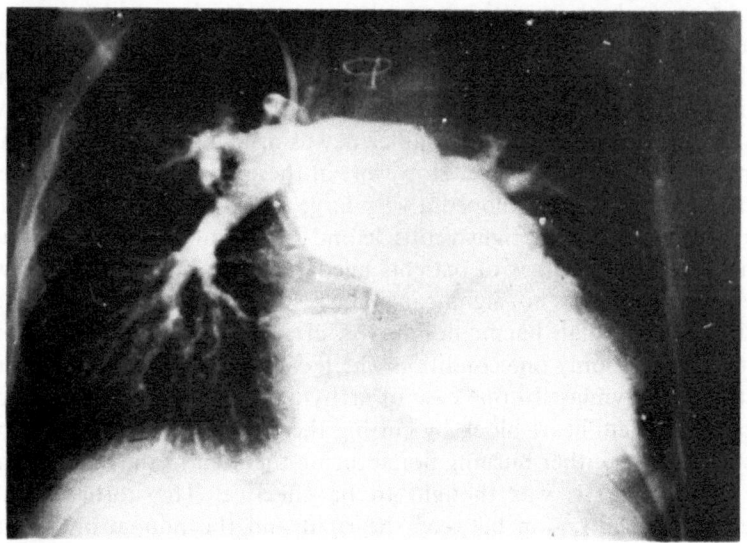

Figure 67.15 Wheat operation performed to correct transposition of the great arteries.

Table 67.2 Results of surgery and severity of the disease

(1) Severity demonstrated before 10 years	
11 cases	7 early deaths
(2) Severity demonstrated between 10 and 20 years ⁝	
2 cases	1 early death
(3) Severity demonstrated after 20 years (or mild)	
7 cases	1 death

There has been little experience at Broussais of replacement of the tricuspid valve using frame-mounted heterografts. Table 67.2 gives the results for this type of valve replacement. There have been a few cases of complete heart block and a few cases of death in desperately ill patients. Fourteen valve replacements were performed, four with Starr ball valve prosthesis and no deaths, and 10 heterografts with four deaths. It is therefore necessary to decide whether or not a patient with Ebstein's disease should be operated on, because the diagnosis of the disease is not synonymous with operation. Many patients with Ebstein's disease are doing very well without operation. They have no arrhythmias and no diastolic murmurs on exertion. In these patients there is no need for operation. Only those patients who have poor circulation, deep cyanosis and numerous arrhthymias are considered for operation. Eleven patients under 10 years of age have been operated on with seven deaths. In these patients, either a Glenn operation was performed or an attempt was made to correct the tricuspid insufficiency using a conservative procedure, or placing an artificial valve. However, in these children who are deeply cyanotic, who have developed a very large heart and in whom the right atrium is a part of the right ventricle and is enormous, any technique is dangerous. The number of patients aged between 10 and 20 years who have been studied, is not significant. The results of operations on cyanotic patients with a high haemoglobin who are over 20 years old are much better. There is only one condition which cannot be improved and this is that of arrhthymias. In one case of arrhythmia the author attempted to obtain complete heart block by cutting the bundle of His, but this was unsuccessful. Neither burning nor suturing the area in the atrium where the bundle of His was thought to be effective. The aorta was then opened and the region between the right and the non-coronary cusps where the bundle is located was sutured. This was also unsuccessful. Then a second attempt to burn all these parts of the right atrium was made, again without success. Finally a sino-auricular block was induced by suturing the bases of the superior vena cava and the patient was returned to the intensive care unit, where after 10 min normal sinus rhythm was restored.

Part 9

Discussion

Discussion

D. B. Longmore

The Fifth Annual Course in Cardiac Surgery was planned such that the sequence of presentation of papers would build up a logical picture of the current status of cardiac surgery. The content of these papers constitutes the first eight parts of this book. Although during the course, each paper was discussed following its presentation, the discussion which from time to time went wide of the point is here presented separately in order not to detract from the main theme of the book. When reading the discussion the reader should bear in mind that this was a course and not a symposium. This means that participants of the course were asked to confine their discussion to the teaching aspects of the subject rather than comparing their results with those of other units. Unfortunately, it has not been possible to include all the points made nor in every case to make specific to individual contributors.

DISCUSSION FOLLOWING THE CARDIAC TRANSPLANTATION SESSION

The discussion was opened by Professor Roy Calne who raised the following points:

1. *Number of potential heart transplantation recipients:* Professor Calne commented on an analysis of the patients in his Unit in Cambridge which suggests that there are few patients suitable for heart transplantation even assuming that comparable results to those of Shumway could be achieved. He therefore feels that there has been an exaggeration in the number of potential recipients who would be suitable for heart transplantation. He also suggested that there is a need for a small number of centres which would combine an experimental background of interest in transplantation with first-class surgical and medical care of patients.

2. *Cardiac* v. *liver transplantation:* In cardiac transplantation there is no doubt that with the immunosuppression that is at present available, around 50% of patients will die from rejection although surgically the operation does not present the difficulties encountered in liver transplantation. The problem of rejection is less severe in cases of liver transplantation but the technical difficulty of joining the bile ducts without leakage often leads to failure. Professor Calne is therefore uncertain which of the two procedures will be the first to be established as a routine.

The discussion was then thrown open to the floor and a number of questions were asked:

Q.   *Cavitation in the media:* Dr Ayoub asked whether this is considered a genuine sign of rejection or just an artefact.

J.F.M.   Dr Mowbray replied that the majority of the cavitation in the media is probably not important and usually its purely an artefact. However, sometimes these vescicles are full of immunoglobulin and are related to the rejection.

Q.   *The technique of endomyocardial biopsy:* Dr. Ayoub asked whether this technique could lead to false negative or false positive results.

J.F.M.   Dr Mowbray replied that the focal nature of lesions is very important as obviously a single endomyocardial biopsy might miss an area of rejection. However, when an area of rejection is located, although the extent of rejection can not be evaluated this positive information is important.

P.K.C.   Dr Caves commented that in Shumway's Unit they usually took two or three biopsy specimens in order to try to avoid the problem of focal rejection. However, there were no false negatives. The policy initially was not to accept the biopsy alone, but it was discovered that in cases where the biopsy revealed rejection but this positive result was not accepted and the rejection not treated, then ultimately other signs of rejection also emerged, e.g. electrocardiographic changes followed within the next two or three days.

Q.   *Enhancement:* Mr Ross asked for a simple explanation of this process.

J.J.V.R.   Dr Van Rood explained that the process of enhancement is not yet fully understood. It is a process which enables an organ graft or a tumour graft to survive much longer than would be expected. This is probably due to an antibody mechanism, since the antibodies directed against antigenic determinants of that graft will in some circumstances not destroy the graft but actually make it possible for the graft to survive. It is not known what types of antibody are involved, nor is it known against which antigenic determinants they are directed – there is a lot of work being done and there is no consensus of opinion on this point. However, at present the Dutch group believes that enhancement might be mainly due to antibodies against MLC determinants. The chromosome which carries the information about transplantation antigens has two types of loci, one of which can be detected by serological techniques – serological-defined determinants. The other can not be detected by serological techniques and can only be found by more complex testing – *in vitro* culturing and the MLC test. These are the so-called MLC loci on the same chromosome and these determinants are called lymphocyte-defined. At the moment the Dutch group believes that enhancement occurs if there is an absence or very small amount of antibodies against these determinants.

Q.   *Heart transplantation in children:* Dr Borde asked whether there is any experience of heart transplantation in children with very complicated heart defects.

P.K.C.   Dr Caves replied that in his opinion organ transplantation should not be performed in children. He explained that this viewpoint is based on his experience of the effects of the long-term steroid administration that follows the operation. This treatment is necessary due to the limitations in the current methods of immunosuppression.

Dr Albert Starr then commented on the need for *diversity of approach.*

Although cardiac transplantation is essentially a research problem that requires an organised team and considerable financial support Dr Starr finds it rather disturbing that a lot of the information on transplantation is being supplied in the main by one group of investigators – the Paulo-Alto group. Obviously much credit is due to this group but Dr Starr believes that diversity leads to more rapid advances in medicine than too much centralisation and concentration of research at one institution. He therefore recommended that an effort be made to obtain adequate financial support to duplicate the efforts of the Palo-Alto group and increase the number of teams and institutions involved in this kind of work.

Following Dr Albert Starr's comments, Dr Caves described the approach to heart transplantation adopted by the Stanford Unit.

Surgical commitment of the team: Heart transplantation does depend very obviously on very meticulous and constant postoperative surveillance. The policy at Stanford has been to make one person responsible for this commitment rather than a team of people. This person can seek the advice and help of anyone but principally he is left in charge and the service for that year stands or falls on what he is able to do.

Expense of transplantation: A survey at Stanford showed that the cost of the medical treatment of patients – the recipients – in the year prior to transplantation was often considerably greater than the cost of their treatment in the year after transplantation. The majority of these patients are so ill that they are often in hospital for many months beforehand.

Selection of the recipient: When a donor became available the Unit was usually faced with the situation of having four or five potential recipients. Usually on moral and clinical grounds the patient who was most likely to die within one or two days was selected for transplantation.

Donor supply: Without a shadow of doubt this is the limiting factor. The Stanford Unit does not do more transplants per year not because it would not like to but because of the limited number of donor hearts available.

Preservation of the donor heart: The best method of preservation is to maintain the heart within the donor's own pericardial cavity. Dr Caves believes that ultimately the concept of brain death will be accepted. It may then be possible, from one tragic death, to bring about the revitalisation of four patients by the donation of two kidneys, the heart and the liver.

Rehabilitation: The vast majority of the patients at Stanford leave hospital two or three months after transplantation and the majority of them are back at work or are enjoying an active retirement.

Finally, Mr Longmore closed the discussion with the following comments:

There are three points that are worthy of note by all cardiac surgeons:

1. At the moment only a very small proportion of the total number of people suffering from heart disease are receiving treatment.
2. A death in a family is a disaster to that particular family.
3. The cost to the community of somebody dying of heart disease is enormous.

Mr Longmore went on to point out that the session on cardiac transplantation had only examined one form of treatment for heart replacement. Other possible forms of treatment were not discussed. The mechanical heart was dismissed as being of no value, the research into animal-to-man transplantation which would overcome the problems of donor acquisition was not discussed nor was the use of foetal material and extracts to cause tissues to replicate themselves. Only one form of treatment was discussed in depth, i.e. the work of Shumway which has been shown to be very effective.

DISCUSSION FOLLOWING THE FALLOT'S TETRALOGY SESSION

The discussion was introduced by Professor Bentall who pointed out that although the best way of treating Fallot's tetralogy has been the subject of research for the past 20 years there is still no final solution to this problem. He then went on to raise a point concerning correct nomenclature.

H.B.   *Conus* v. *crista:* Professor Bentall explained Dr Anderson's reasons for rejecting the term 'crista', which every surgeon has used in the past, in favour of the term 'conus'. It is now clear that that portion of what surgeons are used to calling the crista or more exactly the ascending limb of the crista is called by Dr Anderson the bulbo-ventricular flange. The portion known to most surgeons as the horizontal portion of the crista is called by Dr Anderson the conus septum.

Professor Bentall then asked Dr Anderson to discuss the anatomical considerations of the VSD which becomes a tetralogy.

Q.   *The VSD which becomes a tetralogy:* Professor Bentall commented that it is very difficult to name this situation in embryological terms since the application of embryological terms to a formed situation implies a knowledge of the embryological condition which of course must remain speculative. He then went on to describe the situation of a child with a VSD shunting left to right over a period of time – usually three to five years – gradually develops a balanced shunt and then turns blue in the absence of pulmonary hypertension and finally develops the full situation of tetralogy of Fallot. Dr Anderson was asked to explain the anatomical considerations associated with this change.

R.H.A.   Dr Anderson described Goor's series of measurements which have shown that there is a basic difference between the classic Fallot and the VSD which becomes a tetralogy. In the latter case the conus septum inserts into the anterior septum in line, i.e. the conus septum inserts as in the normal heart between the limbs of the trabecula septo marginalis (septal band). In this situation, increasing ventricular hypertrophy would lead to closure in the area of pulmonary infundibulum, thus being the narrowest point of the right ventricular outflow and a purely muscular structure, whereas the aortic outflow is partly fibrous. In the case of a classical Fallot, the conus septum inserts as a T, leading to more anterior deviation. On the basis of Goor's observations Dr Anderson put forward the theory that the VSD which becomes a tetralogy exhibits conal rotation and therefore right ventricular hypertrophy produces the obstruction whereas the classical Fallot exhibits conal rotation and anterior deviation and is therefore already obstructed due to the conal septal deviation.

Q.   *Conducting tissue paths:* Mr English asked Dr Anderson to explain the difference between the path that the conducting tissue takes in Fallot's tetralogy and the path it takes in an ordinary VSD.

R.H.A.   Dr Anderson explained that the difference lies in the fact that in an isolated VSD, only a small part of the defect, this area has failed to close perhaps due to partial rotation of the conus. In Fallot's tetralogy the entire interventricular foramen constitutes the area of defect. This means that the anterior part of the defect which is normally closed by the conus septum is not blocked in this way in Fallot's tetralogy because the conus septum is deviated. In addition, the presence of the septal band or the trabecula septo marginalis in the inferior rim of the defect covers over the right bundle branch and deviates the left bundle branch to the left side of the defect, whereas in the simple membraneous defect, the trabeculo septo marginalis is still in its normal position. Dr Anderson suggested that the combination of the anterior deviation of conus septum and the presence of a probably hypertrophied trabeculo septo marginalis pushes the conducting tissue away from the defect.

Q.   *Shunt operations in infants:* Professor Bentall asked Mr Waterston to comment on the value of shunt operations particularly in infants under six months old.

D.W.   Mr Waterston replied that he could see no indication for shunting Fallot's tetralogy. In his opinion all infants over six months old (with the exception of unusual cases where it is impossible to correct with a single pulmonary artery) should be corrected. Mr Waterston also suggested that with the high risks associated with shunt closure perhaps even infants under three months should be corrected.

Professor Bentall then asked for comments on *the role of palliation in Fallot's tetralogy.*

I.H.   Mr Hill commented that he would be reluctant to see the departure of the anastomotic era in favour of total correction. He pointed out that although Mr Waterson's figures for total correction were extremely good, they do not include the large number of children who die whilst waiting for corrective surgery.

W.K.   Professor Klinner supported Mr Hill's remarks. He commented that whereas he is able to perform two shunt operations in one day he would not be able to perform two bypass operations in that time. He therefore relies on the shunt procedure when time is limited.

Q.   *Palliative operations:* Mr Donald Ross asked the panels whether they could form an opinion of what is the best anastomosis, i.e. the Brock operation, the Blalock operation or the Waterston operation.

H.D.S. Mr D'Arcy Sutherland commented that he supported the Waterston shunt in preference to the Blalock shunt and the Pott's shunt as the Waterston shunt is particularly suitable for children under the age of one year. He agreed with Professor Klinner that full corrections under the age of one year are not always possible and that when this is the case the Waterston shunt is a valuable operation.

J.S.   Dr Stark pointed out that the number of patients needing operation in the first three or six months of life is very small and that in looking at Fallot's tetralogy several mortality rates have to be considered – the mortality of a shunt (plus the mortality of total correction later on) the mortality of waiting and the mortality of total correction, which may be greater if there has been a previous shunt.

Q.   *Management of the small pulmonary artery:* Mr Parker raised the point that there is little agreement on how Fallot's tetralogy should be managed, particularly with respect to small pulmonary arteries. He asked Dr Starr to explain his programme for managing the problem of the small pulmonary artery and to give details of the type of shunt procedure employed and the timing of the use of total correction.

A.S.   Dr Starr replied that he does not perform total corrections within the first few months of life. A shunt procedure is used in these cases. A shunt procedure is also used if the original lesion is complex, e.g. in cases of pulmonary atresia or marked hypoplasia of the pulmonary artery. The Waterston type of shunt is used in very small babies – in cases as young as 24 hours old, the anterior Waterston shunt has been found to be the most convenient. Dr Starr went on to say that he has only had a few patients who have gone on to the second stage of total correction after this initial shunt procedure. In these cases he has found closing the pulmonary artery from the outside using a patch on the right pulmonary artery, a difficult

	procedure with the added complication of the possibility of haemorrhage when coming off bypass. There is also some doubt as to whether a patch on the right pulmonary artery will grow. In those children that have no severe damage to the right pulmonary artery following the Waterston shunt, Dr Starr has found it very convenient to close the shunt from inside the aorta. Of the two techniques Dr Starr prefers the second.
M.Y.	Mr Yacoub commented that in his opinion the pulmonary artery is rarely so small that it cannot accept the cardiac output. In his patients where a homograft was used to reconstruct the outflow tract, the pulmonary artery pressure always returned to normal. Therefore Mr Yacoub believes that in patients with a hypoplastic pulmonary valve ring or a small pulmonary artery the correct operation is to replace the pulmonary artery with a homograft.
D.N.R.	Mr. Ross agreed with Mr Yacoub's contention that the pulmonary artery will always take the outflow from the right ventricle at a young age but raised doubts as to whether this would be the case at a later age.
A.S.	In Dr Starr's opinion one of the main problems associated with infant cardiac surgery is the training of practitioners. He suggested that where a good training is available then total correction can be used in very young infants but otherwise shunt procedures should be employed.
A.F.F.	Dr Fontan raised the point that in addition to the main pulmonary artery being small, the branches may also be small and this may be a contraindiction to total repair.
Q.	*Patients over two years of age:* Professor Klinner asked Dr Starr whether his work is confined to those children under two years of age.
A.S.	Dr Starr replied that at his Clinic there are very few cases of tetralogy of Fallot in children over two years of age because they now treat this disease within the first two years of life.
Q.	*Patch v. resection:* Dr Starr was asked why a patch is used when greater resection of the outflow tract could avoid this.
A.S.	Dr Starr replied that the aorta is frequently very far forward and no matter how much muscle is taken out just over the aorta it is not possible to obtain the circumference necessary to form a fuse which will not obstruct the right ventricular outflow tract. Therefore in Dr Starr's view there are cases in which it is mandatory to use a patch if the obstruction is to be relieved.

However the use of patches leads to a very high incidence of pulmonary regurgitation unless a homograft valve is used. Therefore the choice lies between residual obstruction of the outflow tract and pulmonary insufficiency due to residual pulmonary regurgitation. Dr Starr has made the choice in favour of the latter.

J.P.   Mr Parker commented that when comparing Dr Starr's series with that of Mr Yacoub the incidence of reconstruction of the whole outflow tract is about the same as the incidence of reconstruction of the right ventricle (10%). A lot of Dr Starr's patches were actually confined to the ventricle and did not go into the pulmonary arteries and therefore would not have created pulmonary incompetence.

A.S.   *Pulmonary valve replacement:* Dr Starr agreed with Mr Parker but mentioned that many patients have pulmonary incompetence because of malformation of the pulmonary valve and only long-term follow up of these patients will reveal whether these malformed valves are functionally important.

Q.   *The use of homografts in very young children:* Dr Somerville asked for comments on the use of homografts in very young children with pulmonary atresia. In her opinion, since the grafts do not grow with the infant it is probably better to use a shunt procedure.

D.N.R.   Mr Ross replied that it is his policy not to try to reconstruct with a homograft as a primary move but rather to do a shunt. In the atresia group he has found a Blalock performed on the left side to be the safest shunt.

A.S.   Dr Starr reported that he had performed total correction of pulmonary atresia in about five or six children between the ages of 18 months to 2½ years without the use of any valvular mechanism in the outflow tract reconstruction. In these cases an outflow tract patch was laid using the denuded but tough tissue of the surrounding pericardium in the back wall of the pulmonary artery as part of the conduit. It was hoped that in this way the patch would be endothelialised with time and so avoid the use of any valvular mechanism in a small child. Dr Starr pointed out that he is unable to judge how this would function in the long-term with respect to aneurysum formation or whether it would hold up. However his experience in doing pulmonary artery reconstructions shows that it takes very little to hold back the pulmonary blood temporarily and then it heals over very well. Dr Starr therefore recommended the use of a simple gusset-type of reconstruction without a valvular mechanism for good long-term results in cases of correcting pulmonary atresia.

M.Y.   Mr Yacoub was interested in Dr Starr's concept but felt that the use of a unicuspid patch with a large homograft cusp is probably better than a patch without a valve mechanism.

Q.   *Cardiopulmonary bypass:* Mr Odeka asked Dr Starr what techniques for cardiopulmonary bypass are being used in total correction for Fallot's tetralogy in infancy.

A.S.   Dr Starr replied that he had only occasionally used the hypothermia surface cooling and core rewarming described by Mr Yacoub for transposition in very small infants. Since tetralogy patients requiring total correction are usually at least 10 weeks of age, Dr Starr has found it convenient to cannulate such a patient for cardiopulmonary bypass. The cannulation sites do not interfere with total correction in any way and in these cases Dr Starr prefers to use total body perfusion with a pump oxygenator rather than circulatory arrest. The bypass time for total correction is not very much greater than the time required to rewarm the child or cool a child from 35 °C or 36 °C down to 22 °C and then to rewarm them. For example, the perfusion times of Barrett-Boyse are between 30 and 40 mins as compared with Dr Starr's times of between 60 and 70 mins for total correction. In addition cardiopulmonary bypass is preferable to the cooling technique when the patient is acidotic. The patient may start bypass with severe acidosis and during the course of a high flow normal cardiopulmonary bypass without the use of bicarbonate, the pH tends towards normal, the buffer base is restored and the child is resuscitated.

Q.   *Management of an acidotic child:* Mr Keith Ross asked the panel how a child who is acidotic after an investigation for Fallot's tetralogy should be managed. Should surgery be undertaken immediately or should an attempt be made to manage the situation?

M.Y.   Mr Yacoub favoured the latter approach, i.e. an attempt to correct acidosis and then proceeding to total correction later. However he felt that repeated cyanotic attacks would be an indication for immediate surgery.

A.S.   Dr Starr disagreed. In his opinion a child doing poorly following catheterisation should be considered for urgent operation. His policy is to intubate the child whilst awaiting operation. Only if the child is clearly on the mend would Dr Starr extubate the child and operate later.

J.K.R.   Mr Ross commented that in his experience angiography often caused the patient's condition to deteriorate presumably due to the sodium load. He would therefore avoid immediate surgery.

DISCUSSION FOLLOWING PROSTHETIC VALVES SESSION

A number of questions were asked following the session.

Q.   Dr Starr asked Dr Gibson whether it is possible to distinguish abnormalities relating to myocardial disease, such as myocardial fibrosis which is so commonly associated with cardiac heart disease, from those artefacts produced by prosthesis.

D.G.G.   Dr Gibson replied that in his opinion abnormal movement is associated in some way with abnormal filling and is not due to disease of the septum.

Q.   *Protection of the myocardium:* Mr Donald Ross asked Mr Sapsford whether or not he would use coronary perfusion in straightforward aortic valve replacement.

R.S.   Mr Sapsford replied that in his series he had cross-clamped the aorta for a time ranging from 33–100 mins, with a mean of 68 mins. In his opinion there is no doubt that cooling of the heart imposes a definite time limit and the evidence suggests that the time limit for coronary perfusion is longer.

A.S.   Dr Starr commented that in his Unit the policy employed for mitral valve surgery is to operate as rapidly as possible and clamp the aorta for a period of 20 mins at the maximum. This is usually long enough for an experienced surgeon to do mitral valve replacement, at least that portion of replacement that requires aortic cross-clamping. However in the case of inexperienced surgeons performing the operation then the policy in Dr Starr's Unit is to cross-clamp the aorta for two separate periods of about 15 mins each with resuscitation in between.

Dr Stalpat from Louvain then discussed *the positioning of the Björk–Shiley prosthesis,* with particular reference to the mitral position.

At the beginning of Dr Stalpat's experience with the Björk–Shiley prosthesis, the procedure was to direct the downward moving part of the disc towards the base of the anterior mirtal leaflet, with an opening angle of 50 degrees of the Delrin disc. From 1973, in order to diminish thromboembolic phenomenon, it was recommended to direct the downward part of the disc, towards the posterior leaflet base with an opening angle of 60 degrees of the pyrolitic disc. Throughout Dr Stalpat's experience, i.e. from the end of 1970 onwards, he has placed a mitral prosthesis so that the downward part opens towards the aortic valve. The middle of the part of the ring which corresponds with this downward moving part of the valve is attached at the transition from anterior to posterior leaflet and four interrupted stitches are used on each quadrant with a running suture in between. For the aortic valve, the opening of the disc is always directed to the left coronary artery. Using this technique, Dr Stalpat's Unit has performed 252 operations with an early mortality rate of 10·7% and a late mortality of 6%. For the scheduled cases this was 7·7% and 6% for late mortality. In the follow-up period of 3385 patient months, the Unit had 448 cases on anticoagulants and only two cases of cerebral emboli at seven months and 36 months postoperatively. There were 33 cases, without anticoagulants and in this group there were fewer cases of thrombosis in the Fallots, three in aortics and two in mitrals. Dr Stalpat therefore drew the following conclusions: The position of the Björk–Shiley valve in the mitral position and perhaps in the aortic position may be of some importance. Putting a mitral opening to the aortic valve, has led to a very low thromboembolic incidence of 1·3% and anticoagulating seems mandatory. As the emboli occurred in mitral replacement alone, Dr Stalpat is uncertain whether these emboli are due to the prosthesis or the oracle appendage, therefore, he now, as was done at the outset of cardiac surgery, ties up the oracle appendage.

Q.   *The small aortic root:* Mr Keith Ross asked the exponents of the cage-ball prosthesis whether they employ a procedure to enlarge the aortic root in order to accommodate the valve.

A.S.   Dr Starr replied that in his opinion the small root is still an un-solved problem. In his series, Dr Starr is very reluctant to use a cloth-covered size 8 valve which corresponds in external diameter to a 21 mm Björk–Shiley valve. Such a prosthesis may be associated with a significant haemolysis and transvalvar gradient in vigorous patients with good cardiac output. He there-fore prefers to use the non-cloth-covered model 1260, in patients who are active and require a size 8 or 21 mm valve.

Sometimes he finds it necessary to enlarge the aortic root with the use of the cage-ball valve. In the animal laboratory and in the autopsy room, he has experimented with methods of enlarging the annulus. However, in Dr Starr's opinion the annulus itself can not be safely enlarged to accommodate a larger prosthesis in patients with hypoplastic annulus and hypoplastic aortic root. Under these circumstances he attempts to place the largest valve possible in the orifices presented to him and then uses a gusset for the aortic root. This is a relatively simple procedure; if a transverse aortotomy is done it is made high enough so that the lower portion of the incision can be opened down into the non-coronary sinus and a gusset placed into the non-coronary sinus. The transverse aortotomy is then closed using the upper portion of the gusset as part of the aortic wall in that closure. If, on the other hand, it is anticipated beforehand that a gusset will be needed because the angiogram showed a very small aortic root, then Dr Starr would use a longitudinal incision as the initial incision, which is the most commonly used incision, and would close it by suturing in place a patch of very tightly woven Teflon that will not bleed in the heparinised state. He also uses reinforcement with a strip of teflon felt on either side of the suture line when a patch is used because even the needle holes at the base of the aorta will bleed in the heparinised patient.

A.S. *Björk–Shiley valve v. ball-valve prosthesis:* Dr Starr compared the hydraulic performance of a 21 mm Björk–Shiley valve with the standard type of ball-valve prosthesis.

The measured orifice of the 21 mm Björk–Shiley valve is 16 mm across, whereas the orifice of the size 8 ball-valve is only 13·5 mm. Therefore there is a definite difference in the effective orifice of the tilting-disc valve compared to the ball-valve, despite the same external diameter. However, with *in vitro* flow studies, it is found that in the range of flows that correspond to resting cardiac output there is no difference in the gradients across the two prostheses. For that reason, Dr Starr continues to use the ball-valve in smaller sizes, at least at the present time.

Q. *The advantages of the ball-valve:* A question frequently put to Dr Starr is, Why, since he has such sophisticated engineers working in his group, does he persist in using the ball-valve which is a relatively crude type of valvular mechanism?

A.S.   Dr Starr replied that he has been aware of other possibilities, along with everyone else, for many years. He mentioned Glen Morrow as an example, who in the early 1960s developed a prosthesis very similar to Professor Björk's which was not quite so elegant a prosthesis in those days but was an asymetrically tilting-disc valve which hydraulically worked very well in the animal laboratory. Dr Starr made the point that a problem with mechanisms other than the simple ball is that these prostheses are susceptible to interference with the poppet motion by a relatively small amount of thrombus. In all of the reports of these valves, including ordinary disc valves as well as tilting-disc valves, there always is a certain percentage of patients (very small in the beginning) in which there is interference with disc motion as a result of thrombus material and this may produce a catastrophic type of valve failure. This is one reason why Dr Starr's Unit prefer not to use a disc valve although they occasionally do so when the ventricle is quite small.

Another aspect of that problem is that these elegant and sophisticated designs of the tilting-disc variety do not lend themselves well to covering the metallic portions with cloth. A neointima in such valves can easily interfere with the motion of the poppet. The design is thus frozen into a non-cloth-covered or non-healing configuration. In Dr Starr's opinion what should be strived for in the long-term in valve replacement is a prosthesis whose surfaces can be completely hidden from the blood stream so that it acts like the tissue valve yet has the mechanical integrity in long-term function of some of the artificial materials. Therefore, despite the obvious excellent results that can be achieved with other valves, Dr Starr still prefers the ball-valve design.

Q.   *Reoperating for leaks:* Mr Cleland commented on the problem of replacing a leaking valve only to find that the replacement valve also leaks. He asked for details of other people's experience with this problem.

V.B.   Professor Björk described his experience with one patient where it has been necessary to reoperate four times. At each reoperation he has been persistent in placing the patch on the aortic side but has moved the valve higher until at the fourth reoperation he placed it in the aorta. This avoided an abscess in the septum.

I.H.   Mr Hill commented that it is very important never to put a vulcellam forcep across a valve because this pinches the muscle and will start a weak area. He also mentioned that it is dangerous to remove calcium from the ventricular wall as this allows ingress of blood to the ventricular muscle and may cause a dissecting aneurysm.

Q. *Position for aortic prosthesis:* Mr English asked Professor Björk two questions. Firstly, whether he had had any other recorded instances of regurgitation through his prosthesis as was described by Mr Smith in his presentation (Chapter 30) and secondly whether he has a preferred position for placing the aortic prosthesis.

V.B. In answer to the first question Professor Björk replied that there was nothing unusual about the regurgitation reported by Mr Smith. The regurgitation is proportional to the pressure difference across the space. In answer to the second question Professor Björk replied that he puts the valve in the aorta so that the downward portion is in the coronary sinus.

DISCUSSION FOLLOWING TISSUE VALVE REPLACEMENT AND REPAIR SESSION

Mr Donald Ross opened the discussion by discussing the advantages and disadvantages of mechanical valves as compared to homograft valves.

D.N.R. *Mechanical v. homograft valves:* Mr Ross pointed out that valve failure does occur in mechanical valves as it does in homograft valves and since there are many different kinds of mechanical valves some of them must have faults. In addition, since new improved valves are still being produced obviously there remain problems associated with the mechanical valves at present available. One of these problems is that the use of mechanical valves leads to subsequent treatment with anticoagulants which carry a mortality rate of 1% per annum. Furthermore anticoagulants are expensive as are the mechanical valves themselves. Therefore Mr Ross feels that there still remains a place for homograft valves in cardiac surgery.

D.N.R. *Sterilisation of valves:* Following Dr Lockey's presentation Mr Ross made the point that initially when antibiotics were used to sterilise homografts valves, the organisms were only killed in about 20% of the valves. When the Barret–Boyse formula was used 47% of the organisms were killed. Therefore Barrett–Boyse's success lies in the fact that he only used sterile valves.

D.N.R.   *The advantages of biological and mechanical prostheses:* Following Dr Carpentier's presentation Mr Ross pointed out that it seems an obvious and logical development to try and combine the advantages of both biological and mechanical prostheses.

Q.   *Constructive reactions in grafts:* Dr Olsen asked Dr Carpentier whether fibroblast hypoplasia and collagen proliferation applies to the surfaces of the valve or to the actual body of the valve that has been transplanted. In Dr Olsen's experience in histopathology of homografts the proliferation straddles the valve cusps rather than the body.

C.   Dr Carpentier replied that in fact two possibilities exist. The first is that the fibroblast of the grafted cell presents an abnormal metabolism leading to abnormal proliferation in some localised area and, at the same time, areas of alienisation or necrosis. The second possibility is one which affects not only living homografts but also non-living homografts and heterografts. In this case proliferation comes from the host. However in neither case does true regeneration of the valve occur.

Q.   *Mechanical tests on valves:* Mr Longmore asked Dr Carpentier whether he had done any mechanical tests on valves. Mr Longmore described his experience at the National Heart Hospital where in the early days of homograft valves a simple mechanical test was carried out to try and assess various methods of preparing and storing valves. A 2·0 suture was placed 1 mm from the edge of the aorta and then pulled to test the strength of the aorta before tear out took place. Mr Longmore found an enormous range of strengths from 250–1000 g. He also discovered that each step of preparation reduced the strength of the valve and concluded that those valves which appeared to give trouble clinically were those that had very poor tear outs.

C.   Dr Carpentier agreed with Mr Longmore. He commented that it is necessary to try and reach a compromise between the necessity of decreasing the antigenicity of the valve and increasing the stability by increasing the number of cross linkages. However by increasing the number of cross-molecular linkages the resistance of the tissue is decreased due to decreased flexibility. Dr Carpentier is therefore trying to enumerate the optimal number of cross-linkages.

Q.   *Anticoagulation:* Following Dr Williams's presentation, Professor Björk asked whether it is necessary to anticoagulate to prevent thrombosis in the superior vena cava.

B.T.W. Dr Williams replied that in the operative procedure he envisaged inserting the anticoagulants just before the cannulation in the ordinary way and using a preclotted prosthesis. In the long-term there is good animal and human evidence that anticoagulation is not required with this prosthesis.

Q. *The diameter of the human SVC:* Mr Sapsford asked Dr Williams whether he had made any measurements in the human as regards the diameter of the human SVC and the normal mitral valve orifice.

B.T.W. Dr Williams replied that most of his work was done on human cadaver hearts and that he had made measurements which do coincide closely, the human SVC being a remarkably distensible structure.

A.S. *Actuarial analysis:* Dr Starr commented on this method of displaying information. The primary interest in actuarial analysis was to provide accurate information rather than to use it as a means of communication between one group and another. Information of this type is needed to determine the direction and speed of progress. However, the use of actuarial displays for complications rather than deaths is a new technique, which is much more complicated than Dr Starr initially realised. For example, there are problems as in the case of a patient who does not complete a full interval? Dr Starr pointed out that the points on an actuarial are at yearly intervals, but that each year when compiling the curves, there are some patients who haven't finished a year-of additional follow-up. Dr Starr pointed out another problem: what do you do with a patient who needs to be removed from the series, for one reason or another, as in the case of patients following aortic valve replacement with a particular prosthesis? The patient has been reoperated on and now has a new prosthesis – is he counted? Does he continue on that same actuarial curve, or is he removed from the curve? When he is removed from the curve, how is that handled mathematically so as not to skew the curve in any way. A further problem in how to construct these curves was then raised by Dr Starr: what do you do with a patient who has been lost to follow-up? Do you assume that he has had the worst possible result and put him in with the complication group; do you assume that he has had the best possible result and assume he has had no complications because you haven't heard anything about it; or, do you assign to him a median position where you make a basic assumption that he has the same course as other patients in the series who have been followed? This is the assumption that Dr Starr has made in those few patients in his group who are lost to follow-up.

Since these curves are constructed by different groups in different ways, Dr Starr feels it is very important that the techniques used in the construction of the curve be standardised. In his opinion these curves are very important. There are two ways of analysing data, either a direct analysis or an actuarial analysis. A direct analysis does not provide the investigator with all of the information which he could achieve from his pool of patients. For example, when considering late survival, e.g. at five years, of patients undergoing a certain operation, there are only a few patients compared to the total series who have reached that five-year level, but there are many patients who are at the time of the analysis in the second- and third-year level. If any complication occurs in that larger group of patients who are only in the second- and third-year level, that will reflect in the five-year figure when those particular patients reach five years; and if only a direct analysis of the data is carried out the effect on the late results (five or six years later) of an increasing sample occurring in the first few years of the operation will be missed. Therefore, by using a direct analysis only, not as much information is squeezed out of the data as is possible.

Dr Starr then commented on the display of operative mortality in these long-term survival curves. He agreed that they can be misleading if one does not use the slope of the curve to indicate the actual survival of patients. The reason why it is preferable to show the operative mortality is that the operative mortality may skew the late death rate. If there is a group that kills most of the sick patients and has an operative mortality, e.g. with aortic valve replacement, of 12 or 16 ($18°_0$), then the first year survival will be relatively flat, i.e. all the patients who in other centres might have lived through operation and died in the first year or two of life as a late death due to congestive failure or arrhythmia have been killed at the time of operation by that initial group. Therefore, if all the curves start at one month after surgery, then it is hard to tell, as an investigator looking at that curve, what sort of patients have been weeded out of the series by inept surgery and, therefore, seem to give a better late result rate because the sick patients have died. In Dr Starr's opinion if the actuarial technique is not used, and instead a direct analysis is used, then the cohorts have to be considered as individual groups.

Q.   *Leaflet failure for individual cohorts:* Dr Starr then asked Mr Ross what happened to the leaflets of patients who were operated on as a cohort in 1962 and 1963 and in 1964 and what percentage of patients who were operated on in 1963 have their original leaflets in place. He pointed out that he was not asking for the percentages of patients in a total series that have had leaflet failure but for figures referring specifically to that particular cohort, i.e. the exact leaflet failure for individual cohorts operated upon early in the series of aortic valve replacement.

D.N.R.   Mr Ross replied that he didn't attempt to show valve survival as opposed to patient survival. He explained that every year represents a group of patients. When taking, for example, all the patients operated on in 1964, which is 18, and then following the whole group until October 1973, there are two figures, one of which is the patient survival, i.e. all the patients who survived – about 50%. This figure also includes the patients who had another operation and had a prosthetic valve, for example, or another homograft. The second figure is one which represents only the valve survival, which is, if early mortality is included, 32. If the early mortality is excluded, it is about 40–50%. This figure is only for 1964. 1965 is the same – 28 patients followed for nine years – therefore it is possible to know exactly what is happening to patients operated on 10 years ago which is not possible with an actuarial curve which mixes patients operated on in 1964 with those operated on in 1973. The patients operated on in 1973 where there is not a long-term follow-up form a very large group. In this case, exactly 50% survive ten years time. If you compare the two curves, for example the 1964 and 1968 curves, in 1968 there was no late mortality. There was a late failure which is about 10% of the patients who had another operation (a prosthetic valve) and they are fine now. So, patient survival is 100% in five years and the valve survival is 90%.

A.S.   In reply to Mr Ross Dr Starr commented that in his Unit, if a patient has had a different valve put in, they are removed from that actuarial curve because they no longer contribute to the

	survival stakes, or to the group of patients to whom the percentages are relegated, as they now have a different prosthesis.
M.	Mr Martelli pointed out that there is an actuarial curve which relates to valve survival, i.e. patients surviving with the same homograft. In 1968 the figure for valve survival was 90°$_0$.

Q.   *Valve repair:* Following Dr Carpentier's presentation Mr Keith Ross asked for details of the technical problems associated with valve repair and whether Dr Carpentier has ever found it necessary to replace a valve after a conservative operation.

C.   Dr Carpentier replied that he checks the quality of the repair by using saline solution in the left ventricle. In his Unit there is an incidence of about 10–15% of residual minimal insufficiency, but this carries no haemodynamic significance and is due to the fact that the surfaces of the valve are not perfectly smooth leading to the possibility of small leaks.

In reply to Mr Ross' second question Dr Carpentier reported that he had reoperated on four patients but these were not in the pure mitral insufficiency group. In two of the cases the ring was detached in part and in the two other cases reoperation was necessary because the original repair was poorly performed. These two patients did not require immediate reoperation but waited for two and three years respectively.

Q.   *Ruptured chordae:* Dr Carpentier was asked whether he would repair ruptured chordae of any aetiology.

C.   Dr Carpentier replied that he would repair all ruptured chordae, even those due to bacterial endocarditis, if the disease is stabilised as far as the bacteriological problem is concerned.

Q.   Dr Carpentier was then asked whether he would repair chordae that had been ruptured due to degenerative changes.

C.   Dr Carpentier commented that he had never seen recurrent insufficiency after a ruptured chordae repair despite the fact that most of the time these chordae are affected by a process of degenerative change.

DISCUSSION FOLLOWING OPEN HEART SURGERY UNDER ONE YEAR OF AGE SESSION

Q.   *Pulmonary valvotomy:* Mr Waterston opened the discussion with some comments on pulmonary stenosis in a very young infant with a large heart and right ventricle under enormous strain. He remarked that these children with a dilated heart, distended ventricle and minimal shunt at the atrial level used to be considered very bad candidates for bypass and that a quick Brock-type valvotomy used to be the preferred procedure. However, in Mr Waterston's experience, even if a satisfactory valvotomy was performed, the presence of any atrial-septal defect or a blown-open foramen ovalis leads to intractable right-to-left shunt at the atrial level with severe cyanosis shortly after operation. This carries a very high mortality. Mr Waterston asked Mr Rees to comment on this problem.

A.R. Mr Rees replied that in his series all the infants had some form of atrial communication; two had a large ASD and all the others had a patent foramen ovalis. One of the advantages of using cardiopulmonary bypass is that the atrial septal communication can be closed completely. Another advantage lies in the relaxation and immediate pinking that can be achieved by bypass in the case of a dilated and very blue heart. However Mr Rees did not have sufficient evidence to be able to say whether a closed pulmonary valvotomy carries a higher or lower mortality than a bypass procedure.

Q. Mr Waterston then asked Dr Starr for his comments on this problem.

A.S. Dr Starr agreed that this is a difficult problem particularly when it occurs in the first week of life. His experience with a group of valvar atresias in the first week of life has led him to believe that a closed valvotomy done rapidly is a good way of decompressing these ventricles. Sometimes it is very hard to make the initial penetration of the valve because there is no opening but a sharp probe can be successfully used. Although Dr Starr has not had 100% success with this procedure, the autopsy of the one child who died (from a group of five) revealed extreme concentric hypertrophy of the right ventricle in addition to pulmonary atresia. It is Dr Starr's opinion that in a child with such a small ventricular chamber, even relief of valvular stenosis could not ensure survival.

C.L. Mr Lincoln remarked that in his opinion a bypass operation is preferable to a closed valvotomy because many people have noticed when reoperating after a pulmonary valvotomy that the original valvotomy is eccentric.

J.S. On the basis of his experience with closed valvotomies Mr Stark agreed with Mr Lincoln but reported that in one of his

	cases with a right-to-left shunt there was a drop in right ventricular pressure after successful valvotomy. The baby was desaturated to the PO_2 of 20/25. A Rushkin balloon catheter was passed through the left atrium, inflated and then held under some tension. At that point the PO_2 went up to 4/500. Unfortunately in this case a clot formed on the catheter, on the tip of the balloon, and the baby died. Mr Stark therefore feels that the ASD is very important.
A.S.	Dr Starr suggested that the solution lies in considering both types of approach. In his opinion a palliative operation should be carried out on children in the first few days of life and a definitive open operation should be reserved for older children. If pulmonary valve stenosis is encountered in any child over the age of three or four months, he uses an open technique without hesitation as this gives a better anatomical result and avoids second bypass. Dr Starr reported that all the infants operated on in his Unit in the first week of life, using a closed approach, have required a subsequent pulmonary valvotomy.
Q.	*The Bentley oxygenator:* Mr Deverall commented that in his Unit the Bentley oxygenator is used. It is felt that the smaller the priming volume the better and therefore Mr Deverall has tried to use this Q130 but has had difficulties with infants around five kilos. He remarked that in the model used by his Unit the venous inlet is restricted to a quarter of an inch whereas Dr Starr mentioned a venous inlet of three-eighths of an inch. Mr Deverall therefore asked for details of the type of oxygenator being used in Dr Starr's Unit.
A.S.	Dr Starr replied that it is important, even in these very small infants, to have a three-eighths inch line free drainage into the oxygenator. He confirmed that such a size of Bentley oxygenator is available and has been used in Dr Starr's Unit without any evidence of venous drainage obstruction.
W.	Mr Waterston commented that in his Unit a standard type of rotating disc oxygenator is used.
Q.	*Aortagrams:* Mr English asked Dr Starr whether he actually dissects out the aorta and whether he has considered asking his radiological colleagues to do aortagrams.
A.S.	Dr Starr replied that in his opinion aortagrams are preferable but in the overwhelming majority of cases, unless there is a very clear delineation of the ductus area on the supravalvular aortagram, he dissects out the area between the pulmonary

artery and aorta, finds the ligamentum and then just puts a little tie around it. However missing this area results in blood in the operative field.

J.S.   Mr Stark agreed with Dr Starr. He commented that even a good technical aortagram sometimes doesn't visualise the duct and that if the pulmonary artery pressure is at systemic level it is possible to miss it.

W.P.C.   Mr Cleland described his method of locating a duct so that dissection down the aortic arch region can be avoided. He suggested that by pressing the root of the pulmonary artery between the right index finger and thumb while at the same time running the left index finger down over the left pulmonary artery, the immediate fall in pulmonary artery pressure will produce a torrential flow through the duct that can easily be felt.

W.   Mr Waterston suggested that it is sometimes not easy to get a finger and thumb into a week old infant.

Q.   *Right ventricular pressure:* Mr Keith Ross asked Mr Stark what procedure he would adopt if the right ventricular pressure remained high after a good valvotomy.

J.S.   Mr Stark replied that his experience was limited but he had found that a small patch across the valve ring is preferable. He would like to do this in more cases and then see the long-term results before coming to any decision as to the procedure's merits.

Q.   Mr Keith Ross then asked whether Mr Stark ever accepts a high residual right ventricular pressure in the hope that the muscle will involute.

J.S.   Mr Stark described his experience with one case of pulmonary atresia where the pressure in the right ventricle dropped from 180–80 mmHg, i.e. to systemic level. At first the patient did very well and it was thought that the hypertrophy would regress, but the patient then re-stenosed and in six weeks there was complete occlusion in the outflow tract again. Therefore Mr Stark would prefer to place an outflow patch than follow this procedure.

A.S.   Dr Starr pointed out that it is possible to change what is really a simple valvotomy into a major damaging operation on the right ventricle. In his opinion many more infants will be lost by extending the operation into the ventricle than by having to do an occasional reoperation on those patients in whom there isn't regression of the right ventricular hypertrophy.

Q.   *Propanolol:* Mr Parker asked Mr Stark how quickly children admitted with hypoxaemia should be operated upon.

J.S.   Mr Stark pointed out that this is a controversial question; some people consider it necessary to wait for one week, others favour a two-week waiting period. He commented that apparently there is a number of products of propanolol that are still active as blockers and that stay in circulation for a longer time. In Mr Stark's Unit if it is possible they admit the child and then use sedation and an oxygen tent and wait for two weeks. Mr Stark suggested that in the hypoxaemia group, early correction before the child is put on propanolol might solve the problem.

A.S.   Dr Starr pointed out that despite the insistence of pharmacological literature that the effect of propanolol disappears within a few days, surgical experience shows that when patients are operated on a few days after discontinuing propanolol treatment, they need enormous amounts of adrenergic drugs to keep them going. He commented that he hadn't seen this problem in Oregon because infants who have had spells with tetralogy of Fallot are not put on propanolol, since the direct resection of the obstructing muscle can be done so safely. Dr Starr prefers urgent operation in patients who have spells.

Q.   *Multiple VSDs in infants:* Mr Orban asked the panel to describe how they would deal, surgically, with multiple VSDs in very young children. He also asked whether they would prefer to go through the left side.

W.   Mr Waterston replied that the difficulty lies in the diagnosis since the angiocardiography does not clearly demonstrate at this age whether the VSD is multiple. In his opinion children suspected of having multiple VSDs, particularly if these are at the apex and in the right ventricle, should be banded in preference to undergoing direct closure.

A.S.   Dr Starr agreed with Mr Waterston and added that he would also insist on having as perfect a ventriculargram as possible before attacking a VSD by direct closure, in infancy Dr Starr commented that he would band the pulmonary artery but would use an elective time for debanding. Whereas in the past he used to deband older children when they became symptomatic or cyanotic, now he would unband the patient at the age of 12 to

18 months, hopefully before severe pulmonary artery injury ensued.

Q.   *Closure of the VSDs:* Mr Orban asked whether a left ventriculotomy should be used in attempting to close these multiple defects.

W.   Mr Waterston replied that in his opinion closure of the VSDs using a left ventricular approach would carry too high a risk in the case of a very sick infant on bypass. He would therefore perform a right ventriculotomy.

A.S.   Dr Starr agreed with Mr Waterston and added that it is a difficult procedure to find most of the openings from the right side and that this approach requires rather deeply-placed mattress sutures to close the VSD. He went on to describe an interesting approach that his Unit have used. This approach involves reattaching the entire anterior septum, with multiple perforations all along the attachment at the septum, to the entry wall. The defect is closed by passing deeply placed mattress sutures through the posterior lip of the septum and then out through the wall of the heart. The sutures are then tied on the outside of the heart in much the same way as a ventricular septum ruptured from a myocardial infarction might be repaired. Dr Starr feels that this approach effectively takes care of quite a few separate defects all lined at the attachment of the anterior septum at the entry of the free wall of the heart.

J.S.   Mr Stark commented that his Unit have been using this technique – Waterston's knitting technique – for a number of years. In his opinion closure of multiple VSDs in older children is very difficult and therefore he would probably use the banding technique in these cases.

Q.   *Transposition of the great arteries:* Mr Mutra asked Dr Starr what sort of approach he would use to close the VSD in correct transposition of the great arteries.

A.S.   Dr Starr replied that he had done a few through the anterior right ventricle and that his youngest case of transposition – about 10 weeks – operated on using this approach, survived. Dr Starr remarked that the patient seemed to tolerate an incision in the anterior systemic ventricle.

DISCUSSION FOLLOWING POSTOPERATIVE CARE SESSION

Dr Starr opened the discussion by expressing interest in Mr Deverall's paper concerning osmolar balance in children. He suggested that in the light of Mr Deverall's information, much of the postoperative discomfort of these patients, which is due to restricted fluids, may be unnecessary. He also commented on the use of computers in managing data in the cardiac recovery rooms and pointed out that this does not seem to interfere with the primary nursing function once it is under .way.

Q.   *Bryn Williams' flow probe:* Mr Lincoln asked the audience in general for details of individual experience with the Bryn Williams' flow probe.

A speaker from Oslo replied that his Unit had used it in 10 cases and found it satisfactory.

B.T.W.   Dr Williams pointed out that there was little zero drift on any of the traces he had shown in his presentation. He explained that there are certain things about blood flow measurement which one needs to pay attention to whether one is using an extractable probe of this kind or any other kind of electro-magnetic flow probe. For example, it is important to get a tight fit on the vessel and to get the electrodes clean. Dr Williams suggested that careful attention to these points would probably give a fairly stable zero, but he pointed out that it is necessary to use a compatible flowmeter and that the unit was specifically designed for the Carolina Medical Electronics flowmeter.

Q.   *Systolic displacement of the probe:* Dr Starr asked Dr Williams if he could explain how to prevent systolic displacement of the probe and therefore ensure a more stable reading.

B.T.W.   Dr Williams replied that the probe is fixed in position using a nylon snare with a rubber outer sheath, which keeps the probe firmly closed around the aorta whilst it is in place. It passes out alongside the probe cable to the exterior of the patient and can be released prior to the removal of the probe.

Q.   *Left ventricular function curves:* Mr Parker referred to the work done by Dr Bradley and Dr Culsson. He pointed out that Dr Bradley's function curves were very flat in the postoperative period and asked why it is necessary to keep the atrial pressure raised at 15 mmHg when this doesn't result in any great increase in ventricular function. Mr Parker also asked whether the curves show any changes during the postoperative period.

R.B.   Dr Bradley replied that very flat function curves are only seen in patients in a critical condition and in these cases, running them at a higher filling pressure doesn't make a great deal of difference. However patients in a less serious condition with good function curves, who raise their stroke output with increased filling pressure, may improve on a slightly higher filling pressure. In reply to the second question Dr Bradley reported that all the function curves were recorded during the first night after operation and that he had no evidence to show whether the curves change or not during the postoperative period. He went on to say that as far as compliance is concerned he has found the relationship between intramural pressure and diameter a very complicated one which depends on when during the cardiac cycle it is measured. Also Dr Bradley feels that the cavity pressure is not the same thing as the transmural pressure and he points out that in any case, Starling's law depends on fibre length rather than pressure. Therefore Dr Bradley takes a greater interest in the dimension rather than the pressure but feels that the relationship between the two is very complex and unpredictable.

Peripheral temperature measurement: A speaker from Leeds commented on the use of peripheral temperature measurement as an aid to postoperative care as described by Dr Matthews. He pointed out that it should be remembered that the environmental temperature and atmospheric humidity conditions of intensive care units in different parts of the world vary.

Q.   *Thermodilution:* Mr Keith Ross asked Mr Rees for his opinion on the future of thermodilution techniques in measuring cardiac output in children.

R.   Mr Rees replied that in his opinion thermodilution is a simple technique which seems to correlate with the Fick principle. Mr Rees intends to continue to use it until he has proof that it is of no use in the postoperative period.

A.S.   Dr Starr commented that in his Unit thermodilution techniques had been found to be very helpful in measuring cardiac output when dealing with very sick patients. He pointed out that when using these techniques it is easy to detect a markedly low cardiac index, e.g. $1 \cdot 8$ litres/m^2 body surface/min and then it is possible to increase the blood volume and bring the cardiac index up to $2 \cdot 5$ or $2 \cdot 8$ litres/m^2 body surface/min, which is compatible with

	survival. Dr Starr also reported that his Unit have not used thermodilution techniques in small children.
R.	Mr Rees pointed out that a low cardiac index, e.g. less than 1·5 litres, is of prognostic value but that figures in higher ranges had no bearing on the mortality or the prognosis of patients.
D.P.	*Devices apparatus:* David Preston, an ex-member of the Clinical Measurement Department at Westminster, commented that this department has used the Devices apparatus for taking measurements during the rewarm period of very tiny children. He went on to raise two points. Firstly he pointed out that the cardiac output in these cases is very small so that it only reaches the first graduation on the apparatus. It is possible to give half the dose so that when the dose is divided by area, the area is half the size and the needle is pushed up away from zero, but Mr Preston did not find this particularly valuable. Secondly he pointed out that the technique requires a certain amount of skill. However in general Mr Preston found the Devices apparatus quite satisfactory in all cases but very small babies.
R.B.	Dr Bradley pointed out that the Devices machine had been designed specifically for adults and it would be necessary to adjust it to make it suitable for children. He went on to explain that in order to get good curves it is necessary that each output determination be the mean of the five squirts of cold, and for reproducable values it may be necessary to take over one hundred measurements of cardiac output in three or four hours. This involves injecting a lot of sugar water and although smaller volumes are injected in children it still may not be possible to take so many readings.
Q.	Mr Lincoln asked Mr Silove for his comments.
E.S.	Mr Silove reported that he has had a lot of difficulty using thermodilution techniques to measure cardiac output in infants and children. He has found that the amount injected has to be so small that it is difficult to compensate for the amount of heat taken up by the indicator from the body while the indicator is passing through the catheter. If larger volumes are injected through a larger catheter as in the case of adults then this problem does not arise.

DISCUSSION FOLLOWING ISCHAEMIC HEART DISEASES SESSION

The discussion was opened by Dr Lennox who asked for questions and comments.

Q.   *Endarterectomy:* Dr Matthews asked for details of any experience with angiographies after endarterectomy.

C.H.   Professor Hahn replied that his Unit had done a small number of angiographies after endarterectomies and found a percentage of patency which was five times higher in the endarterectomised patients than in the others. Professor Hahn pointed out that the number of patients involved was small and therefore the result is perhaps not significant. However it does mean that the patency rate of this type of patient is as good as that of other types.

Q.   Mr Parker asked Professor Hahn whether he decides to do an endarterectomy on the basis of the angiographic appearance or whether he explores the vessel first. Mr Parker then asked Professor Hahn to describe the indications for an endarterectomy which are revealed by vessel exploration.

C.H.   Professor Hahn explained that in his Unit sometimes it is decided to do an endarterectomy before operation but in most cases the vessel is opened and if there are diffuse lesions an endarterectomy is carried out regardless of the size of the vessel. Dr Hahn remarked that when measuring flows after this latter procedure the quality of the results is surprising, with flow rates of up to 150 ml/min.

Q.   Mr Yacoub asked Professor Hahn whether he uses gas when performing an endarterectomy and for details of the indications for operation in patients who did not have aneurysmectomy. Were these patients operated on purely for angina with a good left ventricular function or for congestive failure with angina?

C.H.   Professor Hahn replied that he had no experience with gas endarterectomies. In answer to the second part of Mr Yacoub's question Professor Hahn reported that he had performed endarterectomies in patients where the peripheral vascular bed was very poor, left ventricular function was bad and there had been one or more infarctions.

S.C.L.   Mr Lennox commented that it is difficult to define just what is operable and what is inoperable.

A.S.   In Dr Starr's opinion cardiac surgeons have to decide between the different causes of inoperability in the right coronary artery.

For example, Dr Starr does not think there are many inoperable right dominant coronary arteries. It is usually possible either to do a vein graft or to do an endarterectomy. Dr Starr pointed out that the worse the right coronary artery and the stiffer the core, the easier it is to reconstitute what looks like a normal right coronary system. He added that many of those patients with occluded right coronary arteries have total infarction of the diaphragmatic surface and the amount of retrograde flow, once the core is removed, can be enormous. Dr Starr explained that he is not as familiar with endarterectomy on the left side as his Unit have done only a few cases, but he feels that perhaps there are vessels on the left side that are inoperable. In his opinion the inoperable cases are determined by myocardial factors and the patient with massive cardiomegaly and no angina is probably inoperable, as are patients who have massive infarctions and shock, although it is possible to keep these patients alive with balloon pumping. However Dr Starr pointed out that his Unit is too busy to take on patients who have already lost 60–70 % of the myocardium and suggested that operability be defined primarily in myocardial terms.

Q. *Bypass grafts:* Mr Rees asked Dr Starr to elaborate on his technique of bypass grafts. He asked Dr Starr whether the aorta is cross-clamped and if so how is this effected in the situation of mitral multiple vein grafts.

A.S. Dr Starr replied that he used to use a left ventricular vent and operate on the fibrillating heart, using snares around the vessel. He commented that the method of intermittent aorta cross-clamping without a vent has a great deal to recommend it. Dr Starr went on to describe his most recent technique which involves clamping the aorta and doing a distal anastomosis during the cross-clamping which produces a period of ischaemia varying in time from 10 to 15 mins. It is very rare for this period to be longer than 15 mins. This provides an absolutely perfect field without any danger of injury by using snares. Then Dr Starr defibrillates the heart. He takes the clamp off the aorta, defibrillates the heart and allows the heart to beat for a while. While the heart is beating a proximal anastomosis is carried out with a side-biting clamp. Therefore after each period of ischaemia, there is a period of not only cardiac perfusion but perfusion in the beating heart. In Dr Starr's opinion this is very important as it provides complete resuscitation and under these circumstances it is possible to do a large number of grafts without fear of myocardial injury since the heart is resuscitated after each graft. Dr Starr pointed out that not using a vent is a very important part of this technique because this means that there is no way the air can get inside the heart. In the absence of air in the heart it is easy to defibillate without fear of air embolism and to have a beating heart in between each distal anastomosis.

Q.   Mr Lennox asked Dr Starr whether the reason for putting the aortic on second is that if it is put on first the heart resuscitates immediately when grafted.

A.S.   Dr Starr replied that in his opinion it could be done either way but that he prefers to do the distal anastomosis as the second part of the procedure.

W.P.C. *LV aneurysms and bypass grafting:* Mr Cleland commented that initially his attitude had been coloured by the reported results of bypass grafting and resection of aneurysms. His experience at that time was that coronary bypass grafting alone was carrying a mortality of 5% and LV aneurysm resection a mortality of 10–12%, the combined mortality therefore being 20–25%. Mr Cleland therefore elected to concentrate on LV aneurysms alone. This decision was probably also influenced by the fact that many doctors at that time were reluctant to do coronary arteriography and LV resections for fear of dislodging a clot.

Q.   A speaker from Leeds asked Mr Cleland whether his patients suffered from anginal pain and whether this was relieved by aneurysmectomy.

W.P.C. Mr Cleland replied that only a minority of patients suffered pain, the prime indication being LV failure. He pointed out that the patients with pain are those that ought to be investigated as they probably have a graftable vessel.

Q.   *Intra-aortic balloon pump:* Dr Melrose asked Mr Donnelly to explain the importance of the balloon pump.

R.J.D. Mr Donnelly replied that in his opinion the use is established in post bypass cases where patients will not come off bypass despite full medical treatment and every kind of support. The use of the balloon pump is not yet established in cases with acute complications of the myocardial infarction although it has saved some patients with cardiogenic shock following myocardial infarction. However Mr Donnelly pointed out that this group has to be more clearly identified and that the time from the infarct to the shock, and the duration of the shock is of importance in this respect. With regard to other complications the use of the balloon pump has not yet been evaluated, but Mr Donnelly feels that it does give a greater degree of safety and allows time to stabalise the patient and to reverse cardiogenic shock in the majority of cases. It has also been proved to be of use in cardiac catheterisation and angiography and makes the induction of anaesthetic more safe. Therefore in Mr Donnelly's opinion it can be of use postoperatively in quite a number of these very ill patients.

Q.   Dr Wade asked Mr Donnelly what is meant by the low-volume left ventricle.

R.J.D.   Mr Donnelly explained that this refers to a big thick-walled left ventricle with a small chamber. This type of ventricle has a high oxygen consumption and the balloon pump diminishes the oxygen consumption and gives the ventricle time to recover.

Q.   *Support therapy:* Mr Cleland asked Mr Donnelly in what proportion of patients there arises the problem of having to decide whether to discontinue balloon pumping in order to allow the machine to be used by a waiting patient. He also asked Mr Donnelly how many machines each Unit would need to acquire to avoid this situation.

R.J.D.   Mr Donnelly explained that the cost of the machine – about £6500 – would probably limit the number per Unit in this country to two. Obviously this limited number of machines would lead to the problem described by Dr Cleland. Mr Donnelly therefore stressed that further work on identifying the patients able to come to surgery or to come off the balloon by themselves is needed.

Q.   *Long-term results:* Mr Rees asked Mr Donnelly for details of the long-term results of these patients and whether there is a close correlation between the extent of myocardial damage, the extent of their shock and the requirement for balloon pumping.

R.J.D.   Mr Donnelly replied that he didn't think there was sufficient long-term data to be able to answer the question. However in Mr Donnelly's opinion, it is the amount of residual functioning in the left ventricle after surgery that determines whether or not the patient will survive.

Q.   *Femoral vessels:* Dr Bricco asked Mr Donnelly to enumerate

the cases where it was not possible to fibrillate the femoral
vessels.

R.J.D. Mr Donnelly replied that he did not know the exact number but
that over a period of four years it was still in single figures.

Q. *Renal flow:* Dr Bricco then asked Mr Donnelly whether he had
observed that renal problems are associated with use of a pump.
Dr Bricco described his experimental work which shows that
renal flow definitely decreases with the use of a pump.

R.J.D. Mr Donnelly explained that he had no experience of the data-
scope system being used by Dr Bricco, but that in his opinion
this system might prejudice the renal vessels because it has an
occluding balloon.

M.Y. Mr Yacoub commented that in all his patients on balloon
pumps urinary output immediately improved. This included
one patient who was known to be in chronic renal failure, had
a ruptured intraventricular septum and went into acute renal
failure. This patient had a blood urea of 300 but started
diuresing immediately after being put on the balloon pump.
Therefore in Mr Yacoub's opinion the increase in cardiac
output more than compensates for any drop in renal flow due
to occlusion.

R.J.D. Mr Donnelly suggested that the size of the balloon is perhaps
important and that if a large balloon is put into a small man,
this could occlude the aorta.

M.Y. Mr Yacoub suggested that occlusion of the aorta is desirable
to enable maximum augmentation during diastole and under-
loading of the ventricle. For this reason Mr Yacoub's Unit use
30 and 35 cc balloon pumps all the time. In Mr Yacoub's
opinion studying renal flows in experimental normal animals has
no bearing on the clinical situation where the patients have very
low cardiac outputs. In these patients balloon pumping results
in increased cardiac output which in turn leads to improved
renal circulation. However, in an experimental animal with a
healthy cardiac output, occlusion of the aorta could lead to a
decrease of renal flow.

R.J.D. Mr Donnelly added that in his opinion the major benefit of
balloon pumping is in reducing myocardial oxygen consumption,
thereby reducing the work of the heart. It also has the additional
benefit of diastolic augmentation.

M.Y. Mr Yacoub pointed out that when coronary flow of main
grafts is measured it is found to have almost doubled. Therefore,

apart from reducing myocardial oxygen consumption by reducing end diastolic pressure and shortening isometric ventricular systole, balloon pumping definitely improves myocardial oxygenation.

Q.　　*Mitral insufficiencies:* Dr Melrose asked Mr Yacoub whether he had used a pump on his series of mitral insufficiencies.

M.Y.　Mr Yacoub replied that all the mitral patients were operated on about three years ago and in none of them was a pump used. A pump was used on the ruptured ventricular septum in three patients all of whom improved. One of these patients was on a pump for 16 days and another for 13 days; both were operated on successfuly afterwards.

Q.　　*Arrhythmias:* Dr Melrose asked Mr Donnelly to describe how patients with severe arrhythmias are managed.

R.J.D.　Mr Donnelly replied that in his opinion if it is not possible to control the arrhthymias then it is not advisable to balloon pump patients with the Avco system. He suggested that perhaps another system may be better in dealing with arrhthymias. Mr Donnelly commented that it is essential to control arrhthymias in some way or another even if it is just by pacing them quite fast. He explained that the advantage of helium is that it moves so much faster that it can cope with much faster heart rates – 170–180 beats/min. Mr Donnelly stressed the importance of attempting to establish a regular or relatively regular heart beat.

M Y.　Mr Yacoub pointed out that it is not possible to achieve a regular heart beat in a patient with established atrial fibrillation. He commented that in his Unit this difficulty of irregular fast heart beat in patients requiring balloon support is surmounted by pumping 2 : 1. Mr Yacoub added that he thought this was also possible with the Avco system where there can be deflation pressures dictation so that any QRS will trigger premature deflation of the balloon, thus avoiding a dangerous situation. Mr Yacoub pointed out that although this is not as effective as 1 : 1 augmentation, it will follow the irregular heart beat, particularly 2 : 1.

R.J.D.　Mr Donnelly suggested that it is possible to pace these patients with established atrial fibrillation by digitalising them as heavily as is necessary to restore a regular heart beat.

Index

Absorption, conal 49, 50, 52, 54
Accelerated angina 381, 384
Acid–base balance (monitoring circulation) 331
Acidosis 464, 465
Actinomycin D 36
Acute mitral regurgitation 422–425
Acute myocardial infarctions 370
  balloon pumping 410
  infarctectomy 413, 414
Acute renal damage 331
Acute VSD 428, 429
Advertising for donors 13
Agenesis of the pulmonary valve 444, 445
  Angiogram 443
Allografts 18, 19
  HLA compatability 18
Anaesthesia
  open-heart surgery in infants 298
  total anomalous pulmonary venous damage 308
Anastamosis; see Shunting
Aneurysmal dilations 437, 439, 440
Amneurysmectomy 387–391
  ventricular aneurysm 415–419, 485
Angina 367–372,
  accelerated 381, 384
  aortic valve replacement 385
  chronic disabling 381–385
Angiocardiography
  Carpentier–Edwards xenografts 249
  Fallot's tetralogy 62–68, 81, 86
Angiography 43, 45, 373
  agenesis of the pulmonary valve 443
  Elema angiograms 63
  Fallot's tetralogy 62–69, 84, 85 97
Annulus dilation 279–282, 285

Annulus lesions, mitral 279–282
Antibiotics
  Hank's solution 210–212, 221
  homograft sterilisation 209–218, 221, 255, 266
Antibodies
  enhancement 456, 457
  vessel lesions 20–26
  xenograft recipients 251
Anticoagulants 36, 38, 41, 156, 157, 159, 167, 168, 200, 210, 204, 247, 257, 267, 409–411
Antigens
  HLA matching 14–19
  xenografts 250, 251
Anti-inflammatory drugs 25
Antilymophocyte globulin 36, 41, 43
Antiplatlet drugs 25, 26
Anturan 25
Aorta
  aorta to left ventricular tunnel 442, 443
  coarctation of 435, 436
Aortagrams 476, 477
Aortic flow readings 351–355
Aortic homografts 209–214, 234, 245
  autograft fascia lata 272–274, 276, 277
  inverted 127, 129
  isolated 241–243
  mortality 257
  pulmonary switch operation 239–254
Aortic prosthesis, composite seat 151–153
  Starr—Edwards 192–195, 200
Aortic regurgitation 340
Aortic root, small 466, 467
Aortic stenosis
  Björk—Shiley tilting disc valve

168–170
congenital 435
correction of 320, 321
open-heart surgery 294
surgical results 435
Aortic valve
Autografts 234–245
Carpentier—Edwards xenograft 247–249
homografts; *see* Homografts
mechanics of 123, 124
porcine 246–251
replacement; *see* Aortic valve replacement
Starr—Edwards composite seat prosthesis 192–195
Aortic valve replacement 179–191
angina 385
Björk—Shiley tilting disc valve 160–178
cardiac index 135, 136
intra-aortic balloon pump 406–411
myocardial preservation during 133–143
Aorto-coronary bypass surgery 374–380
endarterectomy 379, 380
mammary artery 379
Arrhythmias 317, 488
balloon pumping 410
infarctectomy 413
Arteriography 368
coronary 383, 384
Arterio-venous O_2 difference 331
Artery disease, coronary; *see* Coronary artery disease
Aspirin 167, 168
Atheroma 22
Atherosclerosis 41–43
Atrial electromyogram 30, 31, 35, 36
Atrial pressure measurement 337, 338
Atrioventricular conduction tissue 59
Auriculo-ventricular block 111, 112
Autografts (aortic valve) 234–245
Autologous tissue 219, 260–270, 272–277
Automation (postoperative care) 357–362
Avcothane 406
Azathioprine 36, 41
vessel lesions 25

Balloon-dependence 408, 409
Balloon pumping 406–411, 485–488
cardiogenic shock 408, 409
intra-aortic balloon pump 406–411, 485, 486
MGH–Avco balloon pump 406–411
mitral incompetence 409, 410
mortality 409
Balloon septostomy 312
Ball-valve prosthesis 467, 468
cage ball prosthesis 144–159
Basic fuchsin staining 402, 403
Bentley oxygenator 298, 476
Bilateral endarterectomy 392
Biliary drainage (transplanted organs) 9, 10
Bioprosthesis 222, 249, 250
Biopsies
endomiocardial 456
serial 32–35
Bioptomes 32–35
Konno—Sakakibari 32–34
Björk—Shiley tilting disc valve 127, 129, 160–178, 191, 196, 202–205, 451, 467
aortic stenosis 168–170
complications 175–178, 202
durability of 160, 161
gradient across valve 164, 165
haemolysis 160–164, 204
infections 175
mortality 202, 204
orientation 176, 178, 465, 466
paraprosthetic leaks 161, 162, 168
regurgitation 166, 167, 202
small aortic root 466
thromboembolism 167–172, 174, 175, 204
Blalock—Taussig shunt 71, 104, 110, 445–447, 461
Blood, filtering 299
Blood flow
coronary index 139
electromagnetic flow meters 347–355, 396
electromagnetic flow probe 347–349, 396–400

parameter (monitoring circulation) 330, 331

Williams–Barefoot flow probe 347–349, 396–400

Blood gas analysis (computers) 359, 360

Braunwald Cutter valve 200, 201, 206

Brock procedure 73–77, 104, 110

Bundle of His 443

Bypass, coronary 381–385

Bypass grafts 484, 485

Bypass surgery, cardiac 38, 39
aorto-coronary; *see* Aorto-coronary bypass surgery
Brock procedure 75
cardiopulmonary; *see* Cardiopulmonary bypass
Fallot's tetralogy 70
surface cooling 97

Cage ball prosthesis 144–159
emboli, incidence of 144–147, 153, 156
mortality 146–148
reoperation 151, 153

Calcification
Carpentier—Edwards xenografts 249, 250
homograft tissue valve 265
mitral valve 282, 283, 287

Cannulation 31, 312, 313

Cardiac bypass surgery; *see* Bypass surgery, cardiac

Cardiac catheterisation 62, 63, 86, 90, 91, 93, 98–100
stress tests 372
valvar stenosis 319, 320
ventricular septal defects 303

Cardiac index (aortic valve replacement) 135, 136

Cardiac output (monitoring circulation) 331, 344–346

Cardiac valves, design characteristics of 123–126

Cardiac volume (revaluation after correction) 111, 116

Cardial decomposition 168

Cardiogenic shock (balloon pump) 408, 409

Cardiopulmonary bypass 92, 93, 4

aortic valve replacement 134–136

atrial pressure measurements 337, 338

balloon pumping 409

mortality 300, 301

open-heart surgery in infants 293, 295, 299–301

right ventriculotomy 429, 430

ventricular aneurysm 415

Cardiothoracic ratio (CTR) 265

Carotid artery, intimal thickening of 21–25

Carpentier—Edwards xenografts 247–250
calcification 249, 250
complications 247–250
histological examination 249, 250
mortality 247
reoperation 249, 250

Catecholamines 296, 314

Cavitation in the preserving media 456

Cells, myocardial
damage 401–404
necrosis 134, 137, 138, 140, 142, 403, 404

Chest X-ray
coronary artery disease 372
intra-aorta balloon pump 407

Cholecystocholedocostomy 10

Chordae tendinae 283–285

Chronic disabling angina 381–385

Chronic mitral regurgitation 423, 425

Cineangiogram (rheumatic mitral valve stenosis) 341, 342

Cloth-covered prosthesis 144–159, 187, 188, 196
cloth tear 148, 149 153, 154
Starr—Edwards 142–145

Coagulation
anticoagulants; *see* Anticoagulants
liver transplants 9

Coarctation of the aorta 435, 436

Collagen degeneration 220–223

Commissure enlargement 279–282

Commissure fusion 283

Commissurotomy 284–286

Compatability (HLA antigens) 14–19

Complications

Björk—Shiley tilting disc valve 175–178, 202
Carpentier—Edwards xenografts 247–250
  homograft replacement 257, 258
  intra-aorta balloon pump 407
  mitral valve replacement 196, 197
  pulmonary switch operation 239–245
  Starr—Edwards composite seat prosthesis 193, 198, 199
  tissue valve replacement 268
  total anomalous pulmonary venous drainage 310
  transposition of the great arteries 316, 317
  ventricular septal defect correction 306
Composite seat aortic prosthesis 151–153
  Starr–Edwards 192–195, 200
Composite seat-trace prosthesis 154
Computer in postoperative care 357–362
Conal absorption 49, 50, 52, 54
Conal invertion (Fallot's tetralogy) 49–52, 60
Concealed haemorrhage 334
Conduits, homograft 118–120
Congenital aortic stenosis (surgical results) 435
Congenital coronary artery disease (surgical results) 436–442
Conoventricular flange (CVF) 54–56
Conus septum 49–51, 54, 55, 60, 62, 63, 89, 103, 459
Cooley's operation 78
Cooling, surface; *see* Surface cooling
Coronary artery disease 38, 381–386
  arteriography 383, 384
  congenital 436–442
  electrocardiography 372
  endarterectomy 386–394
  surgical results 437–442
Coronary blood flow index 139
Coronary bypass operation 381–385
Coronary endarterectomy 379, 380, 386–394, 483, 484
  bilateral 392
  gas 379

left coronary artery 391–392
Mortality 386–394
  right coronary artery 387–391
  triple 393
Coronary insufficiency 370
Coronary perfusion 133–143
Correction
  age-weight relationship 95, 97
  cardiac volume 111, 116
  growth patterns in infants after 98
  indications for 103, 104
  mentation measurements 92, 93
  shuntings *see* Shunting
  total (Fallot's tetralogy) 85, 86, 91–93, 103–116
  total (in infants) 95–102
  ventriculograms 102
Coumadin 156
Creatine phosphokinase (CPK) 134, 137–140, 142
Crista supraventricularis 52, 53, 459
Cyanosis
  Fallot's tetralogy 62, 66, 67, 74, 86, 87, 97, 104
  valvar stenosis 319
Cyclophosphamide 36
Cyproheptadine 26
Cytochrome oxidase 402

Dacron 118–120, 200, 247, 254, 317, 407, 415, 447–449
Death
  definition of cerebral (France) 40, 41
  see also Mortality
Dehydrogenase 401, 402
Delrin prosthetic disc 160, 167, 172, 176, 205
Design characteristics
  cage ball prosthesis 144–159
  heart valves 123–126
Devices apparatus 345, 482
Dextrose 325, 344
Diagnosis of rejection episodes 31, 32, 35
Diastolic murmurs 239, 247, 249, 262, 267
Diastolic pressure time index (DPTI) 137, 139
Dieumarol 167, 169

Digoxin 296, 302, 306, 314
Dilatation, annulus 279–282, 285
Diparydimol 36, 38
Direct revascularisation of the myocardium 386
Diuretics 296, 302, 306, 314, 331
Donors 40, 41, 458
  advertising for 13
  availability of 12–14
  Eurotransplant 12, 14
  related (HLA matching) 17
  reluctance of 12, 13
  selection of 40, 41
Drainage, Biliary 9, 10
Durability
  Björk—Shiley tilting disc valve 160, 161
  tissue valves 219–222
Dypnoea 372
Dysfunction (homografts) 263, 264

Ebstein's disease 450–452
Echocardiography
  left ventricular pressure and dimension 339
  mitral valve replacement 127–132
  Starr—Edwards prosthesis 129–131
Ejection fraction, left ventricular 90, 91
Elastins 221
Electrocardiography
  aortic valve replacement 140, 141
  coronary artery disease 372
  homograft tissue valves 264, 265
  rejection 29, 31, 35, 36
  total correction of Fallot's tetralogy 111, 112
Electromagnetic flowmeters 347–355, 396
Electromagnetic flow probes, Williams—Barefoot 347–349, 396–400
Electromyogram, atrial 30, 31, 35, 36
Elema-angiograms 63
Elongation in vena cava 226
Embolism, incidence of
  cage ball prosthesis 144–147, 153, 156
  homograft operation 239
Starr—Edwards prosthesis 192, 193, 197
  ventricular aneurysm 415
Embryogenesis of Fallot's tetralogy 49–51
Endarterectomy, coronary; see Coronary endarterectomy
Endocarditis, infective 260–262, 266, 274
Endomyocardial biopsy 456
Enhancement 456, 457
Ergometry after total correction of Fallot's tetralogy 112
Erythromycin lactobionate 215
Eurotransplant 12, 14
Evolution of grafts 222–224
Exchange of organs 14
Exercise, effect on valve mechanism 124
Exercise test, preoperative 372, 373

Failure of Homograft tissue valves 263, 264, 267
Fallot's tetralogy
  angiocardiography 62–68, 81, 86
  angiography 62–69, 84, 85, 97
  Blalock—Taussig shunt 71, 72, 445–447, 461
  cardiac volume after correction 111, 116
  categorising patients 86, 87
  classification of 104
  clinical features of 62
  conal inversion 49–52, 60
  conoventricular flange (CVF) 54–56
  cyanosis 62, 66, 67, 74, 86, 87, 97, 104
  development of 49, 103
  electrocardiography after correction 111, 112
  embryogenesis 49–51
  ergometry after correction 112
  Glenn operation 444–449
  haemodynamics after correction 112–115
  Heart block 89
  Infants, total correction in 95–102
  kinking, pulmonary artery 81–83
  management of 84–94
  mentation measurements 92, 93

mortality 69, 70, 86
natural history of 86
palliation of 69, 70, 104, 110, 460, 461
Potts operation 444–449
pulmonary infundibulum 53–56, 62–64, 66
pulmonary insufficiency 92
reoperation 107
revaluation after correction 109–116
surgery technique 87–89
surgical results 445–449
total correction of 85, 86, 91–93, 103–116
ventriculography 102
Waterston shunt 78–83, 85, 445, 446, 460, 461

Fascia lata valves 219, 260–270, 272–277
Fat globules 402
Femoral vessels 486, 487
  vein grafts 374
  Fick method (measuring cardiac output) 334–346, 481
Filtering blood 299
Fistulae 437–442
Flow meters; see Blood flow
Flow parameters (monitoring circulation) 330, 331
Fluid balance (computers) 360, 361
Foetal tissue 5
Foley catheter 174
Formaldehyde 246, 261
France 40–45
Freeze-dried grafts 235–237
Frustrum (fascia lata) 272, 273

Gas analysis, blood (computers) 359, 360
Gas endarterectomy 379
Gentamicin 215, 217
Glenn operation 445–449
Glutaraldehyde 219, 221–224, 261
  xenografts 223, 224, 246, 250
Glycogen depletion 401, 403
Glycoproteins 221, 222
Goor's observations 459
Grafts

bypass 484, 485
evolution of 222–224
freeze-dried 235–237
preparation of 219–222
survival of 17, 18
Growth patterns in infants after total correction 98

Haematoxylin-basic-fuchsin-picric-acid stain (HBFP) 402, 403
Haemodynamics
  cardiac catheterisation in VSD 303
  cardiogenic shock (balloon pumping 408
  Fallot's tetralogy, total correction of 112–115
  homograft tissue valves 265, 266, 268
  mitral valve replacement 259, 265–267
Haemolysis
  Björk—Shiley tilting disc valve 160–164, 204
  homograft operation 239, 262, 263
  mitral valve replacement 148, 155, 156
  Starr—Edwards prosthesis 184, 192, 193
Haemorrhage, concealed 334
Halothane 298
Hancock Laboratories valve 250
Hank's solution (antibodies) 210–212, 221
Hartman's solution (vessel leaks) 374
Heart block (Fallot's tetralogy) 89
Helium 407, 488
Heparin 38
High pulmonary vascular resistance 39
Histocompatibility 41
Histological examination
  Carpentier—Edwards xenografts 249, 250
  homograft tissue valves 264
  myocardial cell damage 401–404
  serial biopsies 32–35
HLA matching 14–19
  antigens 14–19
  graft survival 17, 18
Homografts 469, 470

antibiotics 209–218, 221, 255, 266
aortic valve replacement 234–245
calcification 265
complications 257, 258
conduits 118–120
dysfunction 263, 264
emboli, incidence of 239
evolution of 222, 223
haemolysis 239, 262, 263
inverted aortic 127, 129
isolated aortic 241–243
mitral valve replacement 253–259
mortality 255–258, 260, 261
reconstruction of outflow tract 97, 98, 100, 117–122
sterilisation of 209–218, 253, 266, 469, 470
storage of 209–214, 220, 221
tissue valve preparation 219–224
viability of 211–213, 253
Hyalinization 222, 223
Hypernephroma 7
Hyperperfusion (pulmonary artery) 83
Hypertension, pulmonary; *see* Pulmonary hypertension
Hyponatraemia, plasma 325, 236
Hypo-osmolality, plasma 326–328
Hypoplasia (pulmonary artery) 83, 103, 110, 435, 436
Hypothermia
  Kyoto technique 312
  Mustard's operation 312
  open-heart surgery 293, 295, 298
  profound hypothermic non-perfusion arrest 133–143
  surface cooling; *see* Surface cooling
Hypothermic non-perfusion arrest (HNPA) 133–143

Immunisation 18, 19
Immunosuppression 20, 25–27, 36, 37
  ECG changes during rejection 29, 31, 32, 35
  older patients 39
  postoperative infection 37,38
Impending myocardial infarction (balloon pumping) 410
Imuran 43
Indications for correction of Fallot's tetralogy 103, 104
Indocyanine green dye 349, 351

Infarctectomy 413, 414
Infections, postoperative
  Björk—Shiley tilting disc valve 175
  cage ball prosthesis 144–147, 151
  coronary artery disease 38
  endocarditis 260–262, 266, 274
  homograft operations 239
  pulmonary 37, 38
  Starr—Edwards Prosthesis 182
  total correction after Fallot's tetralogy 106
Inflammatory reactions in xenografts 223
Infundibular stenosis 97, 102–104, 106, 110
Insufficiency
  coronary 370
  mitral valve 279, 280 288
  pulmonary 92
  tricuspid 285–288
Intercalated discs (myocardial cell damage) 404
Intestine transplants 11
Intimal proliferation 38
Intimal thickening 21–26, 43, 44
Intra-aortic balloon pump 406–411, 485, 486
Inverted aortic homograft 127, 129
Isoenzymes 134–143
Isolated aortic homograft 241–243
Isoprenaline, effect of on
  aortic flow 353
  pressure flow derivatives 355

Ketamine 298
Kidney transplants 6, 7, 10, 11, 14
  HLA matching 16, 17
  immunosuppression 27
Kinking of pulmonary artery 81–83
Konno—Sakakibari bioptome 32–34
Kyoto technique (hypothermia) 312

Lactatedehydrogenase (LDH) 134, 138–140, 143, 156, 162, 163
Lactate excretion 137, 140, 141
Laplace Law 422
Leaflet failure 473, 474
Leaks
  Fallot's tetralogy 468, 469
  Hartman's solution 374
  legs, after vein removal 374

mitral paraprosthetic 131
paraprosthetic 161, 162, 168
perivalvular 182, 183, 202, 247, 248, 250
Left coronary artery endarterectomy 391, 392
Left ventricular
aneurysm, surgical treatment of 415–419, 485
ejection fraction 90, 91
function curves 480, 481
outflow tract obstruction (LVOTO) 317
pressure and dimension 339–343
tunnel, aorta to 442, 443
Legs (vein grafts) 374, 486, 487
Lillehei-hunter operation 450, 451
Lillehei—Kaster valve 160, 161
Lipid analysis 372
Liver transplants 7–11, 455
Lone perfusion of right lung (Fallot's tetralogy) 81, 82
Long incision in leg (vein grafts) 374
Long-term results 234–236
balloon pumping 486
Lung transplants 11

Mammary artery 379, 382
Mannitol 298
Manometric studies 351
Mechanics of aortic valves 123, 124
Mentation measurements (total corection of Fallot's tetralogy) 92, 93
6-Mercaptopurine 25
Metallic bead surface prosthesis 157–159
Methicillin 215
Methyl prednisolone 36
MGH–Avco balloon pump 406–411
Millar transducer 351
Mitochondria (myocardial cell damage) 404
Mitral annulus lesions 279–282
Mitral cage ball prosthesis 144–159
Mitral incompetence (balloon pumping) 409, 410
Mitral insufficiency 279, 280, 488
Mitral paraprosthetic leak (echocardiogram) 131
Mitral regurgitation
balloon pumping 409, 410

chronic 424, 425
postinfarction, management of 420–425
subacute 423, 424
Mitral stenosis 339
rheumatic 127, 341, 342
Mitral valve calcification 282, 283, 287
Mitral valve, design criteria for 124–126
Mitral valve insufficiency 279, 280
Mitral valve perforation 282
Mitral valve replacement 127–132, 179–191, 196, 197
aortic flow trace 341
autologous fascia lata 272, 274, 275
Björk—Shiley tilting disc valve 172–174
cage ball prosthesis 144–159
complications 196, 197
echocardiography 127–132
haemodynamic changes 259, 266–267
haemolysis 148, 155, 156
homografts 253–259
Starr—Edwards composite seat prosthesis 192–195
superior vena cava 226–233
Mitral xenografts, Carpentier–Edwards 247–249
Monitoring circulation 330 ff
Mortality 1–5
Aortic valve homografts 257, 258, 260, 261
balloon pumping 409
Björk—Shiley prosthesis 202, 204
Blalock—Taussig shunts 72
Brock procedure 76
cage ball prosthesis 146–148
cardiopulmonary bypass in infants 300, 301
Carpentier—Edwards xenografts 247
composite seat aortic prosthesis 152, 153, 155
coronary bypass 382
coronary endarterectomy 386–394
Fallot's tetralogy 69, 70, 82, 96, 104–107

freeze-drying 236
homograft reconstruction 120
left ventricular aneurysms 418, 419
mitral valve homografts 255, 256, 258, 260, 261
open-heart surgery in infants 294
saphenous vein graft operation 367, 368
Starr—Edwards Prosthesis 179–181, 192–194, 198
total anomalous pulmonary venous drainage 309, 310
total correction of Fallot's tetralogy 96, 104–107
transposition of the great arteries 315, 316
  tricuspid valvuloplasty 286
  valvar stenosis 320
  ventricular septal defect correction 306
  VSD after myocardial infarction 426
  Waterston shunts 79, 80
Mounting tissue valves 220
Mucopolysaccharides 221
Mustard's operation 312–318
Myocardial cell damage 401–404
Myocardial cell necrosis 134, 137, 138, 140, 142, 403, 404
Myocardial infarction
  balloon pumping 410
  postinfarction mitral regurgitation 420–425
  postinfarction VSD 426–433
Myocardial preservation 133–143
Myocardial temperatures 134, 135
Myocardium
  direct revascularisation of 386
  infarctectomy 413, 414
  protection of 465
Myofibrils (myocardial cell damage) 404

Nitro-BT 401
Nomogram 333–335
Normal peripheral warm-up patterns 331–333
Nuclei (myocardial cell damage) 404
Nutrient medium (homograft storage) 210–212
Nystatin 215, 217, 257

Oedema, pulmonary 423
Open anastamosis 303, 310, 311
Open-heart surgery 293–297
  aortic stenosis 294
  atrial pressure measurement 337, 338
cardiopulmonary bypass 293, 295, 299–301
  Osmolar balance 325–329
  toe and rectal temperature 331–336
  warm-up patterns 331–335
Organ exchange 14
Orientation of Björk—Shiley tilting disc valve 176 178, 465, 466
Osmolality, plas na 325–328
Outflow tract
  autologous fascia lata 272, 275, 276
  homograft reconstruction 97, 98, 100, 117–122
  left ventricular outflow tract obstruction 317
  patching 87–92, 106, 107
Oxygenators (open-heart surgery) 298
Oxygen consumption
  arterio-venous O_2 difference 331
  Bentley oxygenator 298, 476
  Fallot's tetralogy, after total correction of 112
  Fick method 344

Palliation
  Fallot's tetralogy 69, 70, 104, 110, 460, 461
  open-heart surgery 293, 294
Pancreas transplants 11
Papillary muscles 420–425
Paraprosthetic leaks (Björk—Shiley tilting disc valve) 161, 162, 168
Patching 462, 463
  annulus 91, 92
  Dacron 317
  infarctectomy 413, 414
  outflow tract 87–89, 106, 107, 305
  Teflon felt 87–89, 106, 107, 305
Paulo—Alto group 457
Penicillin 217, 218
Percentage transmyocardial lactate extraction 137, 140
Perforation, mitral valve 282
Perfusion

coronary 133–143
donor organs 8, 10, 14, 15
lone of right lung 81, 82
myocardial damage 401
open-heart surgery in infants 298–301
Pericardial tamponage 334, 335
Pericardium 118, 120, 254, 260–270, 317, 441
Peripheral pulmonary alteriolar disease 81
Peripheral temperature measurement 330–336, 481
Perivalvular leakage 182, 183, 202, 247, 248, 250
Persantin 26, 167, 168
Physiological monitoring (computers) 358, 359, 361, 362
Plasma hyponatraemia 325, 326
Plasma hypo-osmolality 326–328
Plasma osmolality 325–328
Polymixin B Sulphate 217
Polypropylene 153, 200
Porcine valves 246–251
Potassium supplements (liver transplants) 9
Potts operation 78, 83, 113, 445–449
Practolol 399
Prednisone 36, 41, 43
Preparation of tissue valves 220–222
Preserving donor organs
cavitation 456
freeze-dried grafts 235, 236
heart 14, 31, 458
kidney 6
liver 7, 8
myocardial 133, 143
sterilisation 209–218, 221, 253, 266, 269, 470
storage 209–214, 220, 221
Pressure-dimension loops 339, 340, 342, 343
Profound hypothermic non-perfusion arrest 133–143
Progressive coronary artery disease 381–385
Prolene 374, 376
Propanolol 478
Prosthesis
aortic composite seat 151–153
bioprosthesis 222, 249, 250
Björk—Shiley tilting disc valve; *see* Björk—Shiley
cage ball 144–159
cloth-covered; *see* Cloth-covered composite seat-trace 154
Delrin prosthetic disc 160, 167, 172, 175, 205
metallic bead surface 157–159
mitral paraprosthetic leak 131
Prosthetic mitral valve 179–191
design criteria for 124–126
rings 281, 282, 285
Proteins 221
glycoproteins 221, 222
Pulmonary annulus patch 91, 92
Pulmonary artery
angiography 84
Fallot's tetralogy 49, 51, 52, 62, 66
hyperperfusion 83
hypertension 113
hypoplasia 83, 103, 110, 435, 436
kinking of 81–83
peripheral disease 81
small 461, 462
total correction of Fallot's tetralogy 106
Pulmonary atresias 78, 80–83
Pulmonary hypertension
mitral valve replacement 128
total anomalous pulmonary venous drainage 307, 308
Pulmonary infections 37, 38
Pulmonary infundibulum 53–56, 62–64, 66
Pulmonary insufficiency 92
Pulmonary oedema 423
Pulmonary stenosis 319, 320
Pulmonary switch operation 239–245
Pulmonary valve
agenesis of 444, 445
replacement 463
ring diameter 66, 67
valvotomy 319, 474–476
Pulmonary vascular resistance, high 39
Pulmonary venous drainage, total anomalous (TAPVD) 293, 294, 297, 307–311
Pulmonary venous obstruction 317

Pulmonic stenosis, relief of 90, 91
Pyrolitic carbon disc 160, 161, 166, 167, 172, 173, 176, 205

Radiography
chest X-ray; *see* Chest X-ray
homograft tissue valve 265
Recipients, selection of 29, 30, 40, 455, 458
Rectal temperature 332
Regurgitation
aortic 340
autologous fascia lata 273–276
Björk—Shiley tilting disc valve 166, 167, 202
homografts 262, 263
mitral (balloon pumping) 409, 410
postinfarction mitral 420–425
Rehabilitation
heart transplants 458
kidney transplants 6, 7
Rejection 11, 29, 41–45
diagnosis of 31, 32, 35
electrocardiography 29, 31, 35, 36
HLA matching 15
immunosuppression 29, 31–37
indices of 31, 32
older patients 39
postoperative infection 37, 38
serial biopsy 32–35
vessel damage 20
Related donors (HLA matching) 17
Reluctance of donors 12–14
Renal damage, acute 331
Renal flow 487, 488
Reoperation
cage ball prosthesis 151, 153
Carpentier—Edwards xenografts 249, 250
total correction of Fallot's tetralogy 107
Replacement
aortic valve; *see* Aortic valve replacement
complications 148–159
tissue valve 260–270
Research, computer used in 357
Revascularisation of the myocardium, direct 386
Rheumatic mitral stenosis 127
cineangiography 341, 342

Right coronary artery endarterectomy 387–391
Right ventricular pressure 477, 478
Right ventriculotomy 428–430
Ruptured chordae 283, 474
Rygg canula 312, 313

Saphenous vein graft operation 367–371, 437
aorto-coronary bypass 374–380, 382, 385
mortality 367, 368
postoperative blood flow 396–400
Sarcolemma (myocardial cell damage) 404
Sarcotubular system (myocardial cell damage) 404
Screening (pulmonary infections) 38
Seldinger technique 351
Selection of donors 40, 41
Selection of patients 29, 30
coronary artery surgery 367–371
tissue valves 219, 220
Septal band; *see* Trabecula septo-marginalis
Serial biopsy 32–35
Shumway, Dr. N. E. 18, 20, 28, 29, 41, 455, 456
Shunting
balloon pumping 409, 410
Blalock—Taussig shunt 71, 104, 110, 445–447, 461
Brock procedure 73–77, 104, 110
Cooley's operation 78
Fallot's tetralogy 69, 104, 460
Glenn operation 445–449
infants 460
palliation 460, 461
Potts operation 78, 83, 113, 445–449
total anomalous pulmonary venous drainage 308, 310, 311
Waterston shunt 78–83, 85, 104, 110, 113, 445, 446, 460–462
Silicone rubber prosthesis 226, 228
Single ventricle (surgical results) 443, 444
Sinus of Valsalva 124, 254
Skin; *see* Peripheral temperatures
Skin grafts 11, 16
Small aortic root 466, 467

Small pulmonary artery 461, 462
Staining cells (myocardial damage) 402, 403
Stanford University 28, 31, 34, 37, 457, 458
Starling's Law 340
Starr—Edwards Prosthesis 127, 180–191, 196–200, 235
  composite seat prosthesis 192–195, 200
  echocardiography 129–131
  emboli, incidence of 192, 193, 197
  haemolysis 184, 192, 193
  infections 182
  mortality 179–181, 192–194, 198
Stenosis
  infundibular 97, 102–104, 106, 110
  mitral 339
  pulmonary 319, 320
  pulmonic 90, 91
  rheumatic mitral 127, 341, 342
Step ladder incision in leg (vein grafts) 374
Sterilisation of homografts 209–218, 221, 253, 266, 469, 470
Storage of homografts 209–214, 220, 221
  freeze-dried 235–237
  vein grafts 374
Stress tests 372, 373
Stroke index (aortic valve replacement) 136
Stroke volume
  atrial pressure measurement 337, 338
  derivation of 357
Stroke work (atrial pressure measurement) 337
Stroke-work index (aortic valve replacement) 136, 137
Subacute mitral regurgitation 423, 424
Subacute ventricular septal defect 428
Subvalvular lesions 283–287
Sulphinpyrazone 25
Superior vena cava (SVC) 226–233, 471
Surface cooling
  cardiac bypass surgery 97
  open-heart surgery in infants 295
  total anomalous pulmonary venous drainage 308
  ventricular septal defect correction 303, 305
Surface temperature: *see* Peripheral temperature
Survival
  accelerated angina 384, 385
  aortic valve homografts 257
  aortic valve replacement 187, 188, 234, 235, 238
  Blalock—Taussig shunts 72
  Brock procedure 76, 77
  cage ball prosthesis 144
  chronic disabling angina 382–384
  Fallot's tetralogy in infants 69
  freeze-dried grafts 235–237
  HLA compatibility 17,18
  kidney transplants 6
  liver transplants 7
  mitral valve homografts 255–257
  mitral valve replacement 189
  open-heart surgery in infants 297
  previous cardiac bypass surgery 38, 39
  Starr—Edwards prosthesis 186
  tissue typing 31
  tissue valve replacement 269
Swinnex filter 299
Systemic venous obstruction (Mustard's operation) 317

Teflon
  buttresses 430, 431
  cloth prosthesis tear repair 153, 154
  felt patching 87–89, 106, 107, 305
  felt pledged 232
  infarctectomy 414
  sewing ring 173, 176
Temperature
  myocardial 134, 135
  normal peripheral warm-up patterns 331–333
  peripheral temperature measurements 330–336, 481
  rectal 332
  toe 331–336
  warm-up patterns 331–335
Tension time index (TTI) 137, 139
Tevabi 119
Thermistor 345

Thermodilution 344–346, 358, 481, 482
Thickening, mitral valve 282
Thromboembolism
  Björk—Shiley tilting disc valve 167–172, 174, 175, 204
  cage ball prosthesis 144–146
  homograft replacement 257, 261, 262, 267
  Starr—Edwards prosthesis 188–190, 199, 200
Thymidine uptake 209–211
Tissue encapsulation 200
Tissue typing 11, 31
Tissue valves 179–191
  autologous tissue 219, 260–270, 272–277
  durability 219–222
  electrocardiography 264, 265
  failure of 263, 264, 267
  haemodynamics 265, 266, 268
  histological examination 264
  mounting 220
  preparation of 219–224
Toe temperature 331–336
Total anomalous pulmonary venous drainage (TAPVD) 293, 294, 297, 307–311
  complications 310
  mortality 315, 316
Trabecula septomarginalis 52–56, 59
Transducers 351
Transposition of the great arteries (TGA) 293, 294, 296, 312–318, 479
  complications 316, 317
  Mustard's operation 312–318
  surgical results 450
Tricuspid valve replacement 265, 266, 268, 272, 276
  insufficiency 285–288
  valvuloplasty 285–287
Trinitrin 398, 399
Triple endarterectomy 392, 393
Tubbs dilator 104
Tumour removal (hypernephroma) 7

Unstable angina; *see* Accelerated angina
Urinary output 327, 328
  acute renal damage 331

cardiac output 350, 351
diuretics 296, 302, 306, 314, 331
monitoring circulation 331
renal flow 487, 488

Valvar stenosis 319–321
  cardiac catheterisation 319, 320
Valves
  aortic, mechanics of 123, 124
  Braunwald Cutter 200, 201, 206
  fascia lata 219, 266–270, 272–277
  Hancock Laboratories 250
  Lillehei—Kaster 160, 161
  mitral; *see* Mitral valve
  porcine 246–251
  pulmonary; *see* Pulmonary valve
Valve failure 236, 237
Valve lesions 260
  repair 279, 280, 282, 283
Valve repair 474
Valvotomy, pulmonary 319
Valvuloplasty, mitral 279, 280, 284
  tricuspid 285–287
Vasoconstriction (toe temperatures) 331, 333–336
Vein graft operation, saphenous; *see* Sapheous vein graft operation
Vena cava
  elongation, in 226
  mechanical characteristics of 226
  superior vena cava (SVC) 226–233, 471
Venous cannulation 312, 313
Ventricular aneurysm 415–419
Ventricular septal defect (VSD) 294, 297, 302–306
  balloon pumping 409, 410
  cardiac catheterisation 303
  closure of 479
  complications after correction 306
  Fallot's tetralogy 459, 460
  mortality 306
  multiple in infants 478, 479
  postinfaction 426–431
  subacute 427
  transposition of the great arteries 314
Ventriculography (Fallot's tetralogy) 102
Vessel lesions 20–26
  azathioprine 36, 41

Viability of antibiotic-treated homografts 211–213, 253
Visual Display Unit (VDU) 359–361

Warfarin 36, 156
Warm-up patterns, peripheral
abnormal 333–335
normal 331–333
Waterston shunts 78–83, 85, 104,
110, 113, 445, 446, 460–462
Wheat operation 450, 451
Williams—Barefoot flow probe 347–
349, 396–400, 480
Workbench surgery 7

Xenograft valves 219, 220
antibodies 251
antigens 250, 251
Carpentier—Edwards; *see* Carpentier—Edwards
evolution of 223, 224
gluteraldehyde 223, 224, 246, 250
inflammatory reactions in 223
porcine valves 246–251
preparation of 220–222